D1292530

The Conquest of Malaria

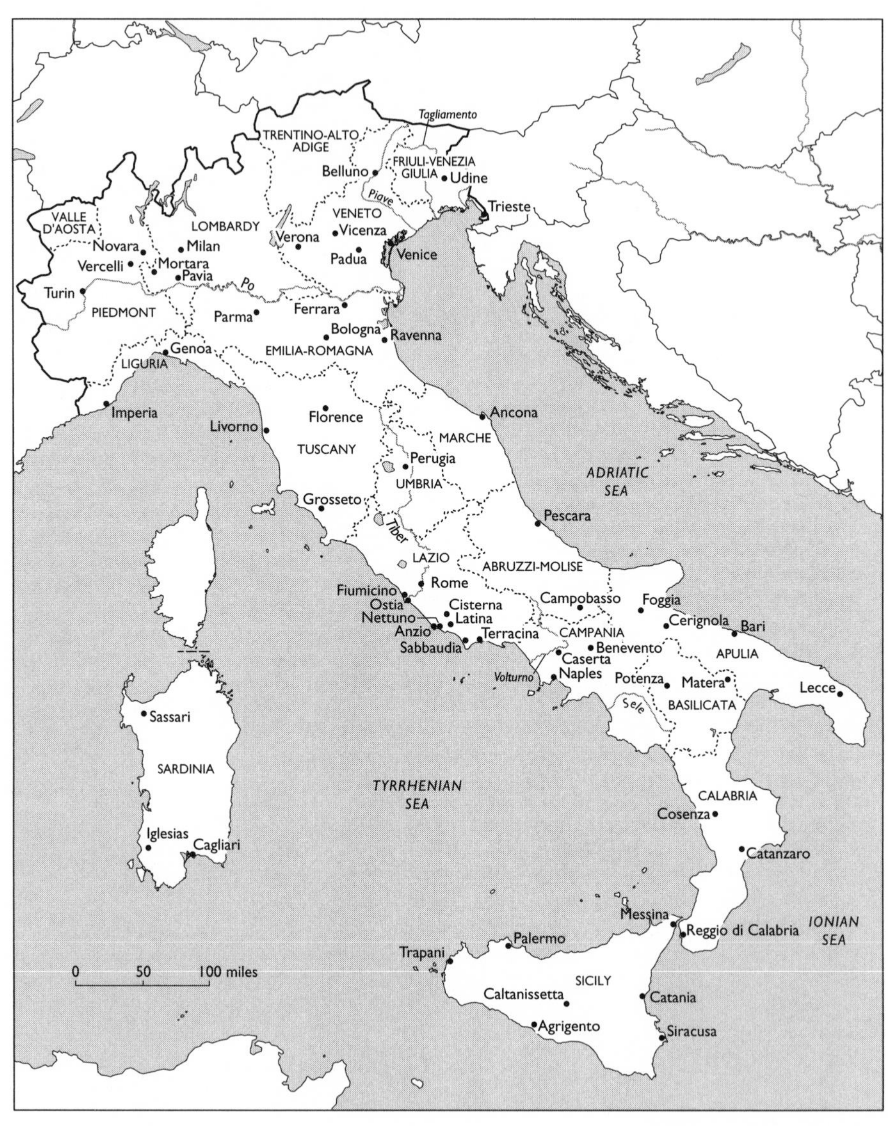

Tagliamento
TRENTINO-ALTO ADIGE
FRIULI-VENEZIA GIULIA
Belluno
Udine
Piave
Trieste
VALLE D'AOSTA
LOMBARDY
VENETO
Vicenza
Verona
Novara
Milan
Padua
Venice
Vercelli
Mortara
Pavia
Po
Turin
PIEDMONT
Ferrara
Parma
Bologna
Ravenna
Genoa
EMILIA-ROMAGNA
LIGURIA
Imperia
Florence
Ancona
Livorno
MARCHE
TUSCANY
Perugia
UMBRIA
ADRIATIC SEA
Grosseto
Pescara
Tiber
LAZIO
ABRUZZI-MOLISE
Rome
Fiumicino
Ostia
Campobasso
Foggia
Cisterna
Nettuno
Latina
Cerignola
Bari
Anzio
Terracina
CAMPANIA
Sabbaudia
Benevento
APULIA
Caserta
Volturno
Naples
Potenza
Matera
Lecce
Sele
BASILICATA
Sassari
SARDINIA
TYRRHENIAN SEA
CALABRIA
Cosenza
Iglesias
Cagliari
Catanzaro
Messina
Reggio di Calabria
IONIAN SEA
Palermo
Trapani
0
50
100 miles
SICILY
Caltanissetta
Catania
Agrigento
Siracusa

FRANK M. SNOWDEN

The Conquest of Malaria

ITALY, 1900–1962

Yale University Press
New Haven
& London

Published with the assistance of the Frederick W. Hilles Publication Fund of Yale University.

Set in Sabon type by Keystone Typesetting, Inc.
Printed in the United States of America.

Library of Congress Cataloging-in-Publication Data
Snowden, Frank M. (Frank Martin), 1946–
The conquest of malaria : Italy, 1900–1962 / Frank M. Snowden.
p. cm.
Includes bibliographical references and index.
ISBN 0-300-10899-0 (alk. paper)
1. Malaria—Italy—History—20th century. 2. Malaria—Treatment—Italy—History—20th century. 3. Mosquitoes—Control—Italy—History—20th century. I. Title.
RC163.I8S56 2006
614.5′32′00945—dc22
2005013483

A catalogue record for this book is available from the British Library.

The paper in this book meets the guidelines for permanence and durability of the Committee on Production Guidelines for Book Longevity of the Council on Library Resources.

10 9 8 7 6 5 4 3 2 1

Frontispiece: Italy, 1962 (Courtesy Bill Nelson)

The illustrations on pages 14, 49 (bottom), 59, 78, and 170 are reproduced courtesy of the Archivio Storico della Croce Rossa Italiana. The illustrations on pages 42, 48, 49 (top), 56, 147, 148, 154 (top), 160, 163, 171, 202, and 210 are reproduced courtesy of the Archivio di Stato di Latina: Comitato Provinciale Antimalarico, Archivio Fotografico. The illustrations on pages 118, 124, and 125 are reproduced from Renato Miracco, ed., *Giulio Aristide Sartorio: Impressioni di guerra (1917–1918)* (Rome, 2002).

Contents

Acknowledgments

This book could have been written only with the help of others, and one of the chief pleasures of being an author is to acknowledge those who have given so generously of their time and knowledge. Most of all, I am grateful to Professor Gilberto Corbellini of the University of Rome "La Sapienza," who encouraged me to undertake this project. He is an inexhaustible fount of information on all things concerning malaria, and he gave wonderful advice on the archives and historical sites in Rome, in Latina, and in the Roman Campagna. Having also read an early draft of the manuscript, he made wise suggestions that have saved me from many pitfalls.

Professor Mario Coluzzi, recipient of the Ross Prize in Malariology, also gave helpful advice at every stage of my research. In addition, near the end of the project, when I thought that I had exhausted his resources and kindness, he informed me of the existence of a diary that his father, also a distinguished malariologist, kept at the end of the Second World War. This diary contains the most definitive available evidence of a major war crime involving biological warfare by the German army at the expense of Italian civilians. I am grateful to Professor Coluzzi for enabling me to consult this diary and to quote from it in Chapter 7.

My work would have been impossible without the expert knowledge of the staffs of a variety of archives and libraries. Professor Ernesto Capanna was a generous and helpful guide to the materials in the Grassi Archive at the University of Rome "La Sapienza." My thanks to the archivists and librarians at the Central State Archive, the Italian Red Cross, the Archivio Capitolino, the National Library, the Library of the History of Medicine, the Museo Storico della Didattica at the University of Rome "La Sapienza," the Archivio di Stato at Latina, the Rockefeller Archive Center in Tarrytown, New York, and the National Library of Medicine in Bethesda, Maryland. I would also like to thank Dr. Giovanna Alatri, who helped me to explore the essential links between antimalarial strategies and education. Marco Fiorilla, the librarian of the Santo Spirito Hospital, gave invaluable assistance in enabling me to gain access to books and patient records at Rome's great malaria hospital.

I have been fortunate to have the support of colleagues, students, and friends at Yale University, where the Whitney Humanities Fund also provided financial support. Professors Henry Turner and Mark Choate carefully read an early draft of the manuscript and gave helpful recommendations. My colleagues Larry Holmes and John Warner provided a number of excellent suggestions of leads to pursue. I am also indebted to Dr. Philip Cooke of the University of Strathclyde, who provided useful bibliographical suggestions.

I was especially fortunate in having a semester as a resident and several periods as a visiting scholar at the American Academy in Rome during the final stages of writing. There is no better environment for the exchange of ideas, and I have benefited from the advice of the director, Professor Lester Little, and the fellows, who provided enthusiasm, insight, and probing questions. Christina Huemer, the librarian, shared my interest in the life and work of Giovanni Battista Grassi, and she assisted me in locating sites and photographs devoted to his memory.

Finally, my thanks to my wife, Margaret, for her generous support and editorial assistance. I am grateful for her willingness to read the manuscript a record number of times.

Introduction

One of the most interesting aspects of historical research is its propensity to lead an author in unexpected directions. The project that produced this book is certainly no exception. It began as an attempt to explore popular political responses to the advance of economic development and modernization during the Italian industrial takeoff in the late nineteenth and early twentieth centuries. I expected to immerse myself in the study of peasant rebellion, political organization, and trade unionism, as well as in the problem of whether economic advances in this period improved the living standards of ordinary men and women. I had no thought of pursuing issues of health and disease, and indeed I had no previous experience in the field.

In the course of researching what began as a topic in social and political history, however, I learned that there were abundant and little used medical sources, which provided more insight into living conditions than the records on which I had originally planned to rely—police files, parliamentary records, court transcripts, and newspaper accounts. Medical sources also furnished more solid bases for making meaningful comparisons of conditions between different historical periods, especially after 1887, when the state began to publish statistics on causes of death. For the purpose of measuring living standards, diseases provided objective and persuasive evidence in a way that wages, for instance, did not. Physicians and public health officials published a vast literature on the afflictions they confronted in their practice and on the circumstances that gave rise to them. The archives of the Department of Health and contemporary medical journals contained an almost inexhaustible —and little used—wealth of investigations into the life of the Italian people, with extensive information on such issues as diet, housing, working conditions, education, social relationships, and religious beliefs. Slowly, my conviction grew that these materials could establish an important and novel vantage point from which to examine modern Italy and especially the life of the poor, who are overrepresented in the attentions of the medical profession and underrepresented in the attentions of almost everyone else.

Such a study would also fill a substantial scholarly gap. Despite the international flourishing of medical history as a discipline during the past generation, its insights remain largely isolated from the historical mainstream. Seldom are diseases acknowledged as an integral part of the "big picture." In the case of Italy, the neglect is particularly stark. Despite the overwhelming burden of diseases that afflicted the country well into the modern period, the study of those diseases is still strikingly underdeveloped. The subject forms no part of the curriculum of Italian medical schools; and issues of health and disease seldom appear in the literature on the development of Italy since unification. Above all, there is no comprehensive history of malaria, even though it was the major public health issue in Italy until the end of the Second World War. There are numerous studies of specific aspects of the problem and of its effects on particular regions of the country, but still no general history. Against this background, my original focus on political history transformed itself into a new interest in the social history of medicine.[1]

Perhaps because of its dramatic and clearly visible effects, cholera first attracted my interest and led to the book *Naples in the Time of Cholera, 1884–1911*.[2] Cholera, however, is an exotic visitor from outside that invaded Italy at irregular intervals. What could one learn, I wondered, by examining instead a major endemic infectious disease that afflicted millions of people year after year? Would such a disease have a more enduring and profound impact, and would its study yield greater insights into the structure of Italian society?

Of all diseases, malaria, the leading problem of public health throughout the modern era, made the strongest claim for attention. Like that exotic and occasional visitor Asiatic cholera, malaria was capable of erupting with epidemic fury within a community and causing mass deaths, widespread illness, and severe social and economic disruption. But, unlike cholera, malaria returned every spring with the grim inevitability of an astronomical event. An endemic as well as an epidemic disease, it held nearly the whole of the peninsula as well as the islands of Sicily and Sardinia under its sway. In the second half of the nineteenth century and the first half of the twentieth, malaria was so enmeshed in the Italian rural society that it was widely regarded as the "Italian national disease"—and, fittingly, the English word itself comes from Italian.

Because of the heavy burden of suffering, poverty, and death that it imposed in every region of the nation, malaria became a leading preoccupation of statesmen, public health officials, and physicians. For this reason it left in its wake an especially rich documentary record. Doctors throughout the nation drafted extensive reports on every aspect of the disease and the conditions that promoted it. It rapidly became clear to me that through the vast and carefully drafted literature that it elicited from Italy's leading scientific, political, and medical figures, malaria cast a revealing shaft of light on the life of the nation. But there was more to it than that. Malaria, I soon learned, is a classic social disease, an occupational disease, and a disease of poverty and societal neglect. Fever thrives on exploitative working conditions, substandard housing and diet, illiteracy, the displacement of people, war, and ecological degradation. For this reason, the history of malaria proved to be also the history of the priorities of Italian statesmanship, of the relationship of the people to their environment, and of that overarching issue known to contemporaries as the "social question"—that is, poverty as revealed in the circumstances of ordinary people. The study of malaria seemed no longer an exotic subspecialty, but rather a central part of understanding modern Italian history.

No issue illustrates this aspect of malaria better than the great sectional issue known as the Southern Question in Italian history. This was the perception that the South formed a semicolonial appendage to the economically advanced North. Although it ravaged the whole of the peninsula, malaria was preeminently an affliction of the South, plus the provinces of Rome and Grosseto in the Center. It was indeed a commonplace among public health authorities that there were "two malarial Italies." As in northern Europe and North America, malaria in northern Italy was prevalent only in its milder strains (now known as vivax). In the South, however, as in the tropics, fever prevailed in its most acute and devastating forms, known at the time as "pernicious" or "malignant" malaria (and now termed falciparum).

Against this background of regional inequality, fever became an important metaphor deployed by southern spokesmen (*meridionalisti*) such as Giustino Fortunato and Francesco Saverio Nitti to describe the plight of the South and to demand redress. Most influential and emphatic of all was Nitti, who attributed the entirety of southern backwardness to this single factor. Malaria, he wrote, "is the basis of all social life. It determines relations of production and the distribution of wealth. Malaria lies at the root of the most important demographic and economic facts. The distribution of property, the prevailing crop systems, and patterns of settlement are under the influence of this one powerful cause."[3]

Among southern spokesmen, Nitti was not alone. Fortunato argued that malaria was "the most terrible of our afflictions" and that its conquest was the necessary precondition for resolving all other problems affecting the region. With a similar emphasis, the physician Giuseppe Tropeano reasoned that "malaria personifies the Southern Question." In confirmation of this conclusion, he painted a full-scale tableau of its social, economic, and medical ravages in his work of 1908, *La malaria nel mezzogiorno d'Italia* (Malaria in the South of Italy).[4] Malaria thus made a major contribution to awakening a consciousness of southern conditions and to mobilizing opinion to redress southern grievances.

It was not only southerners who were mobilized by the issue of malaria. Partly because of the overwhelming presence of the disease, malariology became the glory of Italian medical science and ushered in a period of remarkable intellectual excitement and discovery. In Italy, alone of the European powers, malaria was not a colonial but a domestic problem that confronted its medical faculties with an unending supply of fever patients and thus offered the promise of undying glory for the scientists who could penetrate its mysteries. Accordingly, Italians made most of the discoveries regarding the symptomatology, transmission, and pathology of malaria. Indeed, the study of malaria between 1890 and the Second World War was dominated by the so-called Italian School or Rome School. Its preeminent figure was Giovanni Battista Grassi, who discovered that mosquitoes transmit human malaria but who was unjustly passed over for the Nobel Prize in 1902. An important part of this book became the examination of the great intellectual journey of discovery from the prevailing idea that malaria was a poisoning of the air and soil to the theory of the transmission of parasites by mosquitoes.

On the strength of these discoveries, and because of pressure from the medical profession to transform them into clinical applications, the Italian parliament passed a series of laws between 1900 and 1907 establishing a national campaign — the first of its kind in the world — to eradicate, or at least control, malaria. Here was the most ambitious effort at social welfare ever undertaken by the Liberal regime. This campaign gathered momentum until the First World War and lasted, amid numerous setbacks and vicissitudes, until the eradication of the disease in 1962. The First World War itself undid the achievements of two decades and led to a terrifying recrudescence in malaria throughout Italy. After the Fascist seizure of power in 1922, the conquest of malaria again became a highly publicized national priority (most famously through the draining and settling of the Pontine Marshes), but with radically different priorities, methods, and costs. As Fascist foreign wars overwhelmed domestic policies, however, the program stalled and then collapsed entirely amid military defeat and occupation. A vengeful German campaign of biological warfare at the end of the Second World War helped to unleash a vast malaria epidemic. Final victory against the disease followed the reestablishment of public health infrastructures, the return of peace, and the introduction of DDT and a five-year plan to eradicate fever. The last known epidemic occurred in the Sicilian province of Agrigento in 1955; the last indigenous cases were reported in 1962 from the same province; and the designation of "malarial zone" was officially lifted from the entire peninsula in 1969.

The antimalarial campaign had lasting impacts, however, even beyond the elimination of disease. From the outset, the antimalarial warriors recognized that education and civil rights have great effects on health. The campaign therefore played a major but largely unrecognized role in the promotion of women's rights, the labor movement, and the achievement of universal literacy. A major task of this project became that of tracing the antimalarial campaign's contribution to the expansion of civil liberties and education as well as health. The issue of malaria in Italy was intensely political. Under the Fascist dictatorship, the antimalarial campaign was co-opted by the effort to restrict freedom; to establish totalitarianism, racism, and eugenics; and to prepare the nation for war, empire, and expansion. This book explores these transformations and argues that the effort to combat malaria, particularly in the Pontine Marshes, should hold a central place in the understanding and interpretation of Fascism.

Having adopted the history of malaria and of the campaign to eradicate it as the subject of my work, I attended the Malaria Centenary Conference in November 1998 at the Academia dei Lincei in Rome. In the course of the discussions that followed presentations on the most recent developments in the global fight against the disease, a member of the audience raised a point that altered my topic in a final and unexpected manner. After praising the organizers of the conference for their work, the speaker had one criticism to make: "Where," he asked, "are the historians?" Malaria, he argued, is too important to be left entirely to scientists, physicians, and public health officials. Historians have also studied the experience of societies with the disease, and their insights should become part of the debate. In particular, the study of a national program that successfully eliminated the disease from the entire territory of a nation-state could hold lessons for those dealing with the contemporary world malaria crisis.[5]

Malaria, one of the oldest and most devastating of human diseases, is causing a major global upsurge in illness, suffering, and death. During a wave of euphoria that overwhelmed the World Health Assembly in 1955 and lasted until 1969, the World Health Organization (WHO) confidently planned to eradicate the disease throughout the world. In stark defiance of this premature optimism, however, malaria has reemerged to create a crisis in the tropical world, where it now infects half a billion people annually and kills more than a million. Particularly in sub-Saharan Africa, armed conflicts, population displacement, drug-resistant strains of the malaria parasite, environmental havoc, and climatic change have led to a condition that public health workers describe as a medical catastrophe rivaling and fueling the simultaneous calamities of AIDS and tuberculosis. In Africa a death from malaria—most commonly of a child under five or a pregnant woman—occurs every twelve seconds.

An additional reason to investigate malaria in Italy, then, is the hope for insight. Italy represents the classic case in which endemic malaria was purposefully and successfully eliminated throughout an entire nation. What are the implications for the contemporary world crisis? What factors led to success in Italy? What institutions and programs made a decisive impact? What did Italians learn about the nature of the disease that enabled them to locate key points at which it proved vulnerable to attack? To what extent are the lessons and weapons exportable today as the WHO undertakes the new global antimalarial initiative known as Roll Back Malaria? In 1998 I had no answer to these questions, and I was unable to reply to the malariologist who challenged historians to take part in the global search to control the contemporary medical emergency. But I agreed that it is important to draw lessons from significant past efforts to deal with the disease, and I recognized that the Italian experience was particularly revealing. Generations of Italian physicians confronted malaria in a concerted effort to abolish the disease. They were successful, and they recorded at length their explanations for their victory. This book, in one sense, is my much-delayed attempt to respond to the challenge by reflecting systematically on their achievement and their analyses of its bases.

1

Malaria: The "Italian National Disease"

And truly the malaria gets into you with the bread you eat, or if you open your mouth to speak as you walk, suffocating in the dust and sun of the roads, and you feel your knees give way beneath you, or you sink discouraged on the saddle as your mule ambles along, with its head down. In vain the villages of Lentini and Francoforte and Paternò try to clamber up like strayed sheep onto the first hills that rise from the plain, and surround themselves with orange groves, and vineyards, and evergreen gardens and orchards; the malaria seizes the inhabitants in the depopulated streets, and nails them in front of the doors of their houses whose plaster is all falling with the sun, and there they tremble with fever under their brown cloaks, with all the bed-blankets over their shoulders.

— *Giovanni Verga, "Malaria"*

The full extent of the prevalence of malaria first captured national attention in the decade following 1878. It had been known for centuries, however, that intermittent fever was prevalent in the Italian peninsula. The very term *malaria* (bad air) was Italian, and Italy possessed "the unenviable privilege of having given this word to the world."[1] Before 1861, when "Italy" referred to a peninsula instead of a nation-state, it was as infamous for its lethal fevers as it was famous for its beauty. The radical revolutionary Jessie White Mario reported that midcentury Sardinia had such an evil reputation for malarial fever that "none but those utterly destitute or compelled by the pressure of insurmountable circumstances would think of remaining there."[2]

Camille de Cavour, the first prime minister of the new kingdom of Italy, died tragically of malaria in 1861 just after unification was completed. The Pontine Marshes and the Roman Campagna had been notorious for their insalubrity since ancient times, and for centuries travelers dreaded crossing them during the summer fever season. Henry James and Emile Zola remind us that fever lurked in Rome as well, where hotels in the healthier quarters found it profitable to inform potential customers that their neighborhoods were risk-free. One of the alternative names for the disease, "Roman fever," clearly suggested the danger, and those residents who were sufficiently wealthy fled the city in the summer to avoid the fate of James's Daisy Miller, who perished of fever in the Italian capital. Most famously of all, Giuseppe Garibaldi—the hero of the doomed Roman Republic of 1849 and one of the nation's founding fathers—lost both his wife, Anita, and large numbers of his troops as they retreated across the Roman Campagna during a fearsome epidemic of malaria. The Italian army suffered a similar fate in 1870 after capturing Rome from the Pope, and soldiers filled the wards of the city's fever hospital. Thus stricken, Garibaldi urged the newly united nation to place the fight against malaria high on its list of priorities.[3]

Clearly, then, the fact that malaria existed in the kingdom of Italy surprised no one. Awareness of the disease, however, was partial, imprecise, and anecdotal. For a quarter of a century after unification in 1861, malaria was not reportable, and the official attempt to document and quantify its ravages did not begin until 1887. Furthermore, the rural poor, who suffered disproportionately from malaria, had little or no contact with the medical profession. As a result, their condition was only vaguely apprehended before 1887, and even after the age of health statistics began, the incidence of the disease remained seriously underreported. Greatly limiting public knowledge of the disaster were various additional circumstances: distance, poor communications, the barrier of mutual ignorance dividing North and South, absenteeism, the abyss between city and countryside, and universal uncertainty about the nature of the disease itself, which remained, in the phrase of the Roman physician Francesco Puccinotti, "the darkest of mysteries."[4] The cost of malaria to Italy had never been calculated. Antonio Labranca, inspector general of the Department of Health, recalled in 1928 the imprecise perception of malaria prevailing at the time of national unification: "Only with the establishment of the kingdom of Italy did the problem of the war against malaria begin to be apprehended in its full enormity, but there was still no precise knowledge of its diffusion and severity. In particular, with regard to the prevalence of malaria in the territory of the kingdom, its influence on the physical and sanitary condition of the nation, and its impact on the national economy, there were only vague notions. One was still far from being able to assess all the effects of swamp fever and malaria."[5]

Then, in 1878, an alarm was sounded by an unlikely source: a report from the Parliamentary Railway Commission. One of its leading members, the Tuscan senator Luigi Torelli, the earliest apostle of a nationwide antimalarial program, discovered during his work for the commission that malaria was inseparable from any investigation of the railroad industry because of the appalling rate at which its employees fell ill in vast swathes of the country. For instance, in 1878, 1,455 of the 2,200 railroad workers in Sicily required medical attention for malaria. Torelli proclaimed the emergency in parliament, calling for a systematic investigation of the prevalence of the disease and an assessment of its cost. He sponsored a bill for a national land-reclamation program to combat malaria, and he undertook drainage works on his own estates. In order to substantiate his claims, Torelli also solicited reports on fever from all 259 of the provincial and district health councils (*consigli di sanità*), thereby confirming the urgency of the crisis.[6]

Unwilling to allow so vital an issue to slumber in the halls of parliament at Montecitorio, Torelli launched a campaign to arouse public opinion. In 1882, he began by drafting the first map of malarial Italy. The purpose of this map was to shock the public by dramatically revealing—in yellow and red patches of "severe" and "very severe" prevalence—the full extent of the fever that made Italy a "sick beauty." Then Torelli published *Il curato di campagna e la malaria dell'Italia* (The Country Priest and Italy's Malaria) in 1884. *Il curato di campagna* was an educational document organized in the form of fifteen short dialogues on fever and intended to reach a broad readership. As Torelli patiently explained in the dialogues, malaria was so widespread and so devastating that it ranked chief among the problems facing the Italian nation. He therefore called for an all-out "national war" to liberate Italy from the "tyranny of malaria," and he predicted that the war would pay for itself through reduced health costs and the improved productivity of the Italian workforce.[7]

Torelli's findings were rapidly confirmed by two further fact-finding investigations. The first was the famous parliamentary inquiry into the conditions of Italian agriculture conducted under Stefano Jacini and published between 1881 and 1886.[8] Jacini and his colleagues discovered that, in the dawning era of global competition inaugurated by steamships and railroads, Italian farming was dangerously backward and highly vulnerable to efficient American and Russian competitors. One of the leading reasons for this weakness, the

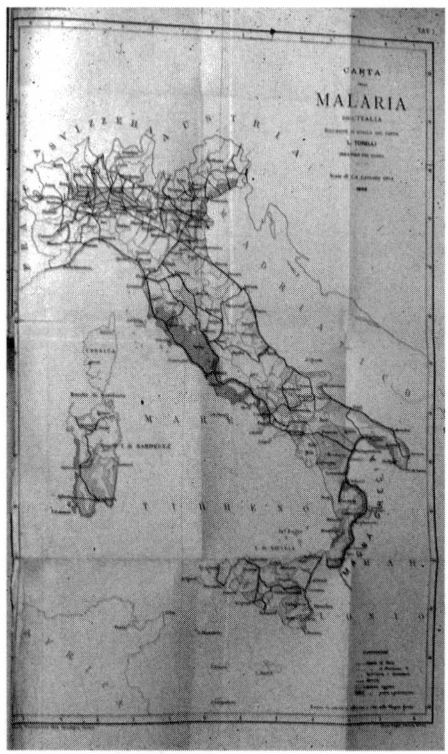

Luigi Torelli, *Carta della malaria dell'Italia* (Map of Malaria in Italy)

inquiry discovered, was the ubiquity of fever, which fatally compromised the health and the productivity of peasants and farmworkers. Jacini himself largely avoided the issue of disease in his final report, but several of the commissioners for specific regions carefully documented its influence. Senator Francesco Nobili-Vitelleschi, for example, reporting on the provinces of Rome and Grosseto, concluded that malaria was a "terrible scourge that covers immense areas of Italian soil with a funeral pall. There it is our great misfortune that only the scythe of death reaps an abundant harvest."[9] Similarly, Baron Giuseppe Andrea Angeloni reported from Apulia and the Abruzzi that, as a result of malaria, "the traveler who crosses our countryside is pained by the squalor in which he finds it." Both Angeloni and Nobili-Vitelleschi explicitly applauded the results of Torelli's labors, endorsed his map, and supported his conclusions.[10] Francesco Salaris, the commissioner for Sardinia, complained that the ravages of malaria were sometimes exaggerated, but he noted of his native island that "in the villages located in these extensive plains, and along the coasts, the poison of malaria lies always insidiously in waiting. In the faces of our men, women, and children one can see the grayish pallor of repeated attacks of fever. It is well known that the dominant disease in many parts of the island is swamp fever, and that neglect and complications can make it serious or even fatal."[11]

In 1887 the Italian state launched a second investigation by beginning to collect and publish health statistics. Declaring malaria a reportable disease, the Department of Health (Direzione Generale della Sanità) produced a statistical profile that illustrated the urgency of taking action.

What did investigators discover about malaria that gave them such a sense of crisis? What was the extent of the Italian malaria problem in the closing quarter of the nineteenth century? Where in the kingdom was it most intense? What was the profile of its victims? What was its seasonality? How did contemporaries understand the disease? This chapter surveys what soon came to be called the "Italian national disease" on the very eve of the great discoveries that unraveled its mysteries and just before the campaign to eradicate it was launched. The intention, however, is to avoid the anachronism of using modern scientific understandings of malaria to explain—or explain away—the great challenge that faced nineteenth-century Italians. It is important instead to sense the alarm that contemporaries felt as the full measure of the problem captured national attention. To that end, it is essential to begin by examining the problem as they saw it, and in their own terms.

Malaria as Miasma

In the 1870s, as Luigi Torelli began to address the crisis, Italians—both scientists and nonscientists—almost universally understood malaria in terms of "miasmatism." According to this interpretation, fever was caused by a "miasma," or poisoning of the air. Francesco Ladelci, a prominent Roman physician and authority on fever, defined miasma as "a disease-causing emanation that rises from wet earth, especially where there is stagnant water and the earth dries out during the heat of the summer."[12] Indeed, here was the etymological origin of the disease's name—"bad air," or *mal'aria.* Opinions diverged over the nature and source of the noxious effluvium. For many, the poison was a chemical that arose from organic material that had fallen into swamp water and then decomposed, releasing pestilential vapors into the atmosphere. In this view, malaria, often called *paludismo* (swamp fever), erupted when susceptible individuals inhaled the gases or absorbed them through their pores. A crucial factor, therefore, in the epidemiology of each locality was the direction of its prevailing winds. In the case of Rome, fever broke out in the late spring and summer when southern trade winds prevailed and wafted deadly swamp gas from Africa, from the nearby Pontine Marshes, or from the swamps at the mouth of the Tiber at Ostia. When autumn returned, cold winds gusted safely again from the north, and the city returned to health.[13]

In the opinion of many, however, it was not necessary for individuals to poison themselves directly from swamp gas in order for epidemic malaria to burst out. A widespread theory was that the lethal swamp material was not a chemical but a living entity, or "germ," that was variously regarded as a microscopic plant or an invisible "animalcule." In this interpretation, winds bore the germs away from the swamps and, even at great distances, seeded the ground as they passed over it. Under the proper conditions of warm temperature, intense humidity, and an impermeable clay topsoil that retained moisture, the germs would ferment in the earth, releasing poisonous fumes. This was the telluric doctrine of malaria, which postulated that not the air but the earth was poisoned. As Corrado Tommasi-Crudeli stated, "Malaria is a production of the earth."[14] Under the influence of the work of Louis Pasteur, Joseph Lister, and Robert Koch, who established the modern "germ theory of disease," some malariologists—most notably Tommasi-Crudeli, Edwin Klebs, and Ettore Marchiafava—even claimed to have isolated the microbe, or *Bacillus malariae,* that infected the soil.[15] The concept of a living organism that could reproduce infinitely seemed the most rational explanation for the sheer magnitude of the malaria problem.

According to this theory, people became infected when they crossed the contaminated "fields of death" and breathed in the poisonous vapors, or when they ingested the germs directly by drinking contaminated swamp water. Men and women were thought to be particularly vulnerable if they found themselves in the open fields at times when sharp changes in atmospheric temperature occurred, causing currents of air to rise vertically from the earth and bear the miasma aloft. For this reason, dawn and dusk—times when swift changes in temperature regularly took place—were exceedingly dangerous. Similarly, there was thought to be great danger in such activities as plowing or excavating, which involved moving the earth and therefore liberating the ferment. In addition, any malodorous task was a cause for disquiet. The retting of hemp and linen, for example, which produced a terrible stench, fell under deep suspicion.[16]

The sway of such miasmatic teaching was powerfully reinforced by the German epidemiologist and sanitarian Max von Pettenkofer, who enjoyed a great vogue in Italy in the closing decades of the nineteenth century even as his authority waned in his native country. Although Pettenkofer concerned himself primarily with Asiatic cholera, the careful attention he devoted to the role of local environmental factors—especially groundwater, temperature, and air—in the etiology of disease was applicable to the study of malaria as well. As with cholera, the implication was that malaria was not a contagious disease. Indeed, malaria was deemed to be the miasmatic disease par excellence because the pathogenic material, having once gained entrance into the body, was not excreted and was therefore not capable of being transmitted from person to person. Malaria was purely a product of local factors of climate and topography. The epidemiology of the disease thus became, in the words of the Roman doctor Francesco Scalzi, a question of "medical meteorology."[17]

Naturally, not everyone exposed to the malarial miasma fell ill. Invoking concepts that had formed part of humoral teaching since antiquity, physicians believed that the individuals who contracted fever were predisposed as a result either of their inborn constitution ("diathesis") or of external "occasional causes" that weakened their resistance. These occasional causes included emotional distress, preexisting infections, dietary excesses and irregularities, severe overwork, and sudden chills that blocked the purifying action of perspiration and allowed the poison to accumulate in the body. In such susceptible individuals, nineteenth-century doctors thought, the miasma produced its effects by attacking the central nervous system. It was this ability to affect the solar plexus, the ganglionic nerves, and the spine that explained the protean variety of malarial symptoms. After a latent period of seven to ten days following exposure, the poison triggered the onset of symptoms. Thereafter, the classic paroxysms of malarial fever occurred—intermittent spikes of temperature, chills, profuse sweating, and violent headaches. Vomiting, diarrhea, and delirium were also common. The subsequent course of the disease was then determined by the specific organs and systems that were affected by the poisoned nerves—the brain, the lungs, the spleen, the gastrointestinal tract, or the circulatory system. In the worse cases of "pernicious" malaria involving vital organs, death resulted swiftly as the patient collapsed into coma, acute respiratory distress, or profound anemia. Pregnant women were subject to miscarriages, premature births, and massive hemorrhage.

In milder or "benign" cases, the disease produced chronic disabilities rather than death—painful enlargement of the spleen (*splenomegaly*), emaciation, anemia, and fatigability that could lead at last to the state of *cachexia*—total apathy and indifference. In the words of the physician Vincenzo Caraffa, "The cachectic patient, having fallen into a state of profound anemia, presents the following features—an ashen color of the skin, severe emaciation, a belly swollen by his massive spleen and liver, and a lifeless stare. He is weak and apathetic; he moves with difficulty; and he suffers from nervous disorders,

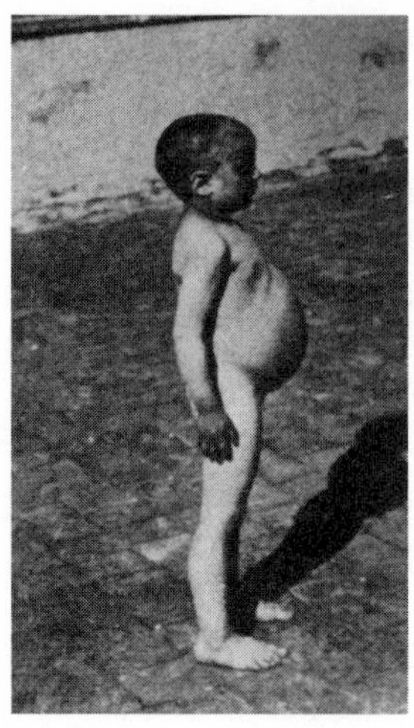

Boy with splenomegaly

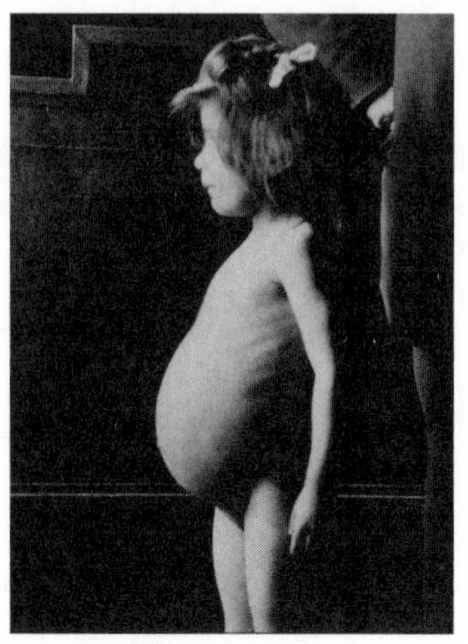

Girl with splenomegaly

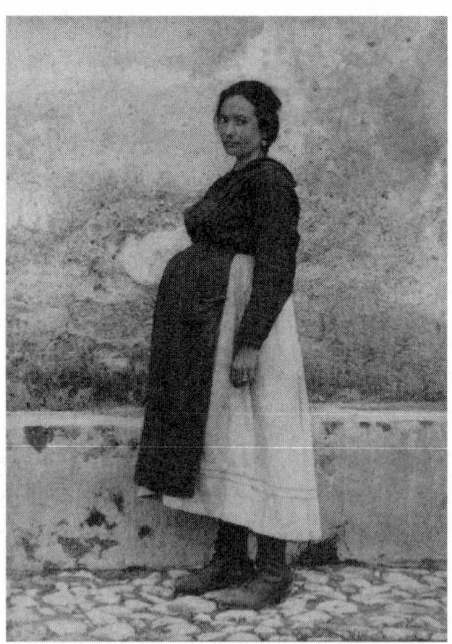

Adult woman with splenomegaly

from bleeding from the nose and gums, from loss of appetite, from dyspepsia, and from diarrhea."[18] In the most fortunate cases, the patient recovered fully, but further episodes of stress could lead to relapses or to assault by what would later be termed "opportunistic" diseases (diseases that prey on weakened organisms), especially catarrhal inflammations of the lungs.[19]

The Scale of the Problem

Miasmatic doctrine, whether in "paludal" or telluric guise, seemed to explain the leading features of the epidemiology of malaria as Torelli and his followers presented them. Of all the revelations made by the Tuscan senator, the most striking was the extent of the red- and yellow-shaded areas on his 1882 map indicating "severe" and "most severe" prevalence. Nearly all of Italy was infected. Indeed, of Italy's sixty-nine provinces, only two—Porto Maurizio (today Imperia) and Macerata—were entirely malaria-free. The shaded areas of the map indicated over 3,300 malarial zones covering nearly a third of the total land area of Italy. Zones of malarial prevalence stretched along the whole of the Po Valley, along the Adriatic littoral from the mouth of the Isonzo River in the north uninterrupted as far as Ravenna and then from the Abruzzi to the southernmost reaches of Apulia, along the whole of the Ionian coast, and along the Tyrrhenian coast except for the gulf of Naples and the northernmost stretch from Livorno to the French border. In addition, the entirety of Sardinia was shaded, as were extensive areas of the river valleys, plains, and coast of Sicily. Of Italy's 8,362 townships (*comuni*), 3,075 were malarial.[20]

In a total population of twenty-five million, therefore, over eleven million people were permanently at risk. Of these, two million were infected, reinfected, or superinfected annually, and at least fifteen thousand died directly from the effects of fever (a figure that later authorities such as Giovanni Battista Grassi revised upward to one hundred thousand).[21] Mortality from malaria varied from year to year, depending on the vagaries of rainfall and temperature, with fearful spikes every five to ten years, as in 1879, 1887, 1895, and 1900.[22] In many zones, virtually everyone was malarious, often from birth and throughout a debilitated and painfully truncated life. The economic cost resulting solely from the diminished productivity of stricken peasants and workers was estimated at several hundred million lire.[23] Longevity and life expectancy data further revealed a terrible toll in radically foreshortened lives. The life expectancy of farmworkers in nonmalarial regions of Italy was 35.7 years on the eve of the First World War. In malarial zones, by contrast, their life expectancy at birth was only 22.5 years.[24] The provinces free of malaria—

Porto Maurizio and Macerata — had the longest life expectancy at birth, while the provinces with the highest rates of infection — Foggia and Rome — had the shortest life expectancy. At Porto Maurizio, for example, 2.3 percent of the population reached the age of seventy-five in the 1880s, as opposed to a national average of 1.3 percent and 0.9 percent at heavily stricken Foggia and Rome.[25]

Malaria, the studies disclosed, was Italy's leading public health problem. Some authorities suggested that Italy was a modern Cinderella, kept in rags and unhappiness by an evil disease personified as the "wicked stepmother" (*la matrigna*). Torelli thought instead of the tale of Sleeping Beauty, declaring the nation a "sick beauty" whom it was his duty to awaken.[26] According to Torelli, the problem of malaria had been steadily increasing since unification, and in 1879 — a year of heavy rains and intense summer heat — the nation suffered the most severe epidemic in living memory.[27]

Those who charted the course of this great scourge noted that its effects on Italian society were profound and manifold. One devastating consequence of so prevalent a disease was economic backwardness. Regarding malaria in the modern world, the World Health Organization (WHO) has defined it as "a disease of poverty" that distorts and "slows a country's economic growth," and it has noted that the nations with severe endemic malaria are among the poorest on the globe.[28] The Italian economy in the nineteenth century, still largely agricultural, supports the characterization of malaria proposed by the WHO. The vision of Cavour and the founders of the Italian Liberal regime was that the new nation should remain predominantly agricultural, but that the agricultural sector should become dynamic, heavily capitalized, and intensive. Cavour and his immediate successors imagined an international division of labor in which Italy would compete with the United States and the industrial countries of northern Europe by specializing in thoroughly modernized farming. The problem with this vision was that productivity in the Italian countryside was too low to compete in a world market unified by the railroad and the steamship. Far from being able to hold its own against the efficient farms of the American Midwest, Italy could not even feed its own population and had to import wheat from abroad.

Because Italy was predominantly a grain-producing nation, it was tragically ironic that its most fertile lands — the coastal plains and river valleys — were precisely the zones where malaria was most intense. Indeed, fever held the countryside so firmly in its grip that, according to Torelli's estimate, fully two million hectares were left totally uncultivated as a direct consequence of malaria, and a further two million were cultivated badly. The height of the annual malaria epidemic in the summer coincided exactly with the peak of the agricultural season, when vast outlays of heavy outdoor labor were required for the tasks of scything, harvesting, and threshing. To survive, farmworkers and peasants had to expose themselves to disease. But disease in turn entailed suffering, days of absence, and low productivity. For some, additional consequences were death and the immiseration of the widows and orphans they left behind. In addition, malaria promoted absenteeism by landlords and farmers, disdain toward manual labor, and an unwillingness to invest in agricultural improvement. It also encouraged peasants to live, if they could, far from the fields they cultivated. Thus, they arrived at work either debilitated by disease or exhausted by the long trek from home. Malaria, therefore, was a coefficient of poverty, undercapitalization, and underdevelopment. It also created long-term international dependence on great industrial powers that were both healthier and more economically advanced. As late as 1918, the Ministry of Agriculture reported that "malaria is the key to all the economic problems of the South, and to the chronic difficulties of Italian agriculture."[29] In 1924, the provincial officer of health for Girgenti (today Agrigento, Sicily) provided a vivid analysis of the disease's impact on the economy of the island and of the nation as a whole:

> The problem of malaria is clearly immense, and it ranks among the most serious and complicated of all. . . . The enormous prevalence of malaria has a great social importance because the infection, which is tenacious and tends to become chronic, damages the human body. It causes a state of debilitation that leads even to total apathy or cachexia, preventing development and even distorting the physical structure of whole populations. A body weakened by malaria is also predisposed to other diseases. In fact, in these malarial populations the rate of death from common diseases is normally very high, even if the rate of death from malaria narrowly defined is low. But what is most important is that malaria undermines the resistance of the body and its capacity to work; it destroys all physical energy; and it makes a people indolent and lethargic. In this manner malaria limits production, it compromises wealth and material wellbeing, and it slows agricultural and industrial progress. Malaria exerts a sinister influence on the whole economy, . . . and it spreads ignorance. The standard of living in these places is lowered with respect to economic, cultural, and moral life. Malaria also makes illiteracy an insoluble problem.[30]

Southern agriculture as a whole was thus deemed to be compromised by disease. Just as in the North, one agricultural institution in particular was widely regarded as emblematic of the plight of the entire region. In the North, this institution was the rice field (*risaia*); in the South, it was the great wheat-producing estate known as a *latifondo*. These estates extended over hundreds, even thousands, of hectares. In the Roman Campagna, one of the classic zones of latifundism, the whole territory of 210,000 hectares was divided in 1885 among only 357 farms that were notorious for both unhealthiness and technical backwardness. Just as with the rice fields, so too with the latifondi there was a strong current of abolitionist opinion demanding their elimination as a measure of public health.

Notorious for backwardness, latifondi practiced only two economic activities, and both were ruinous economically and medically—extensive single-crop wheat farming and the nomadic shepherding known as transhumance. Both enterprises left vast tracts unplanted, thereby promoting the collection of surface water. In addition, the agricultural season peaked on the wheat fields in June and July, just as malaria broke out in full ferocity. Harvesting and threshing at this time generated a sudden, inextinguishable demand for labor. Like rice planters, single-crop wheat growers met their labor needs by massively deploying migrant workers just as the fever season commenced. The great estates of Foggia and Rome, two of the most malarial provinces in the kingdom, exemplified the phenomenon. In the early twentieth century Foggia province experienced an annual summer in-migration of one hundred thousand laborers, primarily from villages high in the Apennines. The population of the Roman Campagna tripled every summer, from nine thousand to thirty thousand.[31]

Since absenteeism was universal among proprietors, estate management was entrusted to a speculative farmer on a short-term lease. A temporary figure in the local economy, the leaseholder had no reason for long-term concern with productivity, labor relations, or the fertility of the land. His activity was purely speculative—the agricultural equivalent of strip-mining. He allowed buildings to deteriorate, ignored the maintenance of roads and the hygiene of wells, overworked farm animals, neglected the drainage of water, failed to remove weeds, and progressively exhausted the soil. The farmer plowed the earth, scattered seed, and then left the rest to nature. Success or failure depended on the elements.

Working conditions under such a system had negative economic and medical consequences. Migrant labor, in the words of two authorities on the Roman Campagna, was "the most fearful ally of malaria."[32] There was no tradition of paternalism, no common stake in the future, no spirit of cooperation. Furthermore, pressed by a high rent, a slack market for wheat, and the acute uncertainties of the harvest, the leaseholder engaged in harsh dealings with his laborers. Labor was the one variable in production over which he could exercise control, and his strategy was to reduce its cost to the minimum. If workers fell ill, it was cheaper to replace them than to invest in prevention or care. Housing was especially inadequate. The undercapitalized estates often provided no accommodations at all, requiring harvesters to bivouac in open fields that were universally thought to be poisoned. Alternatively, workers sheltered in filthy stables or in crowded and unpaved huts such as the notorious *capannoni* of the Roman Campagna built of mud, straw, and bamboo. On some estates the laborers even lived as troglodytes in caves dug into nearby hillsides, as at Grottarossa, which was located only five miles from the capital, still within sight of the dome of St. Peter's Basilica.[33]

On the latifondi, work at the high season fully filled the daylight hours, exposing workers to the well-known dangers of dawn and dusk out of doors. Furthermore, studies of southern farming emphasize other circumstances conducive to disease and poor productivity—low wages, inadequate clothing, unsafe water, poor diet, flogging by overseers, and child labor. On the eve of the First World War, a parliamentary inquiry under Senator Eugenio Faina investigated the conditions of peasants in the South. Both the investigators and the workers themselves frequently invoked the terms *slavery* and *serfdom* to portray life on the great estates.[34]

Similarly, in 1881 the municipal councilor F. Pericoli exposed the conditions endured by laborers just a few miles from Rome—conditions that carried important medical corollaries. "All suppositions," he announced,

> are exceeded by reality. The mind cannot accurately imagine . . . the life they lead. . . . They are transported in . . . foul railroad cars intended for goods and cattle, and they are housed worse than cattle on estates that provide no dormitories. There they lack mattresses, space, and a wholesome diet. And if the summer air is lethal, the water . . . is equally impure. Relations between workers and their recruiters are generally similar to those between slaves and their drivers, who enjoy such an evil reputation in both hemispheres. These relations are deplorable. It is no exaggeration to say that there is no limit to the rapacity of the "corporals" who hire them. Neither the customs of the place nor the terms of contracts permit any resistance to their exactions.
>
> For those workers who fall ill, conditions are still worse. It is not easy for a physician to intervene; medicines are seldom available; . . . and conveyance to the hospitals of our city is both difficult and dangerous.[35]

Production carried out with such methods and by such a workforce was inevitably uncompetitive by international standards. The tragedy for the South was that, if latifundism promoted malaria, so too did malaria promote latifundism. Each was at once cause and effect of the other. Where malaria was hyperendemic (as it was on most southern plains and coasts), there was no incentive to modernize production, to settle the workforce on the land, or to diversify cultivation. Conversely, under conditions of neglect, extensive wheat monoculture, and migrant labor, the sway of malaria was enhanced. Only massive and well-directed intervention from outside could transform the prevailing conditions of health and cultivation.

Great estates also witnessed the little-investigated plight of large numbers of gleaners. In the South and the Roman Campagna they consisted of the most impoverished and marginal groups in Italian society — aged men, widowed or abandoned women, orphans, the disabled, the ill, and the unemployed. To survive, they traveled from distant provinces to gather up the stubble left in the fields after the harvest. There, as the fever season reached its peak, they slept under canvas in the open and with no provision for their welfare. As a consequence, gleaners suffered acutely from malaria.[36]

In the view of the early antimalarial crusaders, the disease was also a major cause of mass transoceanic migration from southern Italy to the United States, Brazil, and Argentina — a movement that got under way in the late 1870s, just as miasmatic fever was reaching new heights of prevalence and virulence. Although the literature on Italian emigration overwhelmingly ignores the role of disease, nineteenth- and early twentieth-century public health reformers regarded malaria — and the poverty it caused — as one of the major factors that led peasants and farmworkers to leave Italy for the Americas. As Torelli commented, "In growing numbers, poverty and malaria supply the annual contingent of Italian emigrants."[37] Later, as the antimalarial movement picked up steam, authorities responsible for combating malaria confirmed Torelli's insight. An example is that of Bartolommeo Gosio, the commissioner sent by the Department of Health to Basilicata and Calabria, two of the regions that contributed most massively to the emigration. Reporting in 1906, Gosio described malaria as an integral part of the circumstances — low wages, underemployment, indebtedness, deforestation, and soil erosion — that drove peasants from the South across the Atlantic.[38] Francesco Saverio Nitti, the deputy from Basilicata who served as a commissioner for the parliamentary inquiry into the conditions of southern peasants published between 1908 and 1911 and later became the Italian prime minister, stressed with greater emphasis that malaria contributed heavily to the decision to depart because of its role in producing pauperism.[39] Finally, looking retrospectively at the great prewar exodus, the Ministry of Agriculture commented in 1918 that "already before the war, the Italian worker refused any longer even to think of going to live on the malarial latifundia" — "even if [workers] went equipped with quinine."[40]

The argument made by Torelli, Gosio, and Nitti was simple. Given the development of cheap and rapid overseas transport in the age of the steamship and steerage passage, peasants from the highland villages of the Apennines for the first time possessed an alternative to the annual summer trek to the wheat fields on the malarial plains. Fearing for their health and even their lives, they engaged in the functional equivalent of a strike for better health conditions by fleeing abroad instead. Here, claimed the antimalarial crusaders, was a major cause of the massive hemorrhage of the most able-bodied and hardworking southern male youths who migrated abroad by the millions between 1880 and the First World War. There they helped to build the economies of Italy's competitors instead of developing productivity at home. G. Ercolani summarized the dilemma when he wrote in 1905, "Ultimately, the malarial regions supply the largest numbers of emigrants. It thus happens that foreign countries profit from the energy of those strong and youthful arms that seek elsewhere what is denied to them in their fatherland by the unhealthiness of the soil."[41]

Inevitably, landlords and farmers looked with alarm on such a massive thinning out of the labor market: it threatened them with labor shortages, high wages, and a weakening of control over the workforce. Therefore, Torelli explained to the Senate, one of the reasons for launching an assault on malaria was to limit that "other evil that afflicts Italy and threatens to grow steadily worse—emigration."[42]

If persistent economic backwardness and mass emigration were two of the by-products of malaria that most troubled nineteenth-century observers, another disturbing consequence was the poor performance of the Italian army. The army was chronically undermined by the high rate at which it rejected recruits, especially from the southern regions where malaria was most severe, as physically unfit for service. In the most afflicted provinces, such as Foggia, the military rejected two-thirds of draftees. Furthermore, malaria debilitated the military and drained its funds. In the 1880s Italy had a standing army of 180,000 men, of whom 10,000 annually fell ill with malaria and were hospitalized for treatment.[43] A substantial burden of malaria still afflicted the army at the turn of the century (Table 1.1).

Such high rates of rejection, illness, and discharge were incompatible with the capacity to wage modern warfare. Furthermore, the army and the primary schools were the chosen means by which Italy sought to "make Italians" by imparting the lessons of civic duty and love of fatherland. Fever, however, greatly complicated the task that the Liberal regime had assumed. By blunting the army, the instrument by which the governing classes intended that patriotism should take root throughout the nation, malaria preserved the distance between the southern masses and the state. Thus the regional disparities that had weakened the Liberal regime since its foundation were perpetuated by disease.

At the same time, malaria made Rome militarily indefensible. It was impossible to staff the fortresses surrounding the capital adequately because of the appalling rate at which defenders fell ill after being stationed in the Roman Campagna. This vulnerability of Rome was one of the chief objections to

Table 1.1 Malaria in the Italian Army, 1898–1914 (cases per 1,000 soldiers on active duty)

1898	38.22
1899	36.33
1900	41.93
1901	49.34
1902	35.78
1903	22.05
1904	24.29
1905	25.23
1906	18.81
1907	13.18
1908	11.91
1909	7.67
1910	10.98
1911	11.75
1912	17.93
1913	10.10
1914	3.77

Source: Data from Ministero dell'Interno, Direzione Generale della Sanità Pubblica, and Ministero dell'Economia Nazionale, Direzione Generale dell'Agricoltura, *La risicoltura e la malaria nelle zone risicole d'Italia* (Rome, 1925), 243.

making it the capital city of the nation after Italian troops successfully captured it from the Papacy in 1870. A source of constant concern to Italian statesmen was the fear that a foreign army could land successfully on Italian soil and take the capital with little resistance. Conquering malaria, therefore, was a vital means of defending the conquests of Italian unification, known as the Risorgimento, and of preserving Italian diplomatic independence.

Furthermore, the disease distorted the life of the new capital and greatly restricted its future prospects for development and expansion. Emile Zola clearly expressed the manner in which the fever-infested Roman Campagna devastated the life of the city it enclosed. In a striking passage in his novel *Rome,* Zola described the Roman Campagna as a formidable impediment to the establishment of Rome as a modern capital:

> The Roman Campagna is a desert of death that a dead river crosses and that forms a belt of sterility encircling Rome. There have been discussions of draining and planting the Campagna, and people have argued idly over the question of whether it was once fertile under the ancients. Meanwhile, Rome abides in the middle of this vast cemetery. A city of bygone days, it is forever separated from the modern world by this steppe where the dust of centuries accumulates.

> Too rapid an effort was made to improvise a capital city. It remains in distress after nearly ruining the nation. The new arrivals—the government, the parliament, and the civil servants—only camp there. They take flight at the first hint of warm weather in order to escape the deadly climate. Then hotels and shops close, while the streets and parks are deserted. Not having a life of its own, the city then falls back into death, while the artificial life that animated it departs.[44]

Finally, malaria was a source of racial panic that augmented military fears. It was a common nineteenth-century belief that the degenerative symptoms of certain diseases, such as consumption and syphilis, could be passed from generation to generation. Malaria was especially conducive to hereditary interpretations because of its effects on pregnant women and their offspring. It led frequently to miscarriages, especially during the second trimester of pregnancy; to premature births; and to maternal death through hemorrhage. It was even possible for the disease to be transmitted from mother to fetus. Infants, therefore, were born with intermittent fever. If they survived, they developed into adults with foreshortened lives, enfeebled physiques, and cognitive disorders.[45]

Such observations suggested that malaria could taint the heredity of an entire population, resulting in a race that was feeble, emaciated, and infertile. As the Rome city council observed in 1873, fever could clearly lead to "the physical degeneration of the nation," and it could cause a "deterioration of the race by producing weak and sickly offspring" who "transmit abortive seeds to future generations."[46] The disease, wrote two officials of the Rome municipal department of health in 1922, "undermines Italy in the integrity of its race."[47] According to the public health officer Antonio Sergi in 1915, malaria had even more serious effects on the human body than either syphilis or tuberculosis, and it therefore had a "ruinous" effect on the life of a people, undermining its strength, destroying its character, and subverting its race.[48] Even Ettore Marchiafava and Amico Bignami, two of Italy's leading malariologists, espoused this view.[49] The fact that malaria was above all a disease of the peasantry heightened such fears because "it is in the countryside that one finds the deepest roots of the race."[50] One of the urgent reasons to attack the malarial problem, therefore, was that the disease threatened the Italian race and its nation with poverty and long-term decline.

North and South

In terms of the nature and severity of the symptoms of malaria, observers in the nineteenth century noted a marked and persistent divergence between North and South. Classifying malaria sufferers according to their most universal and characteristic symptom—intermittent bouts of fever—

Table 1.2 Mortality from Malaria in Italy, 1887

North	1,507
Center (minus Lazio)	696
South (plus Lazio)	18,730
Total (including Sicily and Sardinia)	21,033

Source: Data from *Inchiesta parlamentare sulle condizioni dei contadini nelle provincie meridionali e nella Sicilia,* vol. V, *Basilicata e Calabria, Tomo III, Relazione della sotto giunta parlamentare, Relatore: On. Francesco Nitti* (Rome, 1910), 357.

physicians noted that in the North patients suffered from those milder forms of the disease that were known as "quartan" and "benign tertian" malaria and that had low case fatality rates. In the South, instead, the dominant form of malaria was the virulent and often fatal "pernicious" or "malignant" tertian. For this reason, the southern countryside earned the lugubrious epithet of "the kingdom of death."[51] The reasons underlying this description are readily apparent in the regional mortality statistics for 1887 (Table 1.2). Since few peasants ever consulted a doctor, morbidity statistics were far less reliable than those for mortality. In terms of the sheer prevalence of fever, however, Jacini's parliamentary inquiry in the 1880s made the essential point when it noted that six regions of Italy were especially afflicted, and that all of them were southern — Sardinia, Calabria, Lazio, Basilicata, Apulia, and Abruzzi.[52] Furthermore, in the twentieth century Giovanni Battista Grassi estimated that the danger of infection in the South was ten times greater than in the North.[53]

Among experts who carefully considered the new findings, a consensus soon emerged that there were in fact "two Italies" with regard to malaria — one northern, the other central and southern. Malaria in northern Italy seemed to demonstrate paludal theory; malaria elsewhere conformed to telluric doctrine. The North contained a disproportionate share of Italy's swamplands. These were concentrated in the deltas of the great rivers flowing from the Alps to the Adriatic Sea — the Piave, the Tagliamento, and the Isonzo — and in the flood plain of Italy's greatest river, the Po. Here miasmatists had no difficulty in explaining that in Emilia-Romagna and the Veneto the populations that lived or worked in proximity to the swamps — peasants, fishermen, charcoal burners, and workers on land drainage projects that reclaimed fields for agriculture — suffered from fever. Similarly, when the rivers flooded after heavy rains, the total area subject to fever expanded, just as it contracted in dry years. It was logical, too, that the annual fever or "epidemic" season closely followed the temperature curve. The season began in July, when the combination of moisture and heat favored fermentation and poisonous ex-

Table 1.3 Italian Rice Production, 1901 (in hectoliters)

Lombardy	3,220,000
Piedmont	2,200,000
Veneto	755,000
Emilia	584,000
Sicily	32,000
Tuscany	8,000
Mainland South	600
Total	6,799,600

Source: Data from "La coltura del riso e le diverse operazioni agricole," ACS, MI, DGS (1882–1915), b. 748, fasc. "Legge sulla risicoltura," 14–15.

halations, and it ended in October, when the return of cooler weather brought unfavorable conditions for disease.[54]

More complex was the case of certain northern agrarian systems that were notorious for promoting fever. Most important and complex were the rice fields, or *risaie,* that in 1880 occupied large areas of the whole Po Valley but were concentrated in the provinces of Novara, Pavia, and Milan. Italy was the major rice grower of Europe, and the risaie played a vital role in the economy. Production was concentrated in the regions of Piedmont and Lombardy, although there was also significant cultivation in the Veneto and Emilia-Romagna (Table 1.3).[55]

Italian rice fields, however, were widely blamed for contributing abundantly to the malaria problem of the North. At the heart of the rice belt, for example, the Vercelli city council admitted in 1903 that "to deny the existence of malaria in this district is to deny the light of day. The two words *risaia* and *malaria* are so closely related that they may be considered synonymous." The link between risaie and malaria was occupational. The peak of the agricultural cycle in rice production began in late May and lasted until mid-July. During this period rice fields generated an insatiable demand for labor as a race began to remove the weeds before they destroyed the crop. Each field needed two or three weedings separated by intervals of fifteen to twenty days. Gangs of forty to fifty workers, stretched out in long lines and submerged in water up to their knees, performed the work. Weeding, therefore, set in motion tens of thousands of nomadic laborers, chiefly women whom contractors recruited from distant Apennine villages and deployed in man-made swamps flooded with water to a depth of two feet. Novara and Pavia provinces, for instance, experienced an annual influx of fifty thousand seasonal workers. They began to toil in the open air precisely at the onset of the warm malarial season. Furthermore, under the intense press of time, the workday itself extended from sunrise to sunset, interrupted only by pauses for breakfast and lunch. Thus, the workday encompassed the perilous hours of dawn and dusk, when the cold atmospheric temperature caused noxious vapors to rise from the waters. Miasmatists regarded dawn as especially dangerous because they believed that dew was a virulent miasmatic condensation.

So inevitable was it that large numbers of migrant weeders would succumb to disease that rice cultivation had inspired numerous official inquiries, a wealth of regulations, and an abolitionist literature advocating its ban. Attempts to protect those who worked in, or lived near, rice fields began with the Cantelli Law of 1866. The Cantelli regulations, inspired by miasmatic thinking, sought to protect the population in three ways. First, the law prohibited outdoor labor in rice fields at dawn. Second, it prescribed minimum distances between those fields and human habitations. Finally, it required that all work cease before dusk. This protective framework was supplemented by provincial regulations and by occasional local bans, such as the prohibition decreed by the prefect of Parma in 1893. Unfortunately, since rice was the most profitable of all cereal crops grown in Italy, there was great reluctance to cripple an industry that generated such wealth and created mass employment. For this reason, the Cantelli provisions were not enforced but were allowed to slumber —all but forgotten—until the turn of the new century. Effective measures, however, could not be legislated until science provided a better understanding of the mechanisms of the disease than miasmatic doctrine. Unraveling the mystery of malaria opened new prospects for action.[56]

2

From Miasma to Mosquito: The Rome School of Malariology

The malaria doesn't finish everybody. Sometimes there's one who will live to be a hundred, like Cirino the simpleton, who had neither king nor kingdom, nor wit nor wish, nor father nor mother, nor house to sleep in, nor bread to eat. . . . He neither took sulphate any more, nor medicines, nor did he catch the fever. A hundred times they had found him stretched out across the road, as if he was dead, and picked him up; but at last the malaria had left him, because it could do no more with him. After it had eaten up his brain and the calves of his legs, and had got into his belly till it was swollen like a water-bag, it had left him as happy as an Easter Day, singing in the sun better than a cricket.

—Giovanni Verga, "Malaria"

The Crisis of Miasmatism

Miasmatism persisted as the orthodoxy on malaria until the mid-1880s. Its great appeal to Italians was that it provided a plausible and easily understood explanation for the epidemiology of malaria in the nation. It established a framework for understanding the public health disaster afflicting the kingdom and for galvanizing opinion to combat it. In the late nineteenth century, however, miasmatic theory began to face a gathering intellectual crisis. A clear sign was its inability to accommodate the ever-growing body of information that careful studies such as those commissioned by the Italian parliament were producing. Instead of maintaining intellectual elegance and simplicity, miasmatism became increasingly complex and convoluted. Most obviously, miasmatists reacted to the clear differences between malaria in northern and southern Italy by producing a bifurcated doctrine. Instead of remaining a unitary theory, miasmatism emerged in two different guises: one, in the North, was paludal; the other, in the South, telluric.

Paludal theories asserted that malaria was a form of "swamp fever." Such an interpretation appeared to offer a convincing explanation for malaria in the North, where swamps abounded. The problem arose with malaria in the "other Italy"—the South, plus those neighboring areas of central Italy where southern conditions prevailed (the provinces of Rome and Grosseto). In this "other Italy" the disease was not so readily explicable as a product of marshland. As the Department of Health (Direzione Generale della Sanità) explained, there were three insuperable difficulties with the "swamp fever" interpretation of malaria. The first was that the malarial zones of Italy exceeded the swamplands in area by a factor of 4.6:1. The second difficulty was that malaria was far less prevalent and far less severe in the North, where most Italian swampland was located, than in the rest of the country, where swamps were the exception rather than the rule. Both the prevalence and the virulence of malaria were in inverse proportion to the area of swampland. Comparing the area of swamps and of malarial zones in the various regions of Italy in 1924, the department produced a table to illustrate this point (Table 2.1).[1] The department's conclusion was that it was possible to have swamps without malaria and malaria without swamps. As the American authority Lewis Wendell Hackett expressed the dilemma in 1937, "The name *paludism,* therefore, was as much a misnomer as malaria. In fact the major part of the hyperendemic malaria in Italy occurs in exceptionally dry hilly zones of the South and islands (Sardinia and Sicily). . . . In contrast to this situation, many of the great marshes of north Italy and north Europe were not associated with any malaria at all."[2]

It was in southern Italy, therefore, that an alternative medical philosophy came into its own—the telluric, or "dry earth," variant of miasmatism that the malariologist Corrado Tommasi-Crudeli exemplified. For Tommasi-Crudeli, the northern "marsh prejudice" had to be abandoned when dealing with areas such as the Roman Campagna where swamps were exceptional. Instead, he stressed that malaria could be "dry" as well as "wet." An entire swamp was unnecessary for even the most violent epidemics; heat, small collections of surface water, and impermeable clay topsoil were sufficient to promote fer-

Table 2.1 Swamplands and Malarial Zones in Italy

Region	Area of swamplands (in hectares)	Area of malarial zones (in hectares)
North	1,011,953	1,559,700
Center	113,086	982,200
South (including the islands of Sicily and Sardinia)	690,875	5,862,700
Total	1,815,914	8,404,600

Source: Adapted from Ministero dell'Interno, Direzione Generale della Sanità Pubblica, *Consigli popolari per la difesa individuale contro la malaria* (Rome, 1907), 16.

mentation in the earth and to generate deadly emissions. He concluded that "it is not necessary that there should be swamps of any kind, in order that malaria should exist. If such were the case, Italy would be a much more fortunate country than she is, since at least two-thirds of her soil which produces malaria would be perfectly healthy. A very small amount of humidity is sufficient to stir the noxious production."[3]

Folk wisdom held that malaria in the South burst into epidemic force on the feast of Saint Anthony on 13 June. The fever curve peaked during August and September and then slowly declined to its lowest level in December and January. Then, in January, the "endemic," or "interepidemic," period commenced and lasted for the next six months.[4]

Telluric theorists stressed the role of environmental degradation in creating ideal conditions for fever in the soil of the "other Italy." Thus, for Luigi Torelli, the chief source of Italy's misfortunes was the deforestation of the Apennine Mountains. In Torelli's assessment, topography, climate, and ecological disaster explained the sway of malaria over the Italian South. The topography of the South was determined by the Apennines that ran the whole of its length, so that 50 percent of the area consisted of mountains, 35 percent of hills, and only 15 percent of plains and valleys. Averaging 1,200 meters in altitude, the Apennines were not sufficiently high to be covered in permanent snow. They did not, therefore, replenish southern rivers year-round in the manner that the Alps supplied the Po River and its tributaries in the North. Rainwater alone fed the rivers of the South. Following the downpours of the rainy season in the winter and spring, southern rivers and streams flooded their banks, only to dry up completely during the hot Mediterranean summer. They left stagnant pools both in the adjacent countryside that they overran in the spring and in their beds as they dried out in the summer. Since the topsoil consisted of impermeable clay, pools of water did not readily drain away, but collected in depressions and hollows.

Deforestation further unbalanced this already problematic hydrology. The denuding of the Apennines—a process that stretched over many centuries—reached a climax following unification in 1861. Indeed, the years between 1861 and 1900 marked a critical period of widespread and intense destruction. The 259 reports collected by Torelli from provincial and district health councils are highly suggestive in this respect. Almost unanimously, they indicated that deforestation had proceeded furiously in the aftermath of unification and that, in its wake, malaria had greatly extended its sway. The report of the health council at Oristano in Sardinia was typical. It observed that "Sardinia, which was once rich as a result of its ancient and flourishing forests, is now becoming a desert steppe through the vandalism of greedy speculators. Through love of lucre they are transforming into charcoal an immense number of plants that represent the patient legacy of centuries."[5]

A crucial factor here was overpopulation. The population of the South soared from 3.5 million people in 1740 to 8 million in 1861 and 11 million in 1920. As it grew, the population came to exceed the "carrying capacity" of the mountains, driving peasants to bring ever more areas under the plow. Other influences were also at work, including the desire to make a quick profit by planting virgin soil; the drive to privatize the land at the expense of collective property; the absence of protective forest legislation; and the sale of Church land. Meanwhile, in the famous "crime hysteria" that swept Italy in the late nineteenth century when Cesare Lombroso and his associates developed the science of criminal anthropology, some people even applauded the disappearance of the nation's trees as a measure of law and order. Lombroso himself, for instance, rejoiced at the felling of the forests—those "natural fortresses of malefactors"—and urged that systematic clearing be used as a means of fighting crime.[6]

These factors led to a general invasion of the hills with axes, mattocks, and plows. Frequently, when mountain slopes were cleared with fire, the lumber of the fallen trees was not even exploited. Herds of goats and sheep then completed the destruction. The result was the decimation of the forests of beech, pine, chestnut, and oak that had once performed multiple hydrological functions. The canopy had broken the force of falling water and reduced its volume by providing broad leaf surfaces for evaporation. The roots and undergrowth had anchored the clay topsoil and protected the underlying limestone from the eroding forces of wind and rain. In the absence of the forest's cover, spring downpours generated innumerable torrents that swept away soil and rock, set off landslides, and silted up riverbeds downstream. Fed in this manner by rushes of water and detritus, rivers and streams repeatedly overflowed, creating stagnant ponds in valleys and along the coast, where the action of the waves compounded the havoc by piling up cordons of sand dunes that ran parallel to the shore and were covered in thick scrub. High, wide, and long, these dunes severely obstructed the flow of water to the sea and created shallow inland lagoons. The lagoons were thought to provide perennial opportunities for fermentation and the release of deadly effluvia.

Railways, those potent symbols of modernity, significantly augmented the damage. At unification, Italy possessed only 128 kilometers of track, but in 1881 the figure reached 8,331 kilometers, of which 3,762 were located in malarial zones. The negative impact of the railroads on public health was threefold. First, their elevated embankments supplemented the damage of sand dunes by blocking the drainage of waterways and creating marshes on their inland side. Culverts intended to alleviate the problem were insufficient in number and often improperly sited. At the same time, rainwater collected in the countless unfilled excavation ditches that had been dug during construction of the railways. Second, the demand for wooden ties, stations, bridges, and sheds created an inexhaustible demand for timber. Finally, the rails made Italy's forests vulnerable for the first time by providing a cheap and easy means to remove lumber and transport it to building sites. "The railways," wrote Torelli, "were the death sentence of the forests."[7]

Linking the various processes together, the health council at San Severo in Apulia explained:

> However painful it may be to admit, it is nevertheless certain that, most recently, extensive deforestation has occurred and that it has been tolerated, even authorized, on a vast scale. The loss of the trees has greatly enlarged the area subject to miasmatic air. Furthermore, the all-too-easy clearance of mountain slopes has led to the carrying away of topsoil into the beds of streams until they have been silted up, leading to the flooding of the adjacent plains. Last, the numerous excavation ditches along the railroad lines have led to new foci of infection and to the aggravation of those that already existed.[8]

Similarly, in Calabria, Dr. Carlo Magno lamented the demise of the forests. He wrote that in the three decades preceding 1880, "human greed, aiming at profit and unrestrained by law, began its work of devastation, and proceeded in a barbarian manner until now it is achieving its total objective before our very eyes."[9]

At the same time that miasmatic teaching bifurcated in order to encompass the epidemiology of the South as well as the North, it began to confront rising demands for rigor that it failed to fulfill. These expectations were the result of the revolution in microbiology introduced by Louis Pasteur, Robert Koch, and Joseph Lister. The implication of their work was that a valid medical doctrine should prove capable of guiding public health policy toward effective prophylactic strategies. The most celebrated contemporary examples were Koch's discoveries in 1882 and 1883 of the causative agents for tuberculosis (*Mycobacterium tuberculosis*) and for Asiatic cholera (*Vibrio cholerae*). The implications for public health were clearest in the case of cholera. After Koch had demonstrated that the cause of cholera was a bacterium ingested in contaminated food and water, sanitarians could effectively target for reform those practices that enabled the bacteria to gain access to water supplies and market produce. Understanding the pathogen led to the establishment of sewage systems and clean water supplies, and to the hygienic handling of food, all of which prevented the outbreak of further devastating cholera epidemics. Similarly, Lister, the Scottish surgeon, was not content to use the new germ theory as merely a means of understanding the origins of wound infections. Instead, he made use of the "gospel of germs" to revolutionize surgery. By introducing antiseptic conditions into the operating room, Lister was able to prevent suffering and death from septicemia. His much-publicized success spread a new confidence that scientific knowledge could vanquish diseases. At nearly the same time, Pasteur's pioneering work on anthrax and rabies led rapidly to the adoption of vaccination as a strategy of public health for a wide range of diseases.

Held to such standards, miasmatic teachings on malaria generated ever less conviction, and by the early 1880s the Italian scientific community began to seek alternative explanations. Whether paludal or telluric, miasmatism no longer convinced. To understand this point, one needs to consider the advice miasmatists offered the population as it sought to protect itself from fever.[10] One means of self-defense advocated by miasmatists gained wide acceptance in southern Italy, where infection was most severe and where upland refuges in the Apennines were near to hand. This advice was to flee the lowlands to high ground well above the miasmatic plume that hovered down below. Hilltops were also thought to provide cool temperatures that inhibited fermentation. Escaping the plains and valleys, therefore, constituted a rough-and-ready form of antimalarial prophylaxis.

Adherence to such advice was evident in the pattern of settlement. In northern and central Italy, the majority of the population consisted of peasants who lived in scattered farmhouses, small villages, and hamlets. But the South presented a striking contrast; there, to live dispersed across the countryside at low altitude was to fall victim to disease. Thus, as parliamentary investigators and malariologists explained, malaria was a major factor in the formation of the classic southern landscape of agro-cities perched on elevated sites and inhabited by tens of thousands of urbanized peasants. Such a strategy of prophylactic urbanization was also based on the conviction that the pavements and masonry of towns provided insulation against effluvia rising from the earth beneath. Those compelled to leave such elevated refuges to cultivate the lowlands took care, if possible, to arrive after dawn and to depart again well before dark. If distance made such daily treks impossible, peasants hastened to return to their upland homes immediately after the dangerous weeks of harvesting and threshing were complete.[11]

The prevailing age and gender profile of malaria sufferers in the South suggests that such strategies were partially effective. In southern Italy there was a pronounced division of labor that excluded women and small children from agriculture. In the interior of Sicily, for example, the Italian parliament found that agricultural work was "unthinkable for any women except the most impoverished—wives abandoned by their husbands, widows, and young girls who have experienced some disaster."[12] Tommasi-Crudeli described the medical results with respect to the town of Sezze, located high above the Pontine Marshes in the province of Rome. The men of Sezze, he observed in 1892, "are decimated by the malaria to such an extent that it is unusual to find one of their women who has not had three or four husbands. The town of Sezze itself is comparatively healthy, and it is only the male portion of the population who go down to the fields to work."[13]

Migrant peasants forced to sleep at sea level employed other measures of self-defense. Since malaria-bearing miasma was thought to be absorbed in part through the pores, one widespread protective tactic was to wear wool clothing even in the hottest weather. Woolen garments would stimulate abundant perspiration, ridding the body of the poison and preventing absorption. At the same time the resulting irritation of the skin was thought to act as a tonic on the nerves. Commonly, too, peasants burned fragrant pine needles in their huts or kindled fires in the fields to purify the air. For similar reasons, some employers of outdoor labor, such as the railroad companies, planted eucalyptus trees imported from Australia. These eucalyptus stands gave off a strong resinous odor that was thought to neutralize the effluvia and protect the population. Encouraged by miasmatic thinking, nineteenth-century Italy witnessed a great vogue in the fast-growing and fragrant Australian tree.

Another ploy sanctioned by both tradition and medicine was to drink red wine. Belief in its power to ward off malaria was based on the popular "doctrine of signatures." According to this credo, certain plants were distinctively marked by Providence to indicate their medicinal properties. The two essential operative principles were, first, that like cures like; and, second, that the healer's skill is the ability to read the hidden clues, or "signatures," of nature. Thus identified by the adept practitioner, red wine could prevent afflictions that, like malaria, produced anemia and disorders of the blood. Partly for this reason, and partly for the ability of alcohol to inure workers to privation, it was standard practice for employers to distribute wine abundantly to their laborers. In the 1880s Guido Bacelli, "the dean of Italian medicine," sanctioned this popular wisdom, teaching that red wine and red meat—"barely singed"—had strong protective virtues.[14]

It would be unwise to argue that such prescriptions had no value. They undoubtedly provided reassurance and hope, they probably mitigated the sufferings of southern women and children who avoided low-lying areas, and they may have reduced the burden of disease among nomadic field hands who risked the plains to harvest wheat. On the other hand, their utility was severely limited. Speedy departure, fire, fumigation, and red wine were capricious and unpredictable in their beneficial effects. The larger point was that, despite all such protective practices, malaria continued not only to strike down millions every year but also to expand the area under its sway as the environmental havoc that followed Italian unification created new opportunities for disease.

Apart from the advice it provided for individuals, miasmatism served as a guide for public health policies. Here the doctrine registered its greatest failure. After the revelations of Torelli and of the Jacini investigation, the Italian parliament resolved to take urgent action to combat malaria. The difficulty was that miasmatic theory was incapable of providing a precisely targeted plan of attack. On the contrary, it identified three essential elements as responsible for malaria—air, land, and water. A campaign directed against the disease, therefore, would logically require nothing less than total environmental sanitation if all three elements were to be cleansed of poison. All were ubiquitous, and the nature of the poison remained a mystery.[15]

In passing its first antimalarial legislation—a law for draining the Roman Campagna in 1878 and the so-called Baccarini Law establishing a broad national framework for land reclamation in 1882—parliament chose to concentrate on water. Water was the malarial element that would be easiest to target and that the consensus of medical opinion regarded as most dangerous. Ironically, Italian legislators thereby followed the Old Regime's precedent by attempting through land drainage and reclamation to prevent the formation of miasmatic effluvia and therefore of malaria. Like Pius VI (1775–1799) in the Pontine Marshes, so too parliament attempted to liberate the Roman Campagna from fever by draining the swamps in the Tiber Delta. By 1889, the grand paludal experiment reached completion.[16]

Unfortunately, this experiment failed as miserably as the efforts of the Pope in the eighteenth century. As the year 1900 approached, fever still ruled unabated in the Roman Campagna; the workers on the reclamation projects had sickened and died in discouraging numbers; and the drainage canals, now clogged with vegetation, had become swamps in their own right. The reclamation effort was abandoned as a mistake. More disheartening still was the fact that, apart from draining swamps, miasmatic theory suggested no other guidance for policy, except perhaps the impossible idea of purifying the earth and the air. The 1880s, which had begun with such strong commitment to combat malaria, ended with the conviction that public policy was powerless to protect the nation. Indeed, the Neapolitan physician Giuseppe Tropeano made considerable play on the theme of the unfulfilled promises of the Italian state. Vincenzo Gioberti, one of the founding fathers of the Liberal regime, had proudly proclaimed "the Moral and Civil Primacy of Italians." At the close of the century, however, Tropeano wryly observed that Italy had achieved only the "sad primacy" of illness and death from malaria.[17]

At the same time, physicians began to raise questions that miasmatism was unable to answer in either telluric or paludal form. First, if miasmas rose as telluric effluvia, why did they behave in a manner so different from dust? After a summer rain, for example, malaria normally afflicted a locality with redoubled fury, just as other particulate matter in the air became less plentiful. Similarly, if paludal theory was correct and malaria in the Italian capital was an airborne invader from the Pontine Marshes, why was Rome itself so often afflicted while intermediate localities over which southerly winds gusted were spared? Why were rice fields so dangerous when, logically, the water covering the fields should have formed a protective insulation that sealed off the miasma in the ground beneath and prevented disease? Why was high ground so often unaffected even when wind currents circulated aloft and gusted across hilltop settlements?

Medical researchers of the time (who were less inhibited by regulations than those of today) tried an experiment that raised the most crucial question of all. Why, if the malarial poison originated in the swamps, was it possible to administer liters of swamp water to volunteers without producing any of the usual symptoms of intermittent fever? Frequently the volunteers developed diarrhea, nausea, and continuous fever, but never the classic clinical symptoms of malaria. Just as the ancient doctrine of miasmatism entered a period of intellectual disarray, a puzzling discovery in Algeria opened the way to a new medical philosophy.[18]

The Plasmodium

Posted to Algeria in 1878, the French army physician Alphonse Laveran developed a fruitful hypothesis. Under the lens of his microscope, he noticed that the blood of malaria victims was the one part of their anatomy that was always affected severely by the disease. Other symptoms of malaria were variable, but all patients displayed mysterious pigmented elements in their bloodstreams. Laveran postulated that careful microscopy would reveal the offending pathogen in blood samples. Stationed in a region with an inexhaustible supply of fever patients, he therefore applied himself to the microscopic analysis of their blood serum.

In November 1880, Laveran made an observation that confirmed his hypothesis, inaugurated a new era in malariology, and founded the discipline of parasitology. The military doctor noted that, apart from inanimate pigmented elements, the blood of his patients contained motile filaments that were clearly living organisms. Laveran expected the organisms he had discovered to be bacteria analogous to those found by Pasteur and Koch in their famous work on anthrax. Further observation, however, revealed astonishing novelties. The newly discovered cells were far more complex and protean than bacteria, exhibiting in kaleidoscopic succession round shapes, crescent shapes, and flagella. Laveran reasoned that these were all manifestations of a single organism that he named *Haemamoeba malariae*—the specific cause of malaria.[19]

The very novelty of the newly discovered parasite initially caused disbelief. In the wake of the famous recent discoveries in microbiology, the medical community was predisposed to find bacteria, not Laveran's ever-shifting polymorphs. Indeed, Edwin Klebs, Ettore Marchiafava, and Tommasi-Crudeli promptly announced that they had found the real bacteria responsible for malaria—the *Bacillus malariae*. They believed that they had restored scientific orthodoxy in the matter of infectious diseases. Laveran, meanwhile, weakened the case for his parasite by confining himself entirely to descriptive microscopy, making no attempt to link the different shapes as the successive stages in a complex life cycle.

It was only with the additional research of Marchiafava and Angelo Celli in Rome that Laveran's parasites—renamed *plasmodia*—gained general acceptance. Marchiafava and Celli, using higher magnification and more sophisticated staining techniques than Laveran, began to explain the life cycle of the puzzling shapes Laveran had merely described. In addition, Marchiafava demonstrated that plasmodia were not simply present in the blood of malaria sufferers but were actually the specific cause of the disease. In 1885 he produced rigorous proof of their causative role by successfully inducing malaria in healthy human subjects, thereby fulfilling one of the essential requirements of "Koch's Postulates." His technique was to inoculate healthy volunteers with the blood of malaria sufferers. Since the volunteers regularly developed intermittent fever, plasmodia were clearly responsible for the disease. (Such experiment may shock modern readers, but at the time there were no regulations on human experimentation.)

In bringing the era of miasmatism to an end, however, the most elegant work of all was that of Camillo Golgi. Golgi brought order to the chaos of Laveran's observations by clearly establishing that the multiple forms exhibited by the parasite are successive stages in its complex life cycle. Golgi also revealed that the multiplicity observed under the microscope was partly due to the fact that there were several distinct species of plasmodium in Italy—known eventually as *Plasmodium vivax, Plasmodium falciparum,* and *Plasmodium malariae.* Malaria was not a single disease but a group of related illnesses.

Golgi explained that the parasites, upon gaining entrance to the bloodstream of the sufferer, invade red blood cells, where they multiply in ameba-like fashion until they burst the corpuscles asunder. Then the parasites and their waste—the pigmented material that had so intrigued Laveran—return to the bloodstream. Finally, the parasites attack new red cells and begin the cycle again—a process that occurs simultaneously throughout the circulatory system. Multiplying in geometric progression with a single inoculated parasite capable of generating twenty thousand offspring, the plasmodia rapidly reach sufficient density in the blood to trigger the immune response of the body and the onset of symptoms. The classic paroxysms of malaria recur at regular intervals marked by fever, chills, profuse sweating, and headache. Vomiting, diarrhea, and delirium are common. In falciparum malaria, the most virulent of malarial diseases, the density achieved by plasmodia in the blood is often overwhelming: 40 percent of the red cells of the body can be infected. At the same time, it is now known that the effect of *Plasmodium falciparum* on red corpuscles is to cause them to become sticky, to adhere to the walls of blood vessels, and to agglutinate in the capillaries and venules of internal organs. There they cause occlusion and hemorrhage, with swiftly lethal outcomes if the brain, the lungs, or the gastrointestinal tract is affected. In such pernicious infections, death can also result from hypoglycemia leading to coma, from acute respiratory distress, or from profound anemia.[20]

In less severe falciparum malaria and in most cases of vivax and malariae malaria, the disease is self-limiting. Instead of indiscriminately attacking all red corpuscles, *Plasmodium vivax* and *Plasmodium malariae* demonstrate a marked preference for young and aging erythrocytes. The effect is a much lower level of infection. The immune system of white cells, circulating and fixed, successfully contains and eventually eliminates the parasites from the circulation, although relapses can occur. Relapses are characteristic of *Plasmodium vivax,* which survives in the tissues of the liver, occasionally releasing cells into the bloodstream to resume the infection.

Golgi's greatest discovery was that the regular chronicity of the parasite's life cycle corresponds to the intermittent bouts of fever, chills, and sweating experienced by the patient. The recurring paroxysms coincide with the bursting of the red corpuscles and the release of the parasites into the bloodstream—a process that occurs simultaneously for an entire brood throughout the circulatory system. This was Golgi's Law, established in 1885. Its principles enabled him to predict the onset of fever—at constant intervals of forty-eight or seventy-two hours, depending on the species of plasmodium, or twenty-four hours in the case of superimposed infections of more than one species. For the first time, clinicians understood the bewildering symptoms of intermittent fever thanks to an astonishingly productive group of scientists funded by many interested parties. Among them were the railroad companies, the Ministries of Agriculture and the Interior, the local government of Rome, and a handful of enlightened landlords. Malaria had begun to yield its mysteries.[21]

As a result of the work of Laveran in Algeria, and of Marchiafava, Celli, and Golgi in Italy, the 1880s marked a turning point in understanding malaria, its symptomatology, and its pathology. But simply identifying the pathogen and correlating the phases in its life cycle with the symptoms of patients produced no advances in either treatment or prevention. The plasmodium dwelling in red blood cells rapidly gained acceptance as the pathogen responsible for malaria, but by itself, the discovery of the plasmodium did not elucidate the epidemiology of malaria, explain its etiology, or provide direction for public health policy. The next step would be to determine how the plasmodium reached the bloodstream in the first place. Where did it come from?

The "Rome School" and the Mosquito Theory

During the closing decades of the nineteenth century, malariology became the glory of Italian medical science. Indeed, the study of malaria between 1880 and the Second World War was dominated by the so-called Rome School (or Italian School) whose "Grand Maestros" included Angelo Celli, Camillo Golgi, Ettore Marchiafava, Amico Bignami, Giuseppe Bastianelli, and Giovanni Battista Grassi.[22] In an age of competing scientific nationalisms, the Rome School provided the Italian answer to Louis Pasteur in France, Ronald Ross in Britain, and Robert Koch in Germany. Italians made most of the key discoveries about the symptoms, transmission, and pathology of malaria. They devised the world's first national antimalarial program. The Rome School also made Italy the international center of malariology for nearly a century. As the American expert Paul Russell observed in 1952, "No country has contributed more to malariology than has Italy." He continued:

> So famous have been the Italian activities in malariology that for many years and up to the present time there has been a stream of students coming from overseas to learn from Italy. For instance, Sternberg came from America to study under Marchiafava and Celli in 1880, Laveran came in 1882, Koch in 1898, then William S. Thayer from Johns Hopkins, and many others, especially in the 1920's and 1930's from the United States, South America, the Middle and Far East, and Africa. One can hardly find an outstanding malariologist in the world today who has not visited Italy for the purpose of observation or formal training in this special field. Nowhere has malaria research and training been better developed.[23]

Why did Italy, and especially Rome, play so large a role in the science of malaria? Inevitably, there are factors that defy explanation, such as individual genius and sheer serendipity. But there were also larger processes at work. One was the crucial fact that, in Italy alone of the European powers, malaria was not chiefly a colonial concern but the most important domestic problem of public health. Indeed, the University of Rome was the only major university on earth to be surrounded by a region containing two of the world's most famous malarial areas—the Pontine Marshes and the Roman Campagna. For this reason, Rome possessed a critical mass of physicians devoted to the study of a disease then at the forefront of some of the most exciting developments in medical science. Fame and rewards awaited scientists who made breakthroughs in the field.

Fortuitously for malariologists in the capital, the surrounding province was also an ideal place in which to conduct fieldwork on the epidemiology and etiology of malaria. The province of Rome possessed both northern "wet" malaria and southern "dry" malaria in abundance. The first was characteristic of the Pontine Marshes, where the disease was closely linked to swamps; the second was dominant in the Roman Campagna, where swamps occupied only a limited area. In addition, since the region's mild climate meant that the epidemic season often lasted until December, the supply of patients for study and experimentation continued for most of the year. The climate also permitted the presence of all three species of plasmodium. *Plasmodium falciparum* was dominant, but infections with *Plasmodium vivax* and *Plasmodium malariae* were also common. Roman physicians, therefore, had the broadest possible spectrum of cases and blood samples to examine.[24]

Italian malariology also owed a debt to an important institutional base in Rome—the Hospital of Santo Spirito. Santo Spirito specialized in male malaria patients, most of whom arrived for treatment from the province just beyond the city walls. Given the sexual division of agricultural labor in the region, the malaria patients of the capital consisted predominantly of men. Santo Spirito

Table 2.2 Malaria Patients Hospitalized in the City of Rome, 1892–1895

Year	Male (Santo Spirito Hospital)	Female (San Giovanni Hospital)	Total
1892	4,224	500	4,724
1893	4,810	469	5,279
1894	5,637	664	6,301
1895	6,184	970	7,154
Total	20,855	2,603	23,458

Source: Adapted from Regio Commissariato degli Ospedali Riuniti di Roma, *Statistica sanitaria degli Ospedali per gli anni 1892, 1893, 1894, 1895* (Rome, 1896), table 23, xi.

Hospital therefore played a larger role in the development of malariology than the corresponding malaria hospital for women, San Giovanni.

In the summer, during the peak of the annual malarial season, Santo Spirito was severely overcrowded. Built to accommodate three hundred sufferers, its wards treated up to a thousand patients lined up in cots six rows deep. Santo Spirito and, to a lesser extent, San Giovanni provided Italian physicians with an almost unlimited supply of malaria patients (Table 2.2), which created abundant opportunities for observation, experimentation, and the generation of knowledge. The Rome School could not have existed without its two great fever hospitals.

Another factor in the development of the Italian capital as the world's preeminent center for malariology was the organization of the Rome School itself. The malariologists of the Italian capital were not a formal collective, and they were constantly and bitterly divided by scientific disputes, personal jealousies, and political differences. Nevertheless, the traditional description of them as a school captures the way both the medical profession and the public, in Italy and abroad, regarded them at the time. Furthermore, it correctly indicates that the Roman malariologists were not isolated researchers but part of an intellectual community whose members were constantly—often painfully—aware of the lines of inquiry pursued by the others. Despite the fractiousness and even enmity that divided it, the Rome School rapidly developed a collective presence. At its heart stood the Society for the Study of Malaria (Società per gli Studi della Malaria) founded in 1898. The society adopted its own research agenda; published the latest developments in malariology in its journal, the *Atti;* founded a Malaria Experimental Station at Cervelletta in 1899; and encouraged research in the discipline. It also served as a galvanizing force in the establishment of the antimalarial program, both in the province of

Rome and at the national level. Most of the leading authorities on malaria working in Italy were members of the society, many of them published work in the *Atti,* and all were intellectually indebted to the ongoing stimulation of the competition for preeminence among peers.[25]

Basic research in the sciences requires financial assistance. Members of the Rome School were fortunate in obtaining funds from a variety of sources concerned by the scale of Italy's malaria problem—railroad, mining, and pharmaceutical companies, as well as enlightened individual landlords and philanthropists. The Bank of Naples (Banco di Napoli), which included philanthropy as a central part of its mission, supported the research of Grassi and Celli.[26] The state also made contributions through the Ministry of Agriculture, the Ministry of the Interior, and the city of Rome.[27]

Thus structured, institutionalized, and financed, the Rome malariologists made their most celebrated discovery in December 1898 by answering the central question: How do humans contract malaria? Giovanni Battista Grassi, in close collaboration with Bignami and Bastianelli, unraveled the mode of transmission to reveal an unlikely culprit: the mosquito. The idea that mosquitoes might be involved in transmitting malaria was not new. In the first century BC, Varro suspected that they played a role, as did Lancisi in the eighteenth century. The problem was that the idea itself, unsupported by empirical evidence or an understanding of the mechanisms involved, was neither persuasive nor useful. Indeed, the mosquito hypothesis seemed to be disproved by a simple observation. While mosquitoes were present nearly everywhere in Italy and all over Europe, malaria affected only particular areas. The geographical distribution of malaria did not coincide with that of mosquitoes.[28]

As Grassi explains in his own account of his great discovery, it was only in the 1880s that the idea of mosquito transmission became of scientific interest, following two related developments. The first was Patrick Manson's discovery, in 1876, of the role of mosquitoes in the transmission of elephantiasis, thus proving that vector-borne diseases exist. The second, of course, was Laveran's discovery of the plasmodium. After these discoveries, scientists dissatisfied with miasmatic orthodoxy investigated the hypothesis that the mosquito played a part in the etiology of malaria. Alphonse Laveran advanced the idea in 1891, Robert Koch in 1892, and Patrick Manson in 1894.[29]

Working in India in close epistolary collaboration with Manson, Ronald Ross began the tireless dissection of mosquitoes—"ordinary," "dapple-winged," and "grey"—to locate the malarial parasite in their bodies and to trace its evolution. Since birds were more readily available to him for experimental purposes than human beings, Ross went on to demonstrate that mosquitoes transmit avian malaria and to suggest by analogy that they play a

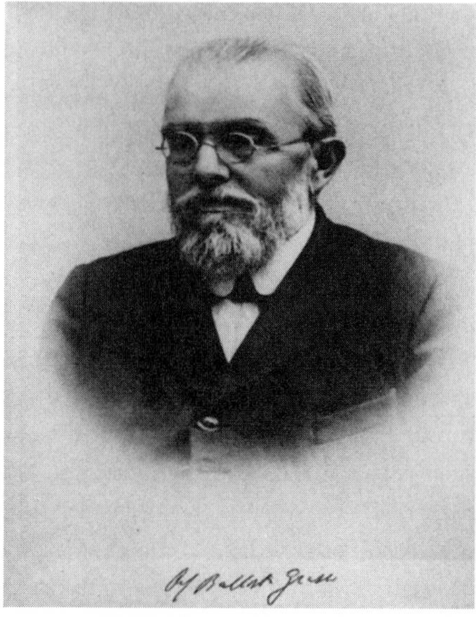

Giovanni Battista Grassi

similar role among humans. This demonstration was epochal, but it left unanswered questions concerning the human disease: Is malaria in humans transmitted in the same manner as among birds? Is transmission by mosquito the only mode by which human malaria can be communicated, or can the disease also be ingested or inhaled? Are all mosquitoes involved or only certain species?[30]

It fell to Grassi, a naturalist with the limitless malarial resources of the Santo Spirito Hospital and the Roman Campagna at his disposal, to establish what he called the "new doctrine" concerning human malaria. Working simultaneously with Ross but independently, Grassi concluded from fieldwork that not all mosquitoes were involved. His suspicions concentrated instead on those mosquitoes he named *Anopheles*. To test his hypothesis, Grassi, along with his associates Bignami and Bastianelli, captured large numbers of anopheles mosquitoes in the Tiber Delta and allowed them to feed on a patient exhibiting Laveran's "crescent-shaped bodies" (*Plasmodium falciparum*) in his bloodstream. Grassi then transported the infected mosquitoes to the wards of the Santo Spirito Hospital and released them into a closed room where a healthy volunteer had agreed to offer his body for their blood meal. Grassi released the mosquitoes into the room on 19 and 20 October, and the volunteer duly developed the classic symptoms of malaria on 1 November. "The experiment," wrote Grassi, "was single, but it was absolute. In the rampart that protected the great mystery of malaria, we had finally made a breach." Human malaria was now positively proven to be transmitted by mosquitoes. Not all mosquitoes, however, were guilty—only females of certain species of anopheles.[31]

To Grassi, this first demonstration of the transmission of malaria by mosquitoes was definitive. He and other members of the Rome School knew, however, that for the idea to win general acceptance they would need to carry out further extensive experimentation. Thus, from 1899 to 1902, they applied themselves to this task. They collected anophelines in the countryside, they allowed them to bite fever patients at Santo Spirito, and then they dissected the mosquitoes and examined them under the microscope. Carefully observing the plasmodium, they demonstrated that it completed its life cycle in the body of the insect. The stages that the plasmodium passed in the human body perfectly complemented and completed the phases achieved in the gut of the mosquito. Anopheline mosquitoes, they concluded, did not transmit malaria as one means of diffusion among many. The mosquito theory they advanced asserted that the plasmodia of human malaria are never found free in the environment at any stage of their existence. Instead, they live their entire lives in a closed circuit between the human body and that of the insect—the "intermediate" and "final" hosts.

The question remained, however, of whether the plasmodia could be transmitted vertically from the adult female mosquito to her offspring. In other words, could the infection of the mosquito predate her blood meal? Exhaustive observation, dissection, and microscopic examination determined that newborn mosquito larvae are never infected with parasites. Even larvae cultivated in the laboratory from anophelines captured in the homes of malaria victims did not contain parasites in their bodies, and humans bitten by the imagoes that emerged from these larvae never developed fever. In addition to these discoveries, Grassi and his colleagues made a series of additional observations that clinched the new mosquito doctrine. They observed that the extent of parasitic development in the gut of the mosquito is proportional to the time elapsed since her infective blood meal, that the parasite that develops in the mosquito is invariably of the same species as that contained in the infected blood she drinks, and that the degree of infection of the insect is proportional to the quantity of blood she ingests.

Grassi further argued that the doctrine solved the puzzle of regions that possess abundant mosquitoes but no malaria, a conundrum known as "anopheles without malaria." Either the mosquitoes involved are not species that are suitable to serve as vectors, or they have not been parasitized by feeding on infected blood. An abundance of mosquitoes is a necessary but insufficient cause of an outbreak of malaria. The crucial point is that, although there are regions with anophelines but no malaria, there are no regions with malaria but no anophelines.[32]

Most famously of all, both Grassi and Celli, working in caustic rivalry, devised experiments to prove that malaria is transmitted only by the mosquito and never by other means. The elegantly simple method they adopted was to send volunteers into the midst of major epidemics of malaria while changing only one factor that set them apart from the afflicted resident population. This crucial distinguishing factor was that the volunteers were rigorously protected from mosquito bites. The intention was to demonstrate that solely by preventing bites by anopheline mosquitoes, one could absolutely prevent malarial fever. This demonstration, wrote Grassi, "was of fundamental importance in order to disprove the widely held opinion that malaria is transmitted not only by anophelines, but by other means as well."[33] Indeed, Grassi admitted that until the great trial of 1899, he too sometimes doubted the validity of his theory. Could plasmodial miasmas, he wondered, infect humans in addition to mosquito bites?

As the site of his experiment, Grassi chose the notorious Capaccio Plain in Campania, where he conducted the trial at the height of the epidemic season, from 26 June to 24 October 1899—a year that proved to be one of the worst epidemic years in modern Italian history. Defined by the lower valley of the Sele River, the Capaccio Plain was one of the most infamously malarial zones in mainland Italy. For the test, Grassi and seven colleagues selected 104 healthy people with no history of fever—railway men and their family members—whom they stationed in sturdily constructed and well-protected housing at the heart of the malarial zone. The subjects of the experiment were at liberty to do as they pleased during daylight hours. Between sunset and sunrise, however, they were under strict orders to remain inside the designated buildings equipped with metal screens on the windows and doors. In order to allow all putative miasmatic vapors to waft freely, the scientists also gave instructions that the windows were to remain wide open except for the screening. What Grassi dubbed "mechanical prophylaxis"—the protective metal barrier between human and mosquito—was the only defense.

The results of the experiment were highly convincing. Of 112 protected subjects (the railway men, their families, and the experiment leaders, including Grassi himself), only five developed fever. All five cases, moreover, were mild, and all five were suspected of serious infractions of the required screening discipline. By contrast, all 415 members of a control group living nearby in unprotected housing contracted malaria, as did nearly the whole population of peasants and field hands who worked on the Capaccio Plain that summer.[34]

Other trials corroborated Grassi's dramatic demonstration at Capaccio. Angelo Celli carried out a famous parallel experiment (also in 1899) using identical means at Cervelletta in the Roman Campagna. Then Grassi repeated the test of mechanical prophylaxis in Salerno province in 1900 and in Dalmatia in 1902. These field tests confirmed that the results on the Capaccio Plain were not anomalous. From 1902, therefore, the mosquito theory grew ever more dominant in the international medical community.[35]

Nevertheless, doubters persisted, and Grassi has written that it was only with the First World War that a consensus emerged with respect to his doctrine. For many Italian clinicians, he explained, the great intellectual barrier to acceptance of the mosquito theory was the rapidity with which the annual epidemic season began. Grassi's doctrine required that there be only one source of plasmodia for the onset of each annual season of disease: the bloodstreams of patients relapsing from the previous year. Given this limited supply, nonbelievers held that there was not sufficient time for mosquitoes to become infected and to inoculate fresh victims widely enough to ignite the mass epidemic that appeared each year. The only possible explanation, they countered, was the operation of multiple sources of infection. Skeptics therefore continued to believe in the vertical transmission of plasmodia from female anophelines to their offspring. They also believed in parasites that live free in the environment and possess the capacity to infect humans by routes other than mosquito bites. Particularly among older physicians, traditional views about malaria receded slowly. As late as 1916, the provincial officer of health for Bari province still qualified as a doctrinal agnostic: he believed neither in parasites nor in mosquitoes. In his opinion, the source of infection was a still-indeterminate "infective element."[36]

Skepticism among the medical profession notwithstanding, Grassi's doctrine swayed parliament rapidly and unanimously. From the standpoint of public policy and legislation, no experiment was more crucial than the one designed by Grassi at Ostia in the Roman Campagna in 1901. Here the idea was to protect volunteers by chemical rather than mechanical means, and the results were no less dramatic than those achieved on the Capaccio Plain with screening. At Ostia, Grassi made prophylactic use of quinine—the first effective "magic bullet" in medical history. The efficacy of quinine as an antimalarial treatment had been known in Europe since the seventeenth century, when the Spanish learned of the ability of the bark of the cinchona, or "fever tree," to treat intermittent fever. The bark's active ingredient—quinine—had even been a central factor in colonial expansion. Quinine, it is said, was just as important to European armies in the tropics as gunpowder.[37]

As a medical resource for mass consumption, however, quinine had always

Table 2.3 Production of Quinine in Java, 1870–1911 (in kilograms)

1870	876
1880	—
1890	124,000
1900	5,237,000
1910	8,325,000
1911	9,558,000

Source: Data from "Relazione circa studi e ricerche per una piantagione di Chinchone (Chine) per conto del Governo Italiano," n.d., ACS, MI, DGS (1886–1934), b. 57, fasc. "Coltivazione dell'albero della china," 2.

been severely limited because of strict and inflexible constraints on world supply. The cinchona was exceedingly fastidious in its requirements for growth, and all attempts to transplant it from its native Andes to other climates had failed. Until the end of the nineteenth century, therefore, quinine was both scarce and prohibitively expensive. Other difficulties further limited quinine's usefulness. First, before the establishment of Grassi's theory, physicians had no understanding of the mechanisms by which the drug acted. Inevitably, therefore, there was great confusion among doctors about the proper use of the medication. Many clinicians regarded quinine as a generic treatment for all fevers rather than an antimalarial specific. Even when they administered quinine to victims of malaria, there was great uncertainty about the correct mode of administration. Was quinine best used preventively or curatively? When should it be administered, for how long, and at what dosage? Repeated attempts to use the medication inappropriately led to poor medical outcomes and undermined confidence in its efficacy. Finally, the high cost of quinine tempted unscrupulous speculators to adulterate or counterfeit the medicine. Physicians, therefore, could have only limited confidence in the potency of the medication they prescribed.

In the second half of the nineteenth century, some of these once insurmountable difficulties were overcome or at least greatly attenuated. In 1852 the Dutch successfully established cinchona plantations in Java, and by the end of the century, production began at last to catch up with demand (Table 2.3). As the supply of quinine expanded, the price per kilogram fell dramatically (Table 2.4). By 1900 quinine had become abundant and affordable.[38]

Moreover, just as the supply of quinine, which Grassi termed the "divine medicine," increased in almost geometric proportion and its cost plummeted, physicians began to comprehend its mode of operation. In light of the discoveries of Laveran, Golgi, and Grassi, they understood that quinine is not a

Table 2.4 Price of Quinine, 1880–1910 (lire per kilogram)

1880	462
1885	163
1890	54
1895	48
1900	42
1905	24
1910	12

Source: Data from "Relazione circa studi e ricerche per una piantagione di Chinchone (Chine) per conto del Governo Italiano," n.d., ACS, MI, DGS (1886–1934), b. 57, fasc. "Coltivazione dell'albero della china,"2–3.

magic panacea for all fevers. Instead, it specifically targets plasmodia in those phases of their life cycle when they swim freely in the blood plasma before invading the next red corpuscles. In this interval they are vulnerable to the action of the bitter alkaloid. Quinine, therefore, is useful both prophylactically and therapeutically. Prophylactically, if quinine is already present in the bloodstream of a healthy person at the time of an infective mosquito bite, the alkaloid destroys the invading parasites before they have time to establish an infection, and symptoms do not develop. Therapeutically, quinine can destroy parasites at each paroxysm of fever when the plasmodia are disgorged into the open bloodstream. If a high level of quinine persists in the blood serum for several accesses of fever, the chemical suppresses the disease and the patient recovers.[39]

A salient feature of the Rome School was the speed with which it transformed discoveries from the laboratory and the field into clinical procedures. The first issue of the *Atti* of the Society for the Study of Malaria announced that a solid "body of doctrine" had been established by Italian scientists. The time had come "for studies to descend from the laboratory into practical application."[40] In compliance with this appeal, Grassi and Celli sought a means to apply the doctrine to the control or eradication of the disease. Here was the special significance of the experiment at Ostia in 1901: it demonstrated the feasibility of chemical rather than mechanical prophylaxis. Mechanical defense had proven on the Capaccio Plain and at Cervelletta that, under carefully controlled conditions, it could protect a population from malaria. But it presupposed two essential conditions that were difficult to meet. First, the populations to be protected mechanically had to transform the routine of their daily lives to match the strict conditions of living indoors from dusk to dawn. Such a transformation was possible with small groups of sol-

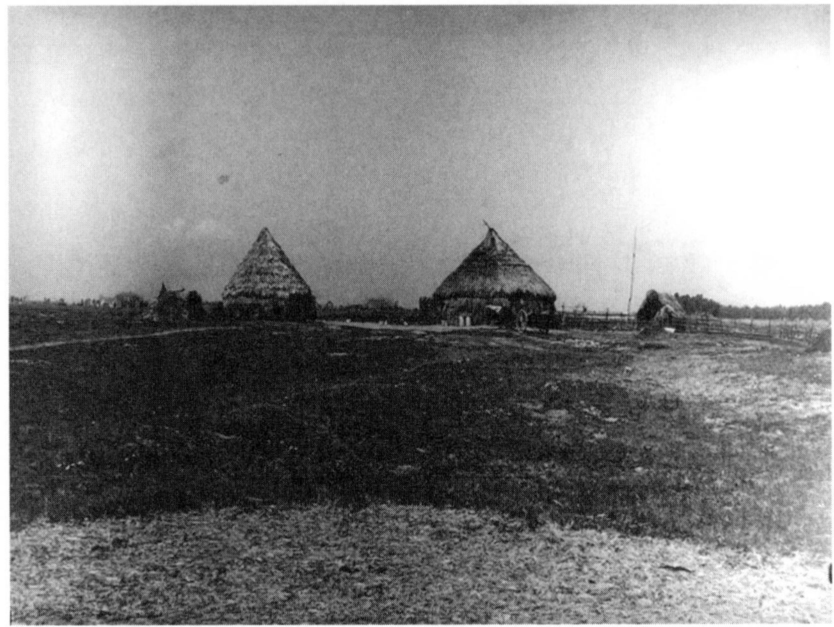

Housing in the Pontine Marshes, ca. 1920

diers and railway men who understood the significance of their actions, who were subject to constant surveillance, and who were free from urgent financial imperatives to extend their time spent out of doors. For the mass of illiterate and nomadic peasants and farm laborers, however, such conditions were impossible.

But even if the entire agricultural population of Italy accepted the regimen devised by Celli and Grassi, a second difficulty would defeat the objective—the impossibility of effective screening under Italian conditions. Mechanical defense presupposed housing of solid masonry with regular window frames, whitewashed interiors, and well-constructed doors. As the Jacini-led parliamentary inquiry and subsequent discussions in parliament revealed, however, substandard housing was one of the most distressing aspects of the "social question" and of public health in Italy. During the height of the malarial season, millions of migrant peasants, farmworkers, and shepherds slept in porous dwellings of straw, reed, or dry stone that allowed free access to all species of flying insect. Countless others spent their nights in caves, like the day laborers at Grottarossa, or under canvas in open fields. To safeguard such people behind a metal barrier would require a housing revolution, a transformation in prevailing patterns of settlement in the South, an end to established

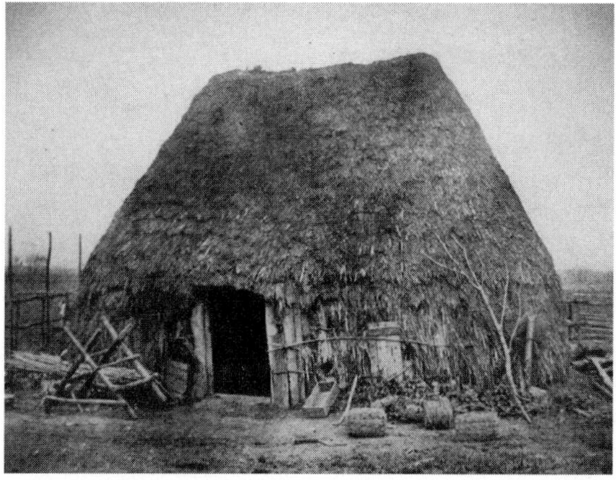

Housing in the Pontine Marshes, ca. 1920

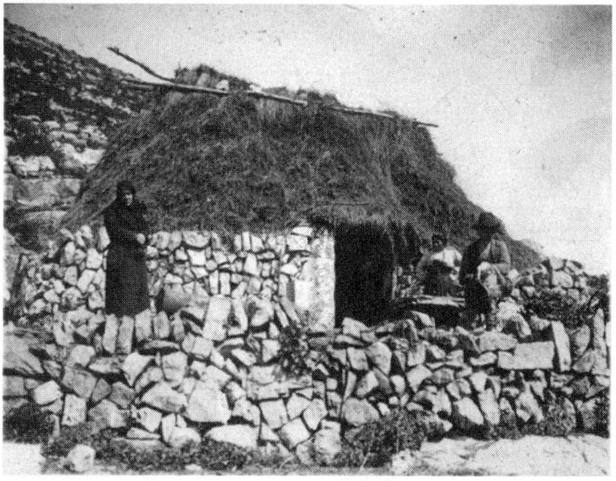

Housing in Sardinia, ca. 1930

patterns of migrant labor and pastoral transhumance, and a massive investment of funds.

Grassi's experiment at Ostia, an intensely malarial zone in the Tiber Delta, served as a pilot project for treating impoverished rural areas. Its purpose was to test the feasibility of replacing mechanical prophylaxis with chemical—of replacing the barrier of metal interposed between human and mosquito with a chemical barrier of quinine. The challenge was to determine whether a small team of doctors could protect many thousands of peasants from infection by administering daily doses of quinine, supplemented with iron and arsenic, which were regarded as tonics that would fortify the patient while quinine attacked the parasites. Grassi and his team persuaded 293 peasants to swallow quinine tablets daily in their presence from the beginning of the malarial season on 1 June until its end on 31 October. The result was that, of the 293 protected people, 239 completed the trial without contracting fever, and 54 developed mild cases that responded well to treatment. Significantly, all 54 of those who contracted mild cases had failed to comply fully with the specified medication regimen. In Grassi's words,

> From the point of view of hygiene and the intention of eradicating malaria, the results we obtained at Ostia have . . . a fundamental importance.
>
> If we compare these results . . . with those observed on the Capaccio Plain, where screening was employed, we see that they are mutually supporting. Our conclusion, therefore, is this: antimalarial prophylaxis can be achieved in two ways—mechanically or chemically.[41]

The experiment resulted in a lifelong and very public enmity between Grassi and Celli. For the Ostia experiment, Grassi made use of the commercial preparation known as Esanofele, which contained—in addition to quinine as its active ingredient—arsenic and iron as tonics. Celli argued that Grassi, by using this product, had become the tool of the Felice Bisleri company, which manufactured Esanofele, and had irresponsibly cast doubt on the efficacy of pure quinine.[42]

Making reference to the Book of Daniel and Nebuchadnezzar's famous dream, Grassi nevertheless proclaimed that he had located the weak point—the "feet of clay"—of the looming Colossus Malaria.[43] Quinine, he maintained, was the weapon of choice, even though he and Celli differed profoundly on whether it should be administered prophylactically or therapeutically. Celli favored the prophylactic strategy, that is, inducing the entire population of malarial Italy to swallow two tablets of the alkaloid a day throughout the epidemic season from June to November. In this manner, it would be possible to prevent new infections and to break the cycle of transmission. If this approach continued for several years in succession, the reservoir of infection in the human population would dry out and the disease would vanish.

Grassi aspired instead to what he termed the "radical cure," or "human reclamation" (*bonifica umana*), of patients by "sterilizing" their blood with quinine during the epidemic off-season from December to May. His strategy was to break the cycle of transmission by curing all patients so that mosquitoes would not be infected and no new cases would develop in the following summer. Summarizing the practical implication of the doctrine he had played so large a role in establishing, Grassi wrote that "the implication of all this knowledge is that it is of great importance to cure the malaria patient, and to take advantage of the interepidemic period to achieve this result. Everyone can understand that, if at the start of the new malaria season, anophelines found no human carriers, then malaria itself would assuredly be completely vanquished."[44] Grassi also reasoned that cure was more feasible than prophylaxis because it reduced the number of people to be dosed with quinine to more manageable proportions. It would not be necessary to locate and treat all the inhabitants of malarial Italy but only the more limited population of people who had actually contracted fever.

Despite the major difference between Celli and Grassi, they both experienced a rush of optimism. Both believed that mass quininization, made possible by the sudden glut of quinine from Java, offered a quick solution to Italy's foremost medical problem. Of the two, Celli was more cautious, calling for malaria control, while Grassi explicitly sought total eradication. The nation would not need, both men initially suggested, to drain swamps, reforest the Apennines, modernize agriculture, revolutionize rural housing, and transform society. All that was required was to dose a sufficient number of human bloodstreams twice daily for several seasons. Grassi estimated the cost at several hundred million lire—a tiny sum, he reasoned, compared with the money annually spent on the military or on far less important public works projects, such as the great Apulian Aqueduct. "That hyperbolic Apulian Aqueduct," he wrote, with reference to the estimated two hundred million lire that it cost to pump water into Apulia from the Sele River in the hills of Campania, "was conceived in an era when people still believed that fevers were spread by water. Therefore, in the opinion of many, it seemed dangerous to seek water in the subsoil of malarial Apulia."[45] The mosquito doctrine would eliminate all such waste in the future. Indeed, Grassi also calculated that the antimalarial program would rapidly pay for itself through enhanced productivity and reduced medical expenses. Success, which he defined as the *finis malariae,* could easily occur, Grassi predicted, during the reign of the newly crowned sovereign, Victor Emmanuel III.[46]

Thus encouraged by science and by an abundance of quinine, parliament passed a series of laws between 1900 and 1907 instituting the great experiment—the first of its kind—to control malaria throughout a nation by chemotherapy. In the words of the *Lancet,* "The sale of quinine by the State is a new and enlightened departure in sanitary legislation of which Italy gives as yet the only example."[47] The simplicity, the frugality, and the scientific authority of the plan suggested by Grassi and Celli made it politically irresistible. The antimalarial campaign was taken up immediately by the Society for the Study of Malaria. Those of the society's members who were deputies, including Celli himself, drafted the bills that were placed before the Chamber of Deputies. Since the Liberal majority under Giovanni Giolitti granted them time for a full parliamentary hearing and the conservative opposition leader Sidney Sonnino sponsored the legislation, the measures all passed unanimously, "with few speeches, and not a single protest from any of the benches."[48]

Celli, a Republican deputy and already a famous advocate of public health in the Chamber, was far more politically influential than Grassi, the pure scientist. Not surprisingly, therefore, the plan enacted was Celli's prophylactic vision rather than Grassi's curative one. In accord with this strategy, the Italian state undertook to purchase quinine of guaranteed quality on the international market, to package it in tablets, and to ship the pills to all designated malarial zones of the peninsula. There the alkaloid would be provided gratis to the poor and to all those who were employed in outdoor labor. Quinine, previously a privilege of the affluent, was suddenly available to all. The objective was that malaria, now precisely targeted, should disappear so that Italy, the "sick beauty," could finally awaken.

3

A Nation Mobilizes

As you watched, O king, you saw a great image. This image, huge and dazzling, towered before you, fearful to behold. The head of the image was of fine gold, its breast and arms of silver, its belly and thighs of bronze, its legs of iron, its feet part iron and part clay. While you looked, a stone was hewn from a mountain, not by human hands; it struck the image on the feet of iron and clay and shattered them. Then the iron, the clay, the bronze, the silver, and the gold, were all shattered to fragments and were swept away like chaff before the wind from a threshing-floor in summer, until no trace of them remained. But the stone which struck the image grew into a great mountain filling the whole earth. That was the dream.

—*Daniel 2:31–36*

Organizing the Antimalarial Crusade

The Italian crusade against malaria, which began in earnest in 1904, involved a close partnership among the state, local governments (*comuni*), and the medical profession. The central government purchased quinine wholesale on the international market, packaged it in tablets at its factory in Turin, and distributed it to municipalities in all the malarial zones in Italy. Bypassing the retail market of pharmacies, local governments provided the alkaloid—dubbed "state quinine"—free to those in need. The network of physicians employed by the campaign supervised the administration of the drug. The intention of the legislature was that every poor Italian at risk would receive regular medication for both prevention and cure at no cost and with the certainty that the chemical was unadulterated.

In the opinion of Giovanni Battista Grassi, who definitively established the mosquito theory of transmission of human malaria, calculations of cost should have played no role at all in the program. Grassi believed that the state should meet all of the expenses involved in the state-quinine campaign because the cost of eradicating malaria would be rapidly recouped through enhanced productivity and reduced medical costs. In malarial areas, he reasoned, quinine was as vital to life as air and water. It should, therefore, be as freely and as plentifully available as those other precious commodities. By collecting any sort of tax to recoup its outlays, the government would only create political opposition, alienate vested interests such as the pharmaceutical industry and pharmacies, foster bureaucratic delays among already demoralized and overworked municipal authorities, and generate complexities that could compromise the final objective.[1]

Parliament, however, balked at the prospect of burdening the exchequer. It preferred to assess blame for the disease and to collect damages from those it determined were responsible. The epidemiological evidence encouraged the politicians because it clearly indicated that malaria was directly linked to the performance of certain forms of outdoor employment. A crucial aspect of the Italian antimalarial legislation, therefore, was that it defined malaria as an occupational disease. In the words of the Ministry of the Interior, "The defining concept behind all the measures is the recognition that malaria is an occupational disease. The reason is that malaria is linked both with work and with work-related residence in unhealthy localities."[2]

Defining malaria as an occupational disease implied that employers were responsible for the illness of their workers and that they should therefore pay for measures of prevention and treatment. Local governments were required to levy a "quinine tax" on landlords and other employers of outdoor labor in malarial zones—contractors on public works projects, mining companies, and railroad companies. For landowners, the amount of the tax was proportional to the total area of the land they held in the designated malarial zones of the township. Other employers paid in proportion to the number of workers they engaged in outdoor projects. The quinine levy was intended to cover the cost of providing chemical prophylaxis to those at risk and of treating the poor for whom prevention failed.

In addition to collecting the quinine tax, local authorities bore the primary responsibility for implementing the Italian antimalarial campaign.[3] Municipalities had legal responsibility for operating health-care facilities and hiring medical personnel to administer quinine to the population. In some measure, delivery fell to an institution that already existed as the basis of public health throughout Italy — the public health clinic (*condotta medica*), which provided medical care to the indigent.

In practice, however, most municipalities, especially in the South, were unable to provide more than a skeletal service. Since regressive local taxation formed the basis of municipal finance, poor townships found themselves in the classic "poverty trap": they had extensive legal obligations to meet the needs of the impoverished, but their resources were severely limited. As a result, health-care provision suffered. Not infrequently, municipalities appointed no public health doctors at all, or paid wages so low — one hundred lire a year in certain localities in Calabria — that the physicians were compelled to become pluralists who devoted little time to their public duties. In addition, since so many peasants were migrants scattered over vast expanses of remote and inaccessible terrain, most were beyond the reach of the public health physicians. Patients who were seriously ill were unable to make the exhausting journey to town to receive care. Even under normal circumstances, public health clinics were unequal to the task of providing medical attention to the rural poor. There was little prospect, therefore, that they could fulfill the onerous new function of administering quinine daily to the whole rural population.[4]

For this reason, the antimalarial campaign established a new institution in the countryside as its sheet anchor — the rural health station (also known as a dispensary). The rural health station was first developed by the city of Rome as a weapon against malaria in the surrounding countryside known as the Roman Campagna soon after Rome became the capital of Italy in 1870. The municipality of Liberal Rome set up five rural health stations in 1874 (at Campomorto, Fiumicino, Isola Farnese, Ostia, and Torrimpietra). Thereafter, the number of rural health stations slowly increased — to seven in 1876, nineteen in 1884, and twenty-five in 1912 — and their functions progressively expanded. Just as the Rome School took the lead in developing the science of malariology, so Rome's city hall provided the initiative in devising institutions to take the new science into the countryside. As early in the campaign as 1906, the provincial officer of health reported that the city had organized a service of prophylaxis and care that was "above all praise," distributing quinine preventively to 9,415 healthy peasants and treating 2,474 fever patients.[5] Roberto Villetti, the alderman in charge of the municipal department of health, wrote with pride in 1922 that "the municipality of Rome was the first to organize the

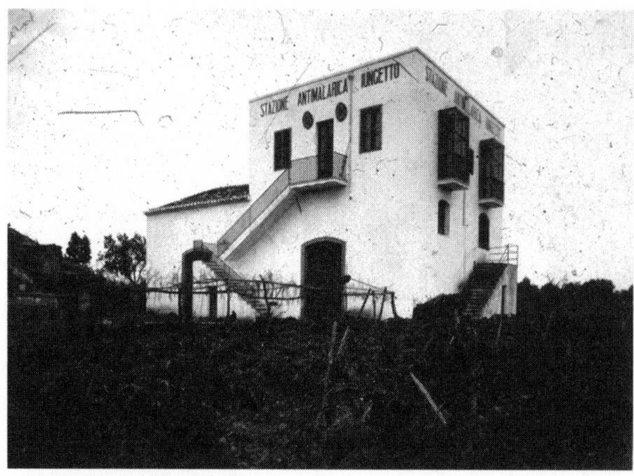

A rural health station, ca. 1930

battle against malaria on the basis of rational scientific methods that . . . served as the model for the Italian legislation passed against malaria and then copied by all civilized nations."[6]

The mission of the rural health stations was to overcome the difficulties that overwhelmed local health facilities and prevented them from providing care to the rural poor. Medical care, concentrated in towns and cities, had long been inaccessible to those most in need. Even the nature and scale of the problem to be addressed were largely unknown. The first phase of activity of a rural health station, therefore, was reconnaissance and orientation. It was essential to base the campaign not on generic impressions but on accurate statistical information—on a reliable estimate of how many people required treatment, what form of malaria they had contracted, and how many healthy people needed chemical prophylaxis. To this end, rural health stations launched the campaign by undertaking a local health census. They examined blood samples for plasmodia, measured spleens, checked temperatures, and established careful records. The medical director at each health station was responsible for maintaining detailed clinical charts, recording how much quinine was prescribed, monitoring what proportion of the quinine prescribed was actually consumed, and providing follow-up care.[7]

In the North, Verona provided a clear demonstration of the methodology by which the campaign was supposed to proceed. At the outset the physicians of the province undertook a "hunt for sufferers," visiting every home in every locality and taking blood samples from all family members. Their chief purpose was to uncover undiagnosed cases, which were widespread. In addition, they hoped to determine the relative prevalence of all three species of plas-

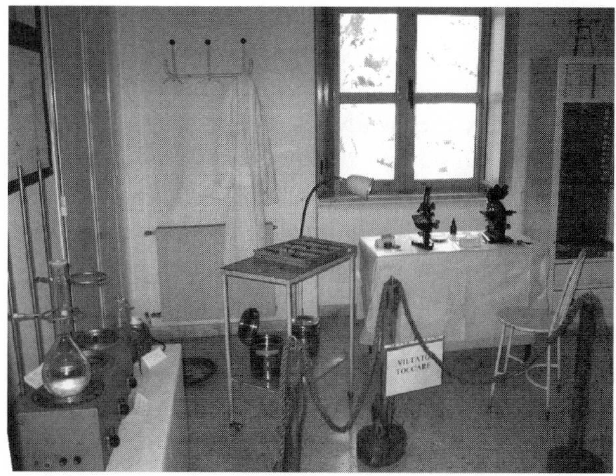

Interior of a model rural health station, ca. 1935

modium, to establish a precise statistical profile of the epidemic, and to map its geography. Having compiled careful data, the physicians sent detailed reports to the provincial officer of health, who in turn produced in 1912 a comprehensive statistical and geographical profile of malaria in Verona. This completed the preparatory phase.

Next, the officer of health for Verona drafted guidelines for the second, or operational, phase of the campaign. On the basis of the information gathered in the house-to-house census, he oversaw the location of health stations, the deployment of medical personnel, the allocation of quinine, and the provision of follow-up care. Where there was a shortage of doctors, the officer recruited teams of medical students and others of proven reliability and intelligence, and he ensured that they were given practical instruction and training. Verona illustrated the system as it was intended to function.[8]

The rural health stations fulfilled their raison d'être by taking aid to those places where its impact could be greatest—along routes frequented by migrant laborers, to workers' quarters on estates, and at strategic locations in the open countryside. Instead of bringing sufferers to the clinic, the health stations took the clinic to the sufferers. By the First World War, Italy possessed 1,200 health stations.[9]

Based on the precedent set by Rome, rural health stations had as their primary function the job of administering quinine. This task, however, required constant contact between the stations' physicians and the populace, providing opportunities for individual persuasion, group instruction, house visits, and inspection tours of workplaces. As a result, young doctors, newly imbued with the doctrine of Grassi and Celli, often supplanted private physicians and public health doctors who were too skeptical of modern science, too old to endure the physical rigors of a demanding rural practice, or too poorly paid to make the effort. Frequently, the health station served as a base of operations for mobile substations that held regular open-air clinics on large estates, at the end of Sunday mass, and at markets and festivals—wherever there were "masses of people to be treated, medicated, and evangelized."[10] Health stations also often operated infirmaries, usually located on the upper floor, where they provided an inpatient service for serious cases. In addition, they organized ambulances for the transport of those too ill to travel. Since remote areas were frequently accessible only over nearly impassable trails, the "ambulances" sometimes consisted of stretchers borne by hand. Finally, the stations served as models to demonstrate the correct installation and use of metal screening.

Those who directed the antimalarial service rapidly discovered, however, that the most important function performed by the health station was to overcome the suspicions of the uneducated. To achieve this goal, the station needed to provide a comprehensive clinical service instead of confining its attentions solely to malaria. Treating a wound, setting a bone, medicating trachoma, or delivering a child was often the essential precondition for the trust that alone made it possible to treat fever. Rural health stations, therefore, normally possessed a fully equipped examining room with facilities for minor surgery, a complete medical armamentarium, a small infirmary, and a diagnostic laboratory equipped with a microscope. Grassi argued that every doctor in the antimalarial campaign rapidly learned the "great truth" that malarial patients would never trust a doctor who referred them to other physicians for every problem except malaria and provided no therapy except quinine. More speculatively, some physicians hoped that establishing a comprehensive medical infrastructure in a malarial area would attract peasant settlers and that the settlers' presence would intensify cultivation and transform the conditions of neglect on which anophelines thrived.[11]

Tullio Rossi-Doria, a gynecologist who served as alderman responsible for health on the Rome city council, drew on his own experience in the Roman Campagna to explain that obstetrical services provided the very best instruments for outreach and the establishment of trust. Women were willing to accept care related to safe motherhood. A physician could then also test their blood for parasites and arrange follow-up visits to their workplaces and homes, explaining all the while the danger of mosquitoes and the utility of quinine. Having established contact with the peasant families, the health station could arrange informal seminars to explain the mechanisms of transmis-

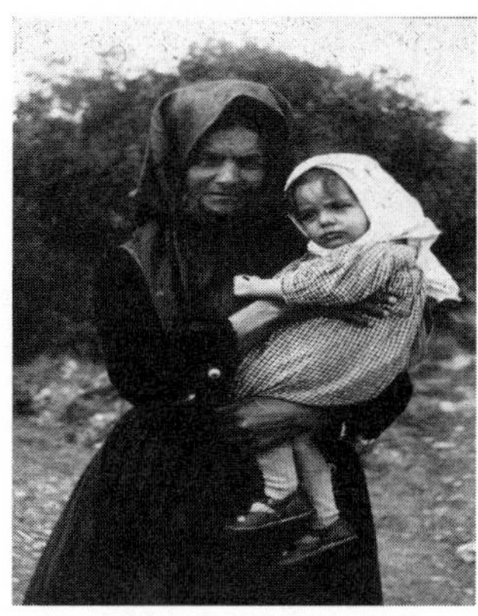

A Sardinian peasant woman bringing her feverish child to the health station, ca. 1930

sion, distribute pamphlets drafted by the Department of Health, collect statistics, arrange public lectures, and inform patients of their rights under the antimalarial legislation. A proper clinic, it was said, should be run not by dispensers of tablets but by the "apostles of health and hygiene."[12]

In the important case of the Roman Campagna, the city of Rome received the support of an outside agency — the Italian Red Cross. Although the constitution of the Red Cross stipulated that its mission was to provide medical care only in time of war, its directors ruled that the campaign against malaria was sufficiently similar to warfare to warrant their involvement. The Red Cross therefore agreed to operate seven health stations, staffing them with a team of forty uniformed doctors assisted by a complement of nurses, ambulance drivers, and stretcher bearers. As with the campaign as a whole, the Red Cross adopted a strategy of not waiting to be summoned. On the contrary, its physicians followed the nomadic farmworkers of the Campagna to their dwellings, seeking fever victims who would otherwise receive no medical attention.[13]

Central government assumed different tasks, which the Department of Health defined as "complementary" to those of municipalities — "direction, supervision, stimulation, coordination, and propaganda."[14] Under the guidance of an advisory committee of leading malariologists, the Italian state operated the quinine factory at Turin for the preparation of tablets, distributed the tablets to townships, and cooperated in recruiting and deploying personnel — doctors, nurses, and scouts — to staff the health stations. Whereas the retail cost of quinine in Italy before the campaign had often reached ten times the cost of production, the state now charged only double. Even these relatively slender profits were set aside to support the eradication effort: the Ministry of Finance used the money to improve the salaries of physicians, to reimburse landlords for installing screens, and to reduce the expenses of municipalities that found themselves severely in debt owing to the cost of administering the program. Furthermore, the state operated a program of "special laws" designed to provide aid for the most disadvantaged regions, such as Basilicata, Calabria, and Sardinia. Under the terms of this legislation, the Italian national government undertook to lessen the burden of purchasing quinine for townships in those regions. The state contributed significantly to the purchase of the alkaloid on their behalf, employing funds from the exchequer. From 1906 the Department of Health also appointed eminent physicians from the universities as commissioners to investigate conditions, superintend the implementation of the program, gather statistical information, and make recommendations to Rome. The commissioners, each of whom was normally charged with overseeing the antimalarial campaign of an entire region, included such medical luminaries as Camillo Golgi, Giovanni Battista Grassi, Bartolommeo Gosio, Errico De Renzi, Giuseppe Cardarelli, and Giuseppe Zagari.[15]

Led by Gosio and Zagari, who directed the campaign in Basilicata, Calabria, and Sardinia, the commissioners advocated a second type of institution to complement the work of the health station—the antimalarial sanatorium for children. Gosio and the other sponsors felt that a special institution was needed to provide for the needs of children, who were particularly susceptible to malaria. Children suffered the highest fatality rates from falciparum malaria, and they experienced the most serious long-term complications and sequelae of chronic malaria. Modeled on the international experience of the struggle against pulmonary tuberculosis, antimalarial sanatoriums were set up in the mountains and by the sea. The first sanatorium opened in 1909 in Calabria at an altitude of 1,200 meters and the second in 1910 at Monte San Giuliano in Sicily. By 1914, nine sanatoriums were operational.[16]

Sanatoriums provided the children of the poor with a refuge from the torment of mosquito bites, a change of climate, and a carefully supervised therapeutic regimen. Since resistance to malaria was widely thought to be compromised by malnutrition, sanatoriums also offered children months of carefully balanced meals to strengthen their immune systems. Meanwhile, nurses and teachers gave lessons on the basics of transmission and self-defense that the children could take home to their families. Finally, to the extent that the sanatoriums physically removed infected children from localities with high rates of transmission, they drained the reservoir of infection and thereby lessened the burden of illness.[17]

Even officials at the highest levels of government assumed important roles. Prefects and provincial officers of health were instructed to educate municipal officials in the purposes of the campaign, to carry out inspection tours to verify their compliance, and to punish obstructionism by those whose vested interests were threatened by state quinine—landlords, pharmacists, taxpayers, and municipal councilors. A vital factor in the involvement of central government was the commitment to the campaign of both prime ministers who held office between 1900 and 1914—the Liberal Giovanni Giolitti and his conservative rival, the Tuscan landlord Sidney Sonnino. Both leaders were convinced that improvements in the living standards of the people were essential to strengthening state authority, bolstering the economy, and countering the appeal of socialism. They were prepared, therefore, to call upon employers to make short-term sacrifices in the long-term interest of political stability and economic development. In their view, the war on malaria was an essential component of enlightened self-interest. Mayors and other municipal officials who disagreed were subject to visits by the police and the provincial officers of health.

Giolitti established the precedent. As the distribution of quinine began for the first time in 1903 and 1904, he telegraphed all the prefects in the kingdom, reminding them of the importance of the "hygienic redemption of our rural population" and instructing them to take vigorous measures to ensure the success of the program. By 1906 Giolitti had earned the unanimous praise of the antimalarial commissioners for his unstinting commitment to the cause. Sonnino, who served more briefly as prime minister, showed an equal enthusiasm for the antimalarial crusade he had helped to launch. In February 1910, for instance, he informed the prefects of Italy that

> the fight against the terrible scourge of malaria constitutes an important economic, social, and public health interest for our nation. It must be pursued this year—even more than in years past—in such a way as to guarantee the fullest possible realization of the intentions . . . of the special laws . . . voted by parliament. . . .
>
> No effort must be neglected. Only the contribution of everyone, no one excepted, and the unremitting employment of every available means . . . will make it possible to achieve significant and lasting results.[18]

The premiers' admonitions often served only to confirm the good intentions of their subordinates. As the highest state official in each province, the prefects were especially important, and many of them were eager supporters of the war against malaria. In Sardinia, for example, the prefect of Cagliari explained in 1911 that, in order to carry out his responsibilities for public order, he had to involve himself actively in the antimalarial effort. Malaria, he wrote, was not simply an issue of health. A "supreme interest" of the poor, it permeated all of the social and economic issues affecting the island. To vanquish malaria was to establish the authority of the state on a firm basis.

In some provinces, therefore, prefects ordered the rural police (*carabinieri*) to assume a prominent antimalarial role by assisting overworked doctors and health-care personnel. In Marsala, Sicily, for example, the police compiled daily lists of all peasants who had failed to take their required dose of prophylactic quinine. They then visited the peasants' homes and escorted them to the police station to receive their tablets. More broadly, the Ministry of Finance urged police everywhere to take advantage of their ascendancy over the rural population to spread the news of state quinine as they made their rounds. In such ways the instruments of law and order played a significant part in public health.[19]

In addition to local and central government, the antimalarial campaign relied on the medical profession. Physicians responded with a zeal that went far beyond the requirements of the law. The antimalarial campaign was the most ambitious public health initiative in Italian history, and the medical profession embraced it wholeheartedly. To reach the population most at risk from malaria, doctors launched what the Socialist paper *Avanti!* described as the most extraordinary movement in the history of the profession—an immense and generous program of "going to the people." Inspired by the vision of the Rome School, doctors and medical students went into the countryside to encounter the poor at their workplaces, homes, and shelters. Their purpose was to educate the people in the fundamentals of the mosquito theory and to administer quinine. Many doctors, however, held the even larger hope of transforming medicine itself. No longer, in their view, should the profession be confined to the care of individual patients. State quinine provided the opportunity for medicine to become "social medicine"—a discipline that was preventive more than curative, ministering to society as a whole by implementing the economic and social reforms essential to health. These reforms constituted the practice of "social prophylaxis." Medical science, explained a leading antimalarial warrior, must assume the collective task of saving nations and humanity as a whole. The "holy crusade" against malaria was the testing ground for this grand purpose.[20]

To describe the campaign, doctors widely resorted to Christian metaphors. They saw themselves as apostles, priests, pilgrims, and disciples charged with spreading the Word, evangelizing the people, and bearing "glad tidings." Their work was a "mission" or "holy crusade" aiming at the redemption, resurrection, and salvation of the people. Furthermore, in the holy battle of good and evil, the weapons of their faith were brotherly love, nonviolence, and the "sanctuary" of the rural health station. Bartolommeo Gosio, who served as commissioner overseeing the campaign in Basilicata and Calabria, noted that the movement was born with a "religious sentiment" and that its institutions could be described as temples for the teaching of a "new consciousness."[21]

Amid the Gospel concepts, there was also a vivid and revolutionary Old Testament motif. Just as bondage was widely used as a metaphor to describe conditions on the rice fields and the latifundia, so the Mosaic concepts of emancipation and abolition recur repeatedly in the medical literature. Many doctors saw themselves as bearing prophetic witness to the sufferings of their people, denouncing the oppression of the powerful, and delivering the poor from the tyranny of disease. An unlikely bureaucratic source provided a powerful description of the religious motivation of the physicians combating malaria in Sardinia. The prefect of Sassari province wrote admiringly of Alessandro Lustig and Achille Sclavo, who directed the antimalarial campaign on the island. "It is my duty," he informed Rome,

> to draw your attention to the disinterested, humanitarian, and intelligent labors of Professors Lustig and Sclavo. They gave up lucrative private practices in order to confront our perilous climate in the fever season. Despite enormous discomfort, they travel tirelessly to health stations everywhere to keep watch over the execution of their program and to encourage the populace. Their intention is to spread the glad tidings of redemption among people who have been too long abandoned and to give them hope of a better future. . . . In the most desolate places . . . they have opened soup kitchens and libraries, using money from their own pockets.[22]

Despite the biblical terminology and sense of Christian mission that motivated many doctors, the political orientation of many was anticlerical, Socialist, and sometimes revolutionary. Among the foremost leaders of the campaign, Angelo Celli, Tullio Rossi-Doria, Pietro Castellino, and Giuseppe Tropeano held views suffused not only with the prophetic tradition but also with the teachings of Karl Marx and Friedrich Engels. They taught that malaria could be successfully defeated only if workers were educated, properly nourished, hygienically housed, guaranteed productive work, and well organized in defense of their rights.[23]

As a counterpart to the Society for the Study of Malaria, the more politically engaged physicians founded a more radical association in 1909. This was the National League against Malaria (Lega Nazionale contro la Malaria), which produced its own journal — *Malaria e malattie dei paesi caldi* (Malaria and the Diseases of Hot Countries) — and a newspaper, the *Giornale della malaria* (Malaria Journal). The league, like the society, galvanized the medical profession, promoted the exchange of information, organized lectures for the general population, and distributed pamphlets. Unlike the society, however, the league claimed to represent the views of clinicians in the field rather than those of elite academic physicians in Rome, and it played little role in furthering basic research. Revealingly, the league chose Foggia province in Apulia rather than the Roman Campagna as the showcase for its organizational efforts. This choice was politically charged since Foggia province was also the stronghold of the most powerful and most revolutionary political movement in the Italian South—the anarcho-syndicalist movement based on the local farmworkers' unions, known as peasant leagues. In addition, the league differed from the society in its therapeutic agenda. The league took a skeptical attitude toward the reliance on quinine alone as the weapon of choice in attacking malaria. Leading figures of the league, such as Castellino and Tropeano, took the radical position that social justice was an even more powerful antimalarial than quinine, and they hoped that land reform and the breaking up of the latifundia would become an integral part of the campaign.[24]

Frequently the findings of the physicians involved in the campaign reinforced such politically advanced conclusions. This trend emerges clearly in the reports that emanated from the antimalarial program in Sardinia, the most malarial of Italian regions. For example, Giuseppe Zagari, the antimalarial commissioner for the province of Sassari, found that malaria was a "pandemic" that afflicted nearly the entire population. All Sardinians, he reported, bore the classic stigmata of chronic malaria—emaciation and a painfully distended spleen. In this context, he observed, careful epidemiological observation revealed that there was a surprisingly direct correlation between poverty on the one hand and fever, its sequelae, and its complications on the other hand. In many villages everyone was infected. But those who were landless and had an impoverished diet consisting of beans, corn meal, and snails suffered more than their comparatively comfortable neighbors. Invariably, the poorest members of the community had the most severe symptoms, the largest spleens, and an intellect dulled by cachexia. For their benefit, Zagari called for the opening of soup kitchens attached to the health stations as an "absolutely necessary" antimalarial measure.[25]

In contrast to the landless poor, landowning peasants of substance ate well, seemed almost in good health—apart from the inevitable Sardinian enlarged spleen (or splenomegaly)—and preserved their capacity for work unimpaired. Zagari followed his observations to highly charged political conclusions. As he wrote in 1909,

> I am therefore perfectly convinced that the malaria question is synonymous with the social question and that it is inseparable from the economic development of Sardinia.
>
> Medical care and pharmaceutical treatment are highly useful, but they are not sufficient to redeem this land from the depression in which it lives, and to which indigence and ignorance make such a contribution. The results of the antimalarial campaign in Sardinia will have better results when (a) the eco-

> nomic conditions of the peasants improve, and (b) the peasants are better educated, and are instructed in the ways of the modern world.[26]

"Indigence" and "ignorance," he concluded, were the two great determinants of malaria. Therefore, he summarized, "it is essential that this population be educated and fed before anything else. Then they will easily follow the precepts of *bonifica umana,* and they will free themselves from malaria."[27]

Furthermore, the provincial officer of health at Sassari observed that oscillations in the severity of the annual malaria epidemic coincided with changes in economic fortunes. In good agricultural years, wages rose, the cost of food declined, and the population was more resistant to malaria. Conversely, in years of dearth, malaria struck with exceptional fury. More generally, the commissioners on the island reported that malaria had experienced a fearful upsurge as a result of two major economic setbacks in the closing decades of the nineteenth century. First, domestic industry on the island collapsed. After unification, the introduction of free trade brought about the destruction of the Sardinian textile industry, which collapsed under the competition from more-developed cotton producers in the North. Second, a major epizootic of anthrax decimated the flocks and herds of the region. As a result of these two disasters, mass unemployment and poverty spread, and in their wake, malnutrition and malaria redoubled their ravages. Defining malaria as a classic "social disease," the commissioners wrote that "it would seriously minimize and trivialize the question to consider it from too simple a standpoint. Malaria is nothing other than the product of the economic, social, and hygienic conditions of the country. And malaria, in its turn, depresses these conditions ever more intensely."[28]

Thus, as it got under way, the campaign gathered intellectual and clinical momentum. The doctrine of Celli and Grassi was an essential starting point: it provided direction and the conviction that malarial control was a practical possibility. But it required modification as clinicians added the insights of their experience. Far from simply or slavishly applying a model devised by the academic medicine of the Rome School, practitioners in the field used their experience in overcoming practical difficulties to take the antimalarial effort into new directions that the Grand Maestros had not envisaged.

The Mines of Sardinia and Sicily

A special case that attracted the attention of the antimalarial crusade was the mining districts of Sardinia and Sicily. An unexpected discovery of the antimalarial commissioners was that, on both of Italy's major islands, malaria was an occupational disease of miners no less than of the agricultural population of peasants, farmworkers, and shepherds.

In Sicily, sulfur mines dotted the whole area from the base of the Madonie Mountains to the southern, or "African," coast of the island. Caltanissetta and Girgenti provinces were the major producers, but deposits stretched into Trapani, Messina, and Palermo provinces as well. All reports described shocking economic and health conditions for a workforce that in the 1870s numbered 19,000 workers in 275 mines. The owners were landlords who contracted out the extraction of the sulfur to entrepreneurs who were the industrial counterparts of the notorious leaseholders (*gabellotti*) on the Sicilian latifundia. The mining contractors were former peasants who had no technical knowledge and carried out the industry "in the greatest possible disorder," with no regard for safety, stable labor relations, or productive rationality. They simply dug improvised shafts and sought to make a profit by minimizing investment in equipment and labor. To that end, they recruited impoverished peasants to dig out the ore. They also employed boys between the ages of ten and fourteen to transport the ore to the surface in sacks weighing as much as forty kilograms (approximately ninety pounds). For minimal wages the boys made innumerable journeys as beasts of burden, stumbling bent double in the semidarkness along low shafts and up steep stairs to the light.[29]

Everyone knew that the life of sulfur miners was harsh and unhealthy. Adult males earned wages slightly higher than those of the surrounding peasantry, but in exchange they endured frightening conditions of violence, industrial accidents, and lung disease. They were also highly anemic, lethargic, and short-lived. Worst of all was the lot of the unhappy sulfur boys, known as *carusi,* who were famous as almost Dickensian symbols of the brutal exploitation of children. Reports described their lot as "attenuated slavery."[30] It was even common knowledge that, like everyone who lived and worked in the lowlands of the Sicilian interior, the miners suffered high rates of malaria. Until the careful investigations of the quinine campaign, however, it was assumed that the malaria of miners resulted not from their working conditions in the pits but from their living in unsanitary peasant villages and from their commuting across the open fields to work and back at perilous times of day. Miasmatic teachings held that sulfur fumigated the mine shafts and purified the air, preventing fever. With regard to malaria, sulfur mines were therefore deemed to be entirely salubrious. After the turn of the century and the establishment of Grassi's mosquito doctrine, however, it was discovered that anophelines infested the warm, humid pits and that their tolerance of sulfur far exceeded that of the workers themselves. Studies carried out "patiently and meticulously" by the physicians of the campaign "strongly supported the hy-

Table 3.1 Output of the Sardinian Mining Industry, 1860–1907

Years	Output (in metric tons)	Miners
1860–1869	42,245	5,235
1870–1879	117,500	9,087
1880–1889	144,212	9,926
1890–1899	164,000	11,286
1900–1907	195,131	14,129

Source: Data from Commissione parlamentare d'inchiesta sulla condizione degli operai delle miniere della Sardegna, *Atti della commissione,* vol. I, *Relazione riassuntiva e allegati* (Rome, 1910), 8.

pothesis that infection occurs in the mine shafts." In Sicily, the surprising conclusion emerged that malaria was an occupational disease of the sulfur industry.[31]

Similar conclusions emerged from Sardinia. Mining in Sardinia experienced a great boom after Italian unification. The free market legislation of the Liberal regime removed the Crown's monopoly over the subsoil of the island, opening it to exploration and enterprise. Substantial deposits of zinc, lead, iron, silver, copper, antimony, and manganese were rapidly discovered in two main areas—the district of Iglesias in the southwest of the island and the district of Sarrabus in the southeast.[32] By the early twentieth century, after decades of high metal prices and exploitation of the profitable virgin deposits of the island, Sardinia produced a quarter of the total mining output of the nation. Conducted by twenty companies, mining, as measured by output and size of the workforce, had expanded at a rapid rate (Table 3.1).

In comparison with the sulfur mines of Sicily, the Sardinian metal industry was heavily capitalized and modernized. Sardinian companies employed modern technology rather than child labor to extract the ore, they employed engineers to construct the shafts and underground galleries, they experienced a low rate of industrial accidents, and they established a network of infirmaries and clinics to attend to the health of the workers. As the price of metals fell between 1880 and 1897 and readily accessible deposits of high-grade ore were exhausted, the companies responded by digging galleries deeper into the earth and extracting low-grade ores.

With the challenge of tighter profit margins, the productivity of the workforce became a major concern for the owners and their association, the Sardinian Mining Association (Associazione Mineraria Sarda). Competition from continental Italian mines was fierce. Given equal levels of technology, Sardinian miners produced less per hour than their mainland counterparts while suffering higher rates of absenteeism and industrial accidents. In the early decades, the mining association responded by importing mainland workers to replace islanders in the pits. Ultimately, however, this recourse to outsiders was costly, complicated, and ineffective. Continental workers rapidly fell ill in their new environment and were no more productive than native islanders.

The dominant issue affecting productivity was health, particularly occupational disease. Studies conducted by the company infirmaries and the commissioners of the antimalarial campaign yielded a surprising conclusion. "The first fact to stress with regard to miners is the high rate of morbidity in Sardinia relative to the other regions of Italy," noted the parliamentary commission that reported on Sardinian conditions in 1910–1911.[33] The leading causes of illness among Sardinian miners were lung diseases related to the inhalation of dust and metal particles, pneumonia, and malaria. Malaria, however, was overwhelmingly the most important health concern, for three reasons. First, there were alarming rates of fever among the workers. The association even passed a resolution noting that "almost our entire population is malarious."[34] A prominent example was the great mine at Montevarchi, where 70 percent of the workers reported in 1902 that they had suffered from malaria in the past year. In response to a questionnaire, the miners at Montevarchi reported having suffered from malaria in far greater proportion to all other diseases (Table 3.2). Second, as a major immunosuppressive illness, malaria increased the susceptibility of the workforce to other diseases, especially "miners' lung" and pneumonia. Finally, the sequelae of chronic malaria included anemia, debilitation, and intellectual impairment. These complications of malaria seriously lowered output and directly contributed to industrial accidents through lack of attention.[35]

Eager to combat so powerful an influence on productivity and profits, the mining association investigated the causes of malaria among its workers. Its conclusion was that the causes of malaria were occupational: they were based, that is, on work and work-related residence. Miners lived in conditions of extreme filth that both promoted swarms of anophelines and deprived the workers of protection from their bites. A notorious example that loomed large in all discussions was the mining village of Gonnesa, which was representative of the conditions prevailing throughout the mining district. Gonnesa was located at the heart of the Iglesias basin just above sea level, and its two thousand inhabitants were transients who moved back and forth from agriculture to mining and from one mining center to another, depending on employment opportunities and wages. When the industry expanded, attracting highland peasants with no immunity to the conditions at Gonnesa, the newcomers

Table 3.2 Diseases Reported by Montevarchi Miners in 1902 (cases per 100 workers)

Malaria	70.3
Rheumatism	5.1
Pneumonia	2.5
Pleuritis	2.5
Influenza	2.1
Saturnism	1.3
Gastric catarrh	1.2
Dysentery	0.4
Nephritis	0.4
Bronchitis	0.4
Scrofula	0.4

Source: Data from Sanfelice and Calvino, "Le miniere della Sardegna," 36.

succumbed to malaria with frightening rapidity. While in Gonnesa, the miners lived in crowded huts with walls of straw and clay and roofs of bamboo, with infinite opportunities for flying insects to enter and depart at will. Furthermore, since the walls were blackened with smoke and there were normally no windows to admit light, mosquitoes sheltered inside, unseen and undisturbed in the half-light. Given such accommodations, many miners preferred to sleep in the pits or outdoors rather than in their homes. Indeed, from June to October—at the height of the malarial season—it was common for miners to drag their straw mats outdoors to sleep in the open air.[36]

Apart from housing, other environmental conditions at Gonnesa directly promoted disease. Since there were no sewers in the village, residents disposed of their waste directly in the streets, creating foul puddles that delighted anophelines. At the same time, Gonnesa boasted seven fountains that ran incessantly into standing basins, thereby creating miniature swamps in the center of the town. The area also possessed the notorious Sa Masa Swamp, which was located at a distance of just 1.5 kilometers from town—well within the flying range of anophelines. Rendering themselves still more vulnerable, villagers cultivated vegetables directly in the fertile ground on the edges of the swamp itself. Finally, a major factor that lowered resistance to fever was the poor diet of the miners, whose wages were undermined by ferocious competition for jobs, by the crisis of the mining industry, and by rampant alcoholism among a demoralized workforce.

Not only did Sardinians earn less than miners elsewhere in Italy, but their daily wages also declined substantially, from 2.98 lire in 1870 to 2.45 lire in

Table 3.3 Cost of Items of Prime Necessity in Sardinia, 1909 (in lire)

Bread of first quality	0.4 per kg
Bread of second quality	0.3 per kg
Pasta	0.42 per kg
Wine	0.25 per liter

Source: Data from Commissione parlamentare d'inchiesta sulla condizione degli operai delle miniere della Sardegna, *Atti della commissione,* vol. III, *Interrogatori* (Rome, 1911), 4.

1907.[37] With such pay scales, miners normally lived on bread, potatoes, and vegetables, with meat reserved as a luxury for special occasions. Despite restricting his diet to the bare essentials, a typical miner spent half his daily salary—1.2 to 1.5 lire—on food alone (Table 3.3).

If work-related living conditions were one factor in the categorization of malaria as an occupational disease, sanitation at work was another. Since the industry relied on the mechanical washing of ore, there were large open-air basins for the collection of rainwater at the entrance to every mine. In the words of the medical officer of health at Cagliari, these basins were transformed in the spring and summer into "nurseries for anopheles mosquitoes." The mine shafts themselves, which were hot, humid, and full of water, provided an additional environment in which mosquitoes thrived, even down to depths of two to three hundred meters.[38]

Given such findings, the Sardinian Mining Association declared officially that malaria was an occupational disease of miners. I. Bertolio, the managing director of a mining company and the spokesman for the association, presented a motion in 1910 to establish an antimalarial campaign throughout the mining districts of Sardinia. Bertolio explained,

> Among the diseases of our miners—both those which are work-related such as pleuritis and bronchitis, and those which are not—the nefarious role of malaria is indisputable. It predisposes the individual to infection, it complicates all pathological processes, and it greatly increases the damage.
>
> There is no doubt that malaria represents the principal basis for the debilitation of Sardinian workers in comparison with the mainlanders who come here to work, and it is reasonable to suppose that it may have an influence in causing industrial accidents.
>
> The question of occupational diseases, therefore, embraces the question of malaria. For us, however, the problem has a direct industrial importance. Everyone knows that, before the actual onset of malaria, the miner undergoes an incubation period of several days during which . . . he cannot work with the usual vigor. Fever itself costs him various workdays, after which he suffers

> a further period of reduced productivity because he recovers his normal strength very slowly. Relapses may then reduce his capacity permanently and significantly, on account of the anemia that they cause.

Therefore, Bertolio concluded, the treatment of miners for malaria was not only a "civic duty" but also the "work of enlightened industrialists."[39]

On the strength of this reasoning, the association voted to establish a comprehensive antimalarial campaign throughout the mineral zones of Sardinia. The mining companies agreed to purchase quinine and to make use of the existing infrastructure of infirmaries and company doctors to distribute the medicine and superintend its use. In addition, since there was already a system of foremen who exercised safety and disciplinary authority, the owners determined that the foremen could also play a role in persuading miners to take their medicine. Thus from 1910 the Sardinian mining entrepreneurs became, along with the Italian railroad owners, the industrialists who took the most active role in supporting the program of state quinine. The association had successfully convinced them of the devastating impact of malaria on their industry, and they took steps to combat it.

In Sicily, the operators of the sulfur industry took an approach that resembled the stance of the island's great absentee landlords. Like the landlords, the sulfur-mine owners had little collective organization or cohesion. They had no stable or personal relationship with the workers in the industry, and they had invested little capital in their operations. The middlemen, known as *capimastri,* were normally uneducated and uninterested in matters of health. For these reasons, the Italian Red Cross intervened from outside to bring the antimalarial campaign to the sulfur districts. Having established in the Roman Campagna the precedent that the campaign against malaria was sufficiently analogous to war to legitimize its involvement, the Red Cross in Sicily assumed the task of opening health stations in the mining villages and providing quinine to their inhabitants.[40]

Poisoners and Teachers

Education became a key aspect of the Italian campaign to control malaria, even though it was not mentioned in the legislation that first established the program. It was introduced pragmatically in response to the problems encountered by physicians in the field. Chief among these problems was the universal distrust with which the poor greeted doctors who asked them to swallow the bitter tablets packed in Turin. A leading theme of the reports written by health officials throughout Italy was that they confronted a serious and unexpected obstacle—the incomprehension, or even implacable hostility, of the populace. When he drew up a list of barriers confronting the "war on malaria" in 1906, for example, Angelo Celli gave first place to the "unconsciousness, ignorance, and apathy of the peasants, and of our workers in general."[41] As the campaign got under way, the countryside teemed with dark rumors of a diabolical plot to rid the nation of its surplus population. Just as in the time of plague and cholera described by Alessandro Manzoni and Giovanni Verga, the land was again filled with tales of poisoners (*untori*) whose mission was to annihilate the unneeded poor. Peasants, doctors anxiously wrote to Rome, suspected that the state had decided to destroy them once and for all. The tablets advertised as quinine were rumored to contain the lethal potion.[42]

For some doctors, such reactions simply reflected "insane" prejudice or represented all that one could expect from backward, illiterate peasants living in "almost savage conditions."[43] Here there was an intriguing irony. One reason that the population viewed quinine as a poison was that the state itself informed them that it was so. In its educational manuals on self-protection against malaria, the Department of Health even taught that "quinine is a most powerful poison for the germs of malaria."[44] Apart from such clumsy and self-defeating instructions from Rome, however, thoughtful medical writers found compelling explanations for the universal suspicion. One reason was simply that rural Italy was not "medicalized," as contacts between peasants and physicians were rare events. To the poor, it seemed implausible that the state had suddenly become interested in their welfare and that its intentions were benign. Medical intentions became all the more suspect when, at the very first visit, health stations routinely performed a disturbing procedure—the blood test. Few peasants had ever seen blood drawn, and they regarded the practice with fright and distrust.

Equally suspect was the requirement, based on Celli's preferred strategy of chemical prophylaxis, that healthy people should ingest tablets and administer them to their children and infants. Such a suggestion could readily seem malevolent, especially in a context in which the dividing line between health and disease was so poorly defined that prevention and cure had little meaning. So many Italians were chronically ill that they had no concept of feeling well. For them, fever, diarrhea, a mildly dilated belly, dyspepsia, and fatigue were not warning symptoms of disease but rather inherent aspects of the peasant condition. Patients whom physicians diagnosed as malarial and dangerously contagious steadfastly considered themselves well until their ability to work, and therefore to survive, was severely impaired. Gustavo Foà, the medical director of the rural health station at Quadrato (now Latina) at the heart of the Pontine

Marshes, wrote that foremost among the difficulties faced by the campaign in his area was "the idea, established in early childhood, that malaria is not a disease but a state inherent in the lot of the peasant, and that it must be endured, along with poverty and filth. Hence the peasants have no desire to treat chronic fevers or to improve their miserable physical condition. These are regarded as of no importance, since there is no role model of the healthy peasant, and since it is impossible to make comparisons with the few wealthy people who are thought to belong to a different caste."[45]

Often, even if doubters were persuaded at last to swallow their medication, they attributed any subsequent symptoms of malaria to the quinine they had taken and not to the disease. Quinine, it was said, caused the spleen to swell and the digestive system to overheat. There was also a common anxiety that if a healthy person took quinine, the medicine would lose its potency when he or she fell ill and really needed it. In addition, pregnant women were convinced that quinine would cause miscarriage.[46]

Often quinine was feared not as poison but as fraud. Peasants suspected that it was a financial ruse devised by the treasury. Since the state had never been known to dispense free gifts, the plausible interpretation was that to consume the tablets was to build up a secret debt that would be settled later by the tax collector. Memories of the grist tax—the most unpopular of levies—gave foundation to such worries. Even peasants who ground their own flour had been presented with a charge for the milling of their wheat. Therefore, even if quinine did not cause death, it might nonetheless entail financial ruin. Such a view was all the more plausible since quinine, before it was suddenly made free in 1900, had been known only as an expensive luxury of the rich. Furthermore, for many farm laborers, the landlord was even more menacing than the tax collector. They feared consuming quinine because they understood that landlords would be assessed for it, and they assumed that workers who caused them such an expense would suffer reprisals and blacklisting.[47]

All such misgivings were reinforced by real medical observations. Quinine has the disadvantage of being discharged from the body through urination in approximately twenty-four hours. Its protective power, therefore, had to be renewed daily throughout the epidemic season. Since the rigorous regimen advocated by the campaign was poorly understood and frequently violated (through ignorance rather than disobedience), everyone knew people who fell victim to fever despite sincere efforts to comply with the physicians. Inevitably, the result was to undermine confidence in quinine and its efficacy. In addition, the claims advanced on behalf of the beneficial effects of quinine reminded many of previous antimalarial vogues that had raised hopes only to dash them later. In recent memory, for instance, eucalyptus trees had been hailed as a means to purify the atmosphere, and arsenic had been touted as a great antimalarial specific. Such disappointing memories fostered skepticism. Any remaining confidence was further diminished by the unanticipated factor of quinine intolerance. Some patients who consumed the alkaloid developed distressing side effects—nausea, blurred vision, headache, and tinnitus leading sometimes to permanent deafness. The sufferings of such patients led easily to suspicions of poison or negligence. In any event, peasants often regarded quinine with suspicion because it was already known to them as a powerful means of inducing medical abortions. That such a drug could now be taken with impunity by the general population tested their faith.[48]

Finally, malaria itself created mental conditions that severely hampered the effort to gain popular support for the campaign to control it. Frequent side effects of chronic malaria are neurological deficit and severe anemia, leading eventually to total torpor and indifference to one's surroundings. Writing from Apulia, where he directed the distribution of quinine in 1906, Pietro Castellino noted that

> if you examine the statistics concerning farmworkers in a malarial zone, you can be certain that every one of them, at least once, has been stricken by the infection. Thus it happens that all the impoverished laborers bear the signs of this terrible disease on their bodies. Almost all of them have emaciated, mask-like faces upon which are permanently imprinted the marks of premature aging, severe malnutrition, idiocy, and indifference.
>
> If to these signs that result directly from the disease . . . you add those still more radical sequelae that have been silently and secretly transmitted from one sickly and enfeebled generation to the next, then you have the ideal type of the worker in a malarial area—weak, undernourished, and, above all, apathetic.
>
> In a malarial land, therefore, one should not then be surprised to find that such apathy and degeneration, transmitted by heredity over the centuries, have bred in the soul of the peasant an unreflecting hopelessness that prevents him from entertaining any idea of improvement.[49]

The apathy of southern life that Edward Banfield has famously termed "amoral familism" and "the moral basis of a backward society" had in fact an overwhelming medical foundation. One of the cruel ironies of malaria was that it made so many of its victims oblivious to the message of hope that they were offered. "How," Castellino asked, "do you expect such a person to understand the benefits of quinine prophylaxis?"[50]

Thus the greatest initial difficulty of the campaign was stubborn resistance by those most in need of its benefits. Peasants, farmworkers, miners, and shepherds refused to attend the newly opened clinics. They barricaded themselves in their homes and turned away visiting physicians and nurses. Alternatively, they accepted the suspect medicine they were offered but then hoarded it for later resale or barter for cigarettes, spat the capsules on the ground after the intruders had departed, or fed the offending tablets to their pigs. A portion of the subsidized Italian quinine made its way to the black market and was exported to the malarial areas of North Africa, where Italian state quinine commanded a high price because of its guaranteed purity. Sometimes parents cautiously swallowed their own medicine but adamantly refused to administer it to their children. Most commonly of all, patients who were seriously ill took quinine just long enough to suppress their fever, after which they ignored the remainder of the required regimen. Thus public health officials estimated in 1909 that the majority of the quinine distributed was not consumed.[51]

Even the less controversial attempt to introduce "mechanical defense" aroused strenuous opposition. Italians of all classes objected that metal screens transformed a house into a cage. Placing metal barriers at windows and doors also made it difficult to dispose of slops, impeded the passage of children and domestic animals, and rendered a building dark and insufferably hot. In any case, it was widely believed, the effort was useless because one or two mosquitoes invariably found their way inside despite the protection. Everyone had heard of someone who had fallen ill despite mechanical prophylaxis. For these reasons, people who urgently needed protection decided instead to rip out the screens, sometimes putting them to alternative use as sieves to make tomato purée and pasta sauce. They also resorted to propping screen doors open intentionally by removing their springs and to defying the regulations by remaining out of doors during the forbidden hours of darkness.[52]

To overcome such resistance, the organizers devised means of outreach and propaganda, some of them strikingly ingenious. Campaigners distributed leaflets printed by the Department of Health and the Society for the Study of Malaria to explain the mechanisms of malaria and the proper role of quinine, and they affixed posters to city walls and post office bulletin boards.[53] Newspapers published articles on all facets of state quinine. Doctors made speaking tours of rural areas, and journals assisted them by publishing lectures explaining basic malariology in simple language. To overcome suspicion, some enterprising campaigners organized public quinine demonstrations. On these occasions, doctors, teachers, and parish priests gathered in village and town piazzas, where they publicly swallowed their tablets as a gesture of good faith. In many places the campaigners made a concerted effort to involve trade-union leaders, who already enjoyed the confidence of their members. Occasionally priests accepted the request of physicians to use the pulpit to preach the gospel of quinine and encourage cooperation with the health campaign.[54]

Unfortunately, the prefect of Sassari observed, such efforts had little effect. The reason was that those who read posters, attended lectures, or watched quinine-swallowing ceremonies were those members of the community who were most educated, open-minded, and informed. Preaching, in other words, reached only those who were already converted. Given the established social conventions regarding gender, such events usually attracted all-male audiences. Most of the population remained "indifferent," "extraneous," and "unprepared to listen." Also, as commissioner Gaetano Rummo observed wryly in Campania, not every peasant had a taste for the pompous speeches of professionals or the sermons of priests.[55]

An alternative method devised by health stations in the Roman Campagna was to recruit the most intelligent and respected workers on an estate as paid, carefully trained quinine distributors. These workers set an example of diligent ingestion of alkaloid tablets, and they used their powers of persuasion to overcome the suspicions of their fellows. In some instances they also practiced surveillance, reporting to the authorities those workers who were hiding symptoms or failing to follow the required prophylactic regimen. Although such model workers were helpful adjuncts to the campaign, they were unable to reverse the strong tides of ignorance and suspicion at work in rural Italy. Too much depended on the personal charisma and commitment of the recruited workers, while the nomadic lifestyle of the work gangs disrupted all continuity. Such a system, moreover, was possible only on large farms where workers gathered in substantial numbers.[56]

Peasant Schools

It was Angelo Celli who first addressed such problems in a systematic manner. On the basis of his practical experience in the Roman Campagna, Celli modified the model of malaria control that he had done so much to embody in the state-quinine legislation of 1900 to 1907. He concluded that education was just as important as quinine in the battle against malaria because neither chemical nor mechanical prophylaxis would ever be possible without it. The absolute necessity of education was a lesson that the American malariologist L. W. Hackett also derived from his dealings with peasant women in the Pontine Marshes in the 1920s. "Now I believe," Hackett reflected,

> that without that minimum amount of learning given by at least the first three elementary classes, nothing can be constructed. The ideology of an illiterate person is almost nil. Her knowledge of language is limited to that which is

> necessary for her daily life and needs. If I ask a mother to "keep the baby to the time-table," I realize that the word "time-table" is too difficult for her. The word does not exist in her mind because the conception does not exist. She has never regulated her daily duties by looking at the clock, or if she has such a thing she cannot tell the time.[57]

Health required more, however, than the passive obedience of patients to medical instruction: it presupposed that they possessed a knowledge of their rights under the new legislation, a basic understanding of the mechanisms of malaria and the action of quinine, and an overall "hygienic consciousness." With these ends in mind, Celli initiated a campaign of "antimalarial education" to support the distribution of quinine and the installation of screens. Under his tutelage, the Roman Campagna again led the way. There his wife, Anna, one of the first female doctors in Italy, established the first "peasant school" in 1904, with the support of the Rome branch of the feminist organization Unione Femminile and with Adele Menghini as its first teacher.[58]

Just as health stations took medicine into the countryside, so the founders of the peasant schools adopted the missionary view that schools should go to the students instead of bringing the students to the schools. Under the slogan "Let's bring literacy to the peasants of the Roman Campagna," Angelo Celli explained that until the late nineteenth century the Catholic Church had been the only organization that reached out to the rural population. Every Sunday priests and monks, accompanied by lay volunteers, set out from Rome to minister to the peasants whom the state neglected. Beginning with the establishment of the first rural health stations in 1874, physicians began to imitate the example set by the Church. In the twentieth century, Celli urged, the time had come for teachers to follow the physicians.[59]

In support of this idea, Celli rapidly gathered a group of educators committed to the cause of taking knowledge into the Roman countryside — Giovanni Cena, Sibilla Aleramo, Alessandro Marcucci, Duilio Cambellotti, and his own wife, Anna. The Cellis, Cena, and Marcucci formed the first executive committee. They took charge of raising funds, recruiting teachers, choosing locations, and drawing up a curriculum. Their project rapidly took root and spread widely. By 1910–1911 the Roman Campagna possessed twenty-two schools with an enrollment of 1,129 students of all ages; and by 1913–1914 it boasted forty-eight schools and an enrollment of 2,519 students. The municipality of Rome provided the necessary supplies of books, notebooks, blackboards, chalk, and pens. In 1908 the schools also began to receive small subsidies from the Ministry of Agriculture and the Ministry of Education. The teachers themselves subsidized the effort by working without compensation,

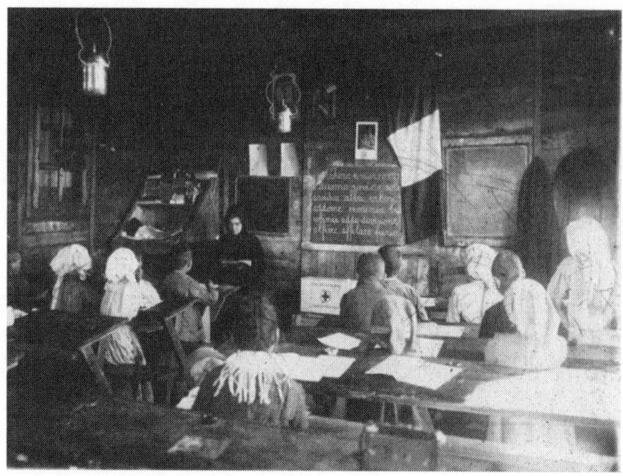

A class at a rural school in the Roman Campagna

claiming only reimbursement for travel expenses. Meanwhile, the initiative that began in Rome inspired similar efforts in other malarial regions.[60]

Celli, the malariologist, and Cena, the first director of the peasant schools, agreed that ignorance and illiteracy played a major role in the etiology of diseases in general and of malaria in particular. Every health station, they suggested, should therefore house a school, affirming the "alliance of the doctor and the *maestro* (teacher)." Cena's successor, Alessandro Marcucci, expressed his belief in the necessity of this alliance. Marcucci wrote, "Angelo Celli and Giovanni Cena complemented each other in their project: the first cared for the body while the second treated the soul. The former employed drugs and medical assistance; the latter made use of books and the word. Thus the school rises next to the health station! But this school is not concerned only with simple technical skills. Its intention is not merely to give its pupils the first instruments of knowledge—reading and writing. This school aims to shape both the mind and the soul."

Marcucci, who directed the schools for most of their formative years before the First World War, was a Socialist. In accord with his belief in social justice, he explained that the mission of his schools was never the purely functional task of spreading basic literacy—the "arid acquisition of instrumental knowledge."[61] Invoking Aldous Huxley, the malariologist Alberto Missiroli captured Marcucci's view when he commented that to provide the three Rs alone was like teaching a hungry man to use a knife and fork while denying him food.[62] The rural schools undertook instead to provide a "spiritual redemption" that was the counterpart of and indispensable precondition for the "physical redemption" to be achieved by the doctors. Through the rural schools, peasants were to learn about their rights as workers and as citizens, about the law, about the "idea of progress," and about the need for emancipation and justice. They were to learn to read while they gathered information about labor contracts, crop systems, plant diseases, and the evils of latifundism. All of these issues were particularly familiar to Marcucci, who had worked as a labor recruiter on behalf of estate managers in the Roman Campagna before experiencing a political conversion. From the moment he responded to Angelo Celli's call, Marcucci espoused a Tolstoyan view of sympathy with the oppressed, whose condition he understood all too well.[63]

Most important, the schools never lost sight of the fundamentals of the new doctrine of malaria. As Ernesto Cacace, the pioneer of peasant schools in the region of Campania, explained, education was "the most important factor in [Italy's antimalarial] campaign and the most powerful weapon for its success." In a report on the methodology of the schools he directed, Cacace carefully illustrated how the findings of malariology were integrated into a curriculum that included instruction in moral education, civics, the Italian language, counting, reading, writing, arithmetic, practical agronomy, geography, and "ideological dictation." In classes on geography, for example, there were numerous opportunities to point out the malarial zones of the nation and of the locality, to explain the seriousness of the problem, and to discuss the mechanisms of transmission and the ways people could protect themselves. Similarly, in adult classes on practical agronomy, the instructors discussed the breeding habits of mosquitoes, the nature of the recent legislation, the function of quinine, and the assistance available to the poor. An understanding of malaria, Cacace held, was more important to a peasant cultivator than information on crop rotations and irrigation.[64]

At Sassari (Sardinia), the provincial officer of health was convinced that only a massive instructional effort in primary and secondary schools at every level would enable the antimalarial campaign to achieve its objectives. His vision was that Italy should model its antimalarial efforts on the campaigns against alcoholism that had been established in other Western nations. "As other nations act in their battle with alcohol," he wrote, "so too we must act in our battle against malaria. In other words, beginning with the first year of primary school and continuing to the final year of our middle schools, classical schools, and technical institutes, we must insert into our curriculum instruction of a kind that will enlighten our young people with regard to the etiology and pathogenesis of malaria, on the economic consequences that it produces, and on the means that exist to protect oneself from it." He envisioned that, to underline the importance of malaria in the school curriculum, there should be compulsory examinations for all students on the subject.[65]

Corriere delle maestre (Teachers' Courier), the newspaper of the teaching profession, provided weekly lesson plans for its members in the rural schools.

These plans illustrate the breadth of subject matter that the schools sought to introduce in the countryside. For example, one issue of the paper suggested such themes as the vine disease *perenospora,* water and its proper management, the constitution, elections, vendettas and forgiveness, the functions of the human body, mutual respect, hygiene, geography, crops, the dangers of greed and unwise spending, cooperation and its uses, the duties of the mayor and the municipality, counting, and the effect of climate on plants. With such a broad syllabus, the schools founded by Celli, Cena, and Marcucci sought to prepare their pupils not only for literacy and health but also for citizenship and participation in civil society. Marcucci recalled that "the work of Giovanni Cena had a social character and purpose; it was almost an act of rebellion!"[66]

A further important aspect of the rural schools was that the teachers were encouraged to live on the premises, so that they became an integral part of the community. After hours, therefore, they continued to remind their students that the health station was near, that quinine was available, and that peasants had a new right—the "right to health." When space was unavailable at the health station, the "apostles of literacy" set up improvised classrooms in cast-off railroad carriages, huts, stables, and inns. Designed to reach a remote and nomadic population, the peasant schools were mobile and flexible, following the laborers in their migrations and offering instruction at times when attendance was possible—on Sundays, on holidays, and in the evenings.

Wherever they existed, the peasant schools assumed a large part in the delivery of state quinine. In Campania, therefore, teachers were given special courses in "antimalarial hygiene." In 1906, Cacace founded an Antimalarial Education Station to train teachers in the basics tenets of practical malariology and to produce its own bulletin of continuing education, *La propaganda antimalarica* (Antimalarial Propaganda). Similarly, in Rome, Anna Celli instituted a course to train schoolteachers as nurses. And at Verona it was the teachers who assumed the primary responsibility for distributing quinine to children, thereby overcoming "the indifference of mothers who were sometimes unintelligent and often stubborn." In 1913, the Verona teachers—those "apostles of civilization, now transformed into so many health-care assistants"—medicated over 2,500 elementary school pupils.[67]

In Cacace's opinion, it was far better for the doctrine of malariology to be taught by teachers rather than by physicians. One reason was that teachers, "living constantly in the midst of their pupils, understand their intellectual powers better. In addition, having greater didactic skills, they are better able to adapt the concepts of the antimalarial campaign to the intellectual level of their students."[68] A second reason that antimalarial education was better provided by teachers was that the schools, unlike the health stations, enjoyed the immediate trust of the population. News that a rural school was to be opened always caused excitement and anticipation. In Marcucci's words, referring to the schools of the Roman Campagna, "Their spirit has spread everywhere, and there is no peasant who does not know of them. The news races from mouth to mouth."[69] Peasants understood that knowledge was power, that illiteracy reinforced their subjection to landlords and moneylenders, and that a better future for their children depended on education. Not infrequently, the peasants of the Roman Campagna referred despairingly to their illiteracy by saying, "We are blind!" Vincenzo Giannelli, who directed a health station in the Pontine Marshes, explained, "Everyone has the desire to learn, and many families . . . complain of nothing so much as of the lack of schools. Their desire to improve the lives of their children is made clear by the fact that two-thirds of the children who assiduously attend school live three, four, even six kilometers away." Furthermore, Giannelli explained, the effect of the school on the antimalarial campaign was immediate and profound. "The foundation of the primary school," he stressed, "was extremely welcome. It was not least among the factors that led the population to have greater trust in the antimalarial campaign and greater gratitude toward it."[70] Similarly, the provincial officer of health at Sassari observed that teachers provided the most reliable means of reaching the Sardinian population and of preparing ground for the subsequent arrival of physicians.[71]

Looking beyond the control of malaria, the founders of the peasant schools saw their mission as one of transforming society as a whole in the interest of justice. Marcucci explained his conception in a passage full of radical political implications. "For the peasant schools," he wrote, "our didactic and civil program is an action of preparation—one might even say the action of an avant-garde. This work precedes the inevitable transformation of rural life and perhaps presupposes a new cultural and economic order, especially in the badly cultivated lands dominated by latifundia. Much, if not everything, will then have to change in the present conditions of production and life in the countryside."[72] Along with halting the ravages of malaria, the peasant schools sought to bring about the end of the "enduring feudalism" that fostered disease. The time had come to change a world in which millions of Italian peasants could name neither the king nor the prime minister of their country; could not comprehend the national language; and, unaccustomed to deploying abstract concepts, observed a habit of silence.[73]

External Factors

In addition to the intentional policies that the campaign put in place to combat malaria, physicians and public health officials stressed the role of spontaneous, external factors in reducing the burden of the disease. In particular, medical authorities highlighted the importance of two major developments that coincided with the implementation of the state-quinine laws and had enormous implications for public health. These factors — rapid industrialization and the commercialization of agriculture on the one hand and mass overseas emigration on the other — were regionally specific, one having major influence in the North and the other in the South.

In a classic pattern of economic dualism, Italian economic growth between 1900 and 1914 largely benefited the North, with industry confined primarily to the "industrial triangle" bounded by Milan, Genoa, and Turin and with modernized agriculture limited chiefly to the Po Valley. Although unevenly distributed, the benefits of economic growth included a thinning out of the labor market and therefore such health-related improvements as better housing, increased wages, and a more sustaining diet. Since the period also witnessed the development of a powerful trade-union movement in the countryside, these gains percolated down the social scale to those sectors of the population most severely at risk of malaria — the peasants and farm laborers of the Po Valley. The attenuation of the malaria epidemic in northern Italy, therefore, reflected the political and economic improvement of the conditions of the rural poor as well as the interventions of the antimalarial campaign. One of the leading figures in the campaign in the Po Valley, Nicola Badaloni, acknowledged the important role of such factors. He criticized Angelo Celli for claiming too much credit for intentional policies and underestimating the role of spontaneous developments. Badaloni wrote,

> As for the decline of mortality in relation to the consumption of state quinine . . . , I have only to refer to the thousands of reports of Celli and his followers to demonstrate how important it is to underline other beneficial factors, which are undoubtedly multiple. Thus, in addition to the import of quinine from abroad and the allocation of state quinine, I have attempted to examine, year by year, from 1888 to 1908, the average wages of farmworkers, the consumption of wheat, the production of the principal agricultural products, deposits in savings banks and post office accounts, the sums spent in land-drainage works. Then I have set these figures side by side with those for general mortality and mortality for malaria. From this comparison it is immediately obvious that factors of an economic nature, which have shown a marked improvement, have had a major role on the progressive decline of rates of death, both in general and from malaria.
>
> Today Celli accepts the role of such factors, but until yesterday he contented himself with comparing two columns of figures, one showing increasing sales of state quinine and the other falling rates of death.[74]

At the same time the advance of land-reclamation projects and the intensification of agriculture in the Po Valley—two major advances of the modern Italian economy—led to the massive draining of swamplands and the disappearance of rice fields employing stagnant water. In provinces near the Po Delta, such as Rovigo and Ravenna, in which malaria had long been associated with stagnant water where anopheline mosquitoes bred, the result was a major attenuation of the disease. In Rovigo province, the medical officer of health reported in 1908,

> In this province there are many townships that, intensely malarial ten or fifteen years ago, are now completely free of infection following land drainage and the intensive cultivation that immediately followed it. . . .
>
> The benefits of land reclamation and the intensification of agriculture are absolutely enormous. Before the introduction of land reclamation, nearly the whole province of Rovigo was intensely malarial. Sanitary improvement everywhere has followed the work of drainage and reclamation.[75]

Other aspects of the modernization of agriculture—mechanization, modern crop rotations, the advance of animal husbandry, and improved housing—were clearly beneficial to the overall health of the people, and they reinforced the spontaneous recession of malaria in the North. Finally, physicians noted that the development of a modern economic infrastructure facilitated their work. Improved means of communication—roads, automobiles, the telephone—made it easier to reach patients, to institute emergency interventions, and to coordinate the follow-up care that was essential to the success of the lengthy quinine regimens for prophylaxis and treatment.[76]

At the highest level of the public health hierarchy, the Superior Health Council (Consiglio Superiore della Sanità) assessed the decline of mortality from malaria between 1888 and 1907. Although the instruments of the state campaign—quinine, health stations, and rural schools—played the principal role in this decline, the council stressed that external factors were also important. All studies, it noted,

> unanimously underline the fundamental importance of the numerous projects of land reclamation and drainage, both big and small, that have been carried out in Italy not only in the past twenty years but also in more distant periods.
>
> Another coefficient worthy of great attention is the transformation from extensive to intensive agriculture and the planting of land that previously had been left abandoned and uncultivated.
>
> One should also consider the economic and social progress made by a significant part of our rural population. Their living standards, diet, and housing are no longer as meager as they once were.[77]

Table 3.4 Average Annual Number of Transoceanic Emigrants, 1876–1910

1876–1880	25,596
1881–1885	58,995
1886–1890	131,283
1891–1895	147,444
1896–1900	161,901
1901–1905	309,242
1906–1910	393,694

Source: Adapted from Foerster, *The Italian Emigration of Our Times*, 7.

The second major external factor stressed by the antimalarial campaigners was emigration, whose effects were primarily felt in the South. The exodus of southern Italians to North and South America between 1880 and the First World War is one of the great mass movements of population in modern times. As the outward flood gathered momentum after 1876, the Italian Bureau of Statistics (Direzione Generale della Statistica) charted its course (Table 3.4). Extensive in its effects on both sides of the Atlantic, this migration has attracted an abundance of scholarly attention. Scholars have carefully analyzed the economic, social, and political ramifications of this phenomenon.[78] To date, however, they have paid scant attention to the effects it produced on malaria in the land from which the migrants departed. We have already examined the causes of this movement—desperate poverty and ill health.[79] The conditions that resulted from the mass departure, however, led to vastly improved living conditions and a declining burden of disease.

A clear and authoritative contemporary analysis of the contribution of emigration to the attenuation of the malaria epidemic is provided by the parliamentary inquiry, led by Senator Eugenio Faina, that investigated the conditions of peasants in the Italian South. The commissioners for the various regional volumes that composed the investigation reported between 1908 and 1911—that is, precisely at the moment when emigration was reaching its peak and when the attenuation of the malarial epidemic was becoming apparent. The parliamentary investigators were therefore in an ideal position to notice and assess the link between the two phenomena, and the medical officers of health responsible for the antimalarial campaign corroborated their conclusions.

Most revealing of all were the two volumes dedicated to the Abruzzi-Molise region, which was an especially indicative case because mass emigration there had begun at an early date, had achieved enormous proportions, and had left profound effects. Cesare Jarach, the commissioner for the Abruzzi, noted that the decision of so many peasants to escape abroad had transformed the life of the rural poor in the region. By departing, the emigrants radically reduced the pressure of population on resources and revolutionized the labor market. Having for the first time to compete for scarce workers, landlords decided to mechanize their farms, introducing steam-powered harvesters and threshers. Such modernization of production decreased the numbers of workers employed outdoors at the height of the malarial season and shortened the workday of those who remained to perform the imperative tasks of the agricultural cycle. Vastly reduced in numbers, farmworkers were in an effective position to demand higher wages, better diets, and improved accommodations. Peasants from the Abruzzi also began refusing to make the long treks to the great estates of the Roman Campagna and of Apulia, where so many of their predecessors had contracted fever and had been compelled to return seriously ill to their homes. As the Giolittian era advanced, they also paid off their debts and accumulated savings, which they deposited in post office savings accounts.[80]

At the same time, a majority of emigrants returned from the Americas to their homes, most of them with significant savings. These returning "Americans," as they were called, showered money—the "rain of gold"—on their native region to transform the property market.[81] Jarach noted that the early twentieth century witnessed a massive expansion in small peasant landownership and that the new owners practiced intensive cultivation, built sturdy houses impervious to insects, ate abundantly, and wore adequate clothing. For the first time in the history of the region, the standard of living of the poor improved immeasurably, and as it did, such indexes of poverty and high medical risk as morbidity and mortality from infectious diseases, including malaria, began to plummet. Naturally, the assiduous efforts of the antimalarial campaigners were a major factor as well. Jarach, however, clearly explained that the spontaneous improvements introduced by mass emigration provided the favoring context within which quinine, education, and health stations could achieve positive results most effectively.[82]

The Abruzzi region exemplified a pattern that prevailed in much of the South at the height of the Giolittian period. Commissioners for other regions—Calabria, Basilicata, Campania, and Sicily—reported similar effects of emigration on the economy, on labor relations, on standards of living, and on the prevalence of malaria. In Sicily, for example, Giovanni Lorenzoni noted that emigration effected fundamental transformations in the Sicilian countryside that had implications for public health. In his words,

> Emigration is the cause of a transformation. Emigration took the Sicilian peasant, who had lived for centuries in the harshest form of serfdom, and transported him to new worlds where the most ample freedom prevails,

> where the worth of a man is measured by his productivity, and where labor is the highest value. Thus the former social pariah acquired a consciousness of his human dignity, a certain comfortable standard of living, and an education. He was now in a position to refuse humiliating conditions of employment.
>
> Thus emigration has caused a deep revolution to occur in Sicilian society. Through this change the parasitic and idle classes . . . must renew themselves or perish, giving way to the new classes of peasants whose money accumulated in America has turned [them] into small landlords.[83]

Emigration, in short, was the "only ray of hope that, after many centuries, has appeared on the horizon of the peasants—the true outcasts of Sicilian society."[84] Linking the improvements noted by the parliamentary commissioner explicitly to malaria, the provincial officer of health for Messina observed in 1907 that there had been a substantial decline in the prevalence of malaria—a decline that he attributed primarily to emigration, which "depopulated the malarial zones" and "removed the most important factor in transmission—nighttime residence in malarious areas."[85]

So great were the effects of emigration that there were debates about whether the overseas movement of poor southern peasants was the long-awaited solution to the Southern Question in Italian history and a shortcut to the control of malaria. Unfortunately, the changes brought about by emigration would not last. Within a few years of the Faina investigation, the movement his commission described came to an end as the First World War initiated a new period of immigration quotas, controls, and restrictions that halted the flow or reduced it to a trickle. Furthermore, the new structures of peasant proprietorship, and the conditions of life and health that they supported, were fragile and impossible to sustain in the long term. Small peasant proprietors possessed holdings that were often marginal in size or location, and they lacked access to agricultural credit, technical expertise, and marketing experience. Many peasants were doomed, therefore, to be expropriated in the face of competition, sudden misfortune, the onset of renewed economic crises, or the implementation of unfavorable state policies.

Malaria and the crises of the southern countryside were alleviated for a time by the unplanned consequences of the mass movement of people. In the long run, however, this "spontaneous" solution was to falter, and the problems of the region—like those of the nation as a whole—would require remedies that were more sustained, multifaceted, and intentional. It was imperative that the antimalarial campaign, which made its own unprecedented contributions to the advances of the Giolittian period, be continued, strengthened, and provided with new knowledge and more-effective tools.

4

From Quinine to Women's Rights: Hopes, Illusions, and Victories

Malarial fever is perhaps the most important of human diseases. Though it is not often directly fatal, its wide prevalence in [most] warm climates produces in the aggregate an enormous amount of sickness and mortality. . . . Unlike many epidemic diseases it is not transient, but remains for ever in the areas which it has once invaded. It tends to abound most in the most fertile countries, and at the season most suitable for agriculture. Very malarious places cannot be prosperous. . . . Malaria . . . has, I believe, profoundly modified the world's history by tending to render the whole of the tropics comparatively unsuitable for the full development of civilisation. It is essentially a political disease—one which affects the welfare of whole countries, and the prevention of it should therefore be an important branch of public administration. For the state as for the individual, health is the first postulate of prosperity. And prosperity should be the first object of scientific government.

—*Ronald Ross,* The Prevention of Malaria

The years between 1900 and the First World War marked a distinctive and important period in Italy's protracted struggle against its greatest national enemy, malaria. In this phase, all hopes rested on quinine and the ability of health stations to distribute it to the people. It was also a period of euphoric belief that control or even eradication could be achieved within a few epidemic seasons. But how successful was the antimalarial campaign in this first period? How close was Italy to vanquishing malaria when the First World War severely disrupted the effort? What were the major obstacles and setbacks it encountered? What major lessons did its organizers draw from the experience? What were the consequences for Italian political life?

Early Lessons

Contemporary sources provide abundant evidence of the achievements of the state-quinine campaign up to the First World War. The campaign itself generated detailed annual progress reports from nearly every malarial province. The Society for the Study of Malaria and the National League against Malaria published journals dedicated to the issue. In addition, between 1910 and 1912 the commissioners appointed by Prime Minister Giovanni Giolitti drafted studies addressing the effects of the program on public health and making proposals for the future. Finally, leading figures in the crusade—Alberto Lutrario and Alessandro Messea, who succeeded one another as director-general of public health, as well as Angelo Celli, Anna Celli, and Giovanni Battista Grassi—wrote extensive retrospective commentaries.

All accounts suggest that the great prewar eradication program succeeded in ways that it had not initially envisaged, while failing to approach the ultimate goal of eradication. Everyone agreed that the great achievement of the campaign was that it succeeded, for the first time in Italian history, in making quinine, the specific remedy for malaria, available without cost to all impoverished sufferers. Although patients were reluctant to swallow tablets preventively when they felt well or to continue to take them in the interest of "radical cure" after their symptoms had passed, they were invariably eager to take quinine while in the throes of serious infections. In ever-increasing numbers, the victims of severe malarial infections received chemotherapy and medical attention. The dramatic result was a rapid and sustained fall in mortality from the disease.

In Grassi's last article, written two months before his death in 1925, he surveyed the consequences of the campaign he had done so much to fashion.[1] He noted that "pernicious infections"—the greatest causes of death from malaria—had become "infinitely less frequent" as a result of state quinine.[2] Mortality statistics confirm Grassi's assertion. Since malaria is a great immunosuppressive disease (like AIDS, though by entirely different mechanisms), most of the deaths it causes are indirect through its many complications, especially pneumonia. In the annual epidemic, therefore, two major waves of mortality

Table 4.1 Mortality from Malaria in Italy, 1900–1914

Year	Deaths	Deaths per million inhabitants
1900	15,865	490
1901	13,358	417
1902	9,908	303
1903	8,517	259
1904	8,463	256
1905	7,845	236
1906	4,871	146
1907	4,231	126
1908	3,478	103
1909	3,533	104
1910	3,621	105
1911	4,420	127
1912	3,161	90
1913	2,664	75
1914	2,045	57

Source: Data from Ministero dell'Interno, Direzione Generale della Sanità Pubblica, *La malaria in Italia ed i risultati della lotta antimalarica* (Rome, 1924), 20–21.

occurred. The first crested in the summer and consisted of deaths directly caused by malaria; the second wave followed in the winter and resulted from deaths attributable to the respiratory complications of the disease. Grassi estimated that, at the turn of the century, the direct deaths from malaria in Italy numbered approximately twenty thousand a year, while total mortality —direct and indirect—reached one hundred thousand a year. Official mortality figures, however, registered the first wave, not the second. Measured in these terms, the official graph of mortality from malaria between 1900 and 1915 showed a remarkable and nearly steady decline, interrupted only by occasional recrudescences.

By 1914 annual malaria mortality as reported by the state had fallen to one-eighth of its total in 1900—from approximately sixteen thousand to two thousand, and from 490 deaths per million inhabitants to 57 (Table 4.1).[3] In evaluating these figures, one must allow for underreporting, as many deaths from malaria were not properly diagnosed, especially among children.[4] Nevertheless, the overall trend was striking, and all authorities acknowledged it.

This decline in mortality coincided with the progressive expansion in quinine distribution as the work of health stations and rural schools reached an ever-larger percentage of the population. A good example is the highly malar-

Table 4.2 Malaria Deaths and Quinine in Siracusa, 1903–1912

Year	Deaths	Quinine distributed (kg)
1903	491	63
1904	443	121
1905	447	167
1906	480	205
1907	390	309
1908	297	391
1909	244	402
1910	220	408
1911	292	338
1912	158	392

Source: Data from Medico Provinciale di Siracusa, "Relazione sulla campagna antimalarica del 1912," ACS, MI, DGS (1910–1920), b. 116 bis, fasc. "Siracusa."

ial province of Siracusa in Sicily, where figures for mortality from malaria dropped dramatically between 1903 and 1912 as the amount of quinine distributed increased significantly (Table 4.2).[5]

Surveying these figures, Alberto Lutrario, the director-general of public health, wondered whether the explanation for the decline could have little to do with the quinine program. The Giolittian period (1900–1914) witnessed great economic expansion and amelioration in standards of living. Mortality from all high-impact infectious diseases in Italy, therefore, declined substantially. Could it be that the progress made against malaria was merely a reflection of a general improvement in sanitary well-being and that the quinine campaign was of little importance? Lutrario's answer to this question was negative. In his words, "The rates of death from general mortality and from infectious diseases continued their slow and steady decline. By contrast, after 1902, mortality from malaria plummeted steeply, so that by 1914 it reached an extremely low level—so low that it was less than that of any other infectious disease."[6] In his view, the chain of causation worked in the opposite direction. Aggregate deaths and deaths from all infectious diseases declined in significant part because of the sharp fall in malaria-related deaths, including the many "opportunistic infections" that were complications of malaria. As mortality from malaria plummeted, however, the rate of death from all causes declined far more slowly (Table 4.3).

Alberto Albertazzi, the medical officer of health for Foggia province in Apulia, made a closely related point. With reference to the enormous local improvement in mortality from malaria—from 1,329 deaths in 1900 to 172 in

Table 4.3 Average Annual Deaths in Italy per 1,000 Inhabitants, 1896–1913

1896–1900	22.93
1901–1905	21.88
1906–1910	21.08
1910–1913	19.44

Source: Data from Mortara, *La salute pubblica,* 16.

1908 — Albertazzi asked whether this advance was due to causes other than the antimalarial campaign. On the one hand, there had been significant improvements during this period in the workday, diet, living conditions, and general sanitation. On the other hand, these gains were not evenly distributed throughout the province, whereas the decline in mortality from malaria was universal. He concluded that only one factor was sufficiently generalized that it could account for the ubiquitous fall in malarial deaths. This factor was the state-quinine campaign.[7]

It was not mortality statistics alone that demonstrated the progress made by the campaign with respect to deaths from malaria. In the Roman Campagna, the model zone where the antimalarial program was first and most powerfully established, physicians reported impressionistically that there was a dramatic qualitative change in the patient populations they encountered. Writing from Fiumicino in 1925, Grassi noted, "A quarter of a century ago, anyone who traveled in the Roman Campagna during the malarial season before the end of the agricultural year met at every step individuals stretched out on the ground wrapped in their coats and shivering from fever. Sometimes, if, moved to pity, one attempted to transport them to hospital, they died on the spot. This sad spectacle, which I shall have forever before my eyes, no longer occurs!"[8]

There was a consensus that the annual malaria epidemic had become milder. An indication of the change was that physicians holding clinics on the eve of the First World War rarely encountered those cases of extreme splenomegaly and cachexia that had once been so common.[9] Infections tended to be less severe, to last for shorter periods, and to lead to fewer complications. Errico De Renzi, the commissioner for Campania, was representative of the profession when he concluded, "One cannot fail to acknowledge that the antimalarial campaign has brought about a substantial attenuation of the epidemic."[10]

In addition to such attenuation, the commissioners noted a second important result — the geographical recession of the disease. Certain zones, once malarial, had become malaria-free. A clear example was the province of Rovigo in the Po Valley. Malaria, formerly prevalent throughout Rovigo's three districts, had retreated from the upper and middle districts to its final stronghold in Lower Rovigo. In 1909, the provincial officer of health reported that many townships, "intensely malarial ten or fifteen years ago, are now completely free of infection."[11] Similarly, in Campania, the district of San Bartolomeo in Galdo celebrated the fact that it no longer produced indigenous malaria. The few remaining cases there all involved migrant workers who had contracted the disease in their travels. Places once known as "fields of death" were settled and cultivated. In such places, the campaign produced the very condition that had once so perplexed physicians—*anofelismo senza malaria* (anopheline mosquitoes without malaria).[12]

For Grassi, such progress rewarded the efforts of a lifetime. Although eradication had not taken place with the speed he had originally expected, Grassi still believed that the campaign would ultimately achieve this ambitious goal. Indeed, he stipulated in his will that he wished to be buried at Fiumicino, where he had directed the campaign, so that he could witness eradication in person when it finally came about. What had already been done, he wrote, "exceeded all reasonable expectations" and fell short only of the euphoria that followed the great scientific breakthroughs of the turn of the century.[13]

Despite all advances in preventing death from malaria, however, Grassi wrote that the disease remained Italy's leading problem of public health because of the "limitless area" that it still affected and because of the "massive damages that it continues to cause." Messea, the director-general of public health, commented, "The problem of eradicating malaria is far more arduous and complex than it might seem at first sight."[14] Indeed, it was possible for some authorities to accept the facts presented by Grassi, Messea, and Lutrario while reaching far more somber conclusions. In 1925, just as Grassi was penning his final optimistic assessment, the malariologist Giuseppe Sanarelli harbored gloomy misgivings. Sanarelli was Grassi's colleague both at the University of Rome and in the leadership of the antimalarial campaign then advancing in the Pontine Marshes. Although he agreed with Grassi that malaria remained Italy's "greatest and most urgent problem," Sanarelli also thought that "our situation remains very pitiful" and that the hope of eradication was a "pure utopia."[15]

How was it possible for experts to reach such contrasting conclusions on the basis of the same facts? The explanation involved two sobering aspects of the great malarial challenge. The first was that the founders of the campaign had underestimated the devastating impact not of death but of sickness. Ronald Ross was prescient in observing that chronic malaria is synonymous with poverty and economic stagnation. "Very malarious places," he wrote, "cannot be prosperous. . . . For the state as for the individual, health is the first postulate of prosperity."[16] As the campaign unfolded in Italy, those responsible for combating the epidemic learned the disease's full cost to society. The prefect of Girgenti, in Sicily, provided a cogent assessment. "The problem of malaria," he wrote in 1908,

> is immense . . . and complicated. The enormous prevalence of the disease has the most serious social consequences because the infection—tenacious and lasting—undermines the body. Malaria causes physical decline . . . , it prevents growth, and it alters the very structure of the population. . . . Fever destroys the capacity to work, annihilates energy, and renders a people sluggish and indifferent. Inevitably, therefore, malaria stunts productivity, wealth, and well-being. Malaria shackles the development of industry and agriculture. Malaria casts a pall over the whole society. The misery arising from this malady produces ignorance, a low standard of culture and morality, and ineradicable illiteracy.[17]

In other words, as the American malariologist Fred Soper later reflected, malaria enslaves those it does not kill. The drama for Italy was that even as malaria ceased to kill, it continued to enslave.[18]

Here the second aspect of the malaria challenge demonstrated its full importance. Although mortality from fever plummeted as a result of the quinine campaign, the caseload confronted by the campaigners remained almost unchanged. On this point the reports of health officials are unanimous. Sanarelli, for example, argued that in 1925 two million Italians continued to run the annual gauntlet of infection, reinfection, superinfection, and relapse just as they had in 1900. Furthermore, he observed pessimistically, morbidity is "socially more important" than mortality. A major difficulty with the eradication program in its first twenty-five years was that it had produced a stark divergence between a rapidly declining mortality and a stubbornly resistant morbidity.[19]

Here, unfortunately, the figures published by the state lead only to confusion. The official statistical profile of the prevalence of malaria after 1900 is one of a steady decline that mirrored the fall in mortality. Foggia province, for instance, produced figures that clearly suggest parallel declines in cases of and deaths from malaria (Table 4.4). The authorities who gathered these reassuring statistics, however, argued that the data were seriously misleading. Reports from experts stationed in three regions—Campania, Sicily, and Sardinia—clearly establish the point. Gaetano Rummo, commissioner for Benevento province in Campania, wrote in 1909 that data for cases were useless. In his view, "Grand statistics, collected and aggregated, make a great impression. But there are so many sources of inaccuracy and of error that they have no value. People have forgotten that, even in ideal conditions, . . . exact statistics regarding cases of malaria are impossible."[20] Similarly, the provincial officer of

Table 4.4 Malaria in Foggia Province, 1905–1914

Year	Cases	Deaths
1905	15,593	609
1906	8,574	312
1907	10,779	262
1908	5,605	283
1909	8,031	200
1910	9,469	192
1911	7,653	290
1912	8,939	156
1913	8,050	132
1914	6,333	75

Source: Data from "Relazione sull'applicazione delle leggi contro la malaria durante il 1914," ACS, MI, DGS (1910–1920), b. 114, fasc. "Foggia: Relazioni, 1914–1916."

health at Siracusa, in Sicily, declared flatly that "it is not possible to take into consideration the data for morbidity . . . because they do not convey the true extent of malaria in this region."[21] Finally, attempting to measure the difference between officially reported cases and real malaria prevalence, the prefect of Cagliari, in Sardinia, noted that the reported cases for the province in 1905 numbered 24,046, but the real total was at least twice as great—over 50,000.[22]

Explanations for such serious inaccuracy abounded. A first factor was that the malaria afflicting infants was commonly misdiagnosed. As Grassi explained, infants with malaria do not present the same symptomatology as adults because babies have fever without chills or sweating. As a result, in a milieu in which most doctors practiced without a microscope, infants' illnesses were frequently attributed to indigestion, teething, worms, or rheumatic fever. Alternatively, he noted, their malaise was often simply neglected. In addition, most mild malaria cases in people of all ages went unreported because such patients preferred either to ignore the disease or to medicate themselves without consulting a physician. In many places medical attention was simply unavailable. Even patients with severe symptoms often found medical care inaccessible because of distance, poor communications, and distrust. At the same time, since physicians felt overwhelmed by the workload confronting them, they normally favored the treatment of patients over the completion of the paperwork required by law. The very length and complexity of the forms demanded by Rome encouraged doctors to practice deception and evasion.[23]

Such circumstances produced anomalous results such as those described by

Table 4.5 Cases of Malaria at Cerignola, 1902–1906

1902	245
1903	178
1904	403
1905	206
1906	255

Source: Data from G. Tropeano, "Per la lotta contro la malaria," 40–42.

Giuseppe Tropeano in Foggia province, in Apulia. Cerignola, a city of thirty-five thousand inhabitants at the heart of this infamously malarial province, officially reported very low rates of malaria (Table 4.5). To anyone familiar with malaria in Apulia, Tropeano reasoned, such figures were so absurdly low as to demonstrate that "statistics, as they are presently compiled, have no value whatsoever." Indeed, to verify his conclusion, Tropeano carried out an investigation to discover the magnitude of the difference between officially reported cases and actual cases. He concluded that "we can state loudly, and without the least exaggeration, that no township officially reports as many as ten of every hundred actual cases of malaria."[24]

Expressing the progress of the campaign against malaria in geographical terms, the Department of Health also reached ambiguous conclusions. Between 1902 and 1924, Italy had made tangible advances. At the outset of the campaign, only eleven of sixty-nine provinces had been malaria-free. By 1924 the disease had been eliminated from a further six provinces, and the number of zones officially designated as malarial had been reduced from 3,349 to 3,270. Similarly, 2,647 of the nation's 8,362 townships had been malarial in 1902, and by 1924 that number was down to 2,616. This progress was noteworthy, but it was overshadowed by the enormity of the problem that remained. Of the total area of the nation — 286,610 square kilometers — 84,046 square kilometers, or 29.3 percent, remained infested and dangerous. Moreover, advances had been registered primarily in the North and Center, leaving the more severely afflicted South just as extensively diseased as it had been at the turn of the century. Of the seventeen provinces that the Department of Health proclaimed malaria-free in 1924, not one was located in the South.[25]

Thus by the First World War, Grassi rightly rejoiced at the decline in deaths from malaria, while Sanarelli worried with equal reason that the goal of eradication seemed to be an ever-receding mirage. Since both took eradication rather than control as the standard by which to assess what had been achieved, the potential for a negative assessment was enhanced. Grassi was more sanguine than Sanarelli in part because he came late in his career to regard control

—the attenuation of the epidemic—as at least a valid interim accomplishment. For both scientists, however, the persistent burden of morbidity remained a fundamental and troubling issue. Making quinine universally available had dramatically lowered mortality, but it had not significantly affected morbidity. Why was the campaign so unable to reduce the burden of illness as well as the burden of death? What were the main problems that it encountered?

Human Obstacles Facing the Campaign

At the outset, the principal problem reported by physicians was the ignorance of the rural population. But with growing numbers of health stations and peasant schools, and with the increasing contact of peasants with physicians and their doctrine, views began to change substantially. By the eve of the First World War, campaigners reported that peasants, once diffident, had come to regard quinine as a right and as an effective remedy for serious illness. This success in convincing a once-hostile populace that quinine was beneficial helped to reduce mortality, but it was insufficient to bring the ultimate goals of Celli and Grassi—control and eradication, respectively—much closer. Their strategy was that victims of malaria would take quinine daily for months, either preventively before the onset of the epidemic season (Celli) or curatively after contracting fever (Grassi). Their optimism rested on experimental results obtained at Capaccio, Ostia, and Cervelletta under carefully managed circumstances.

The quinine legislation was thus enacted on the basis of tightly controlled experiments without tests of its feasibility in the real world. Commissioner Gaetano Rummo commented,

> This question has taken a strange course. First we hastily enshrined a theoretical solution in the law, . . . and only then did we turn to the clinicians to find a real remedy for the problem.
>
> We began by extolling the preventive use of quinine without testing it, as if the enactment of a law were sufficient to ensure its triumph. We rejoiced too soon in the law as the means to redeem malarial Italy.[26]

In practice, the complex reality of the clinic confounded the abstract logic of laboratory science. Patients did not behave in the disciplined, rational manner that the strategy of the Rome School demanded. Once convinced that quinine was available and effective, they made use of it, but only to the extent necessary for the purpose of ridding themselves of painful symptoms. In overwhelming numbers, fever victims with mild symptoms avoided the rigorous treatment needed to avoid infecting others. Similarly, patients who were sufficiently ill to seek medical attention refused to continue taking quinine after their symptoms had ceased. Four days of quinine at the "therapeutic dose" of 1 to 1.5 grams a day were normally adequate to end all chills and fever, but months of treatment were considered necessary to "sterilize" the bloodstream.[27] In a report presented to the Superior Health Council (Consiglio Superiore della Sanità), the antimalarial commissioner Nicola Badaloni observed that real adherence to the strict official quinine regimen was exceptional, and that a large proportion of the quinine distributed was never actually consumed.[28] Thus asymptomatic but still infectious patients disappeared from health-station infirmaries and discharged themselves from hospitals. No longer suffering, they paid no heed to the fact that, with plasmodia remaining in their bloodstreams, they could maintain the cycle of transmission.

Of the two strategies of malaria control by quinine — Grassi's path of radical cure and Celli's path of chemical prophylaxis — Celli's proved the more problematic. Grassi's policy of radical cure at least targeted actual patients — that is, people with undeniable motivation to ingest quinine tablets. Celli's alternative of universal quinine prophylaxis committed the campaign to medicating the whole population of every malarial zone — even those who were healthy or at least asymptomatic and therefore found no reason to comply with public health requirements. Physicians in the field rapidly concluded that chemical prophylaxis set an impossible goal for the antimalarial program. In addition, the medical training that physicians received prepared them to accept Grassi's strategy more easily than Celli's. After the early years, therefore, health stations everywhere quietly abandoned universal prophylaxis as an aim, replacing it with the radical cure of sufferers.[29] In 1929, under the chairmanship of Ettore Marchiafava, the Superior Health Council announced officially that cure, not prophylaxis, was the proper use of quinine, which could neither prevent malaria nor lower morbidity.[30] As the malariologist Claudio Fermi explained, chemical prophylaxis was a theoretical concept that was impractical in large settings. It served a useful purpose only with carefully selected and well-disciplined populations — sailors, armies on the march, colonizers. To attempt it with the general population of a sizable country was merely to waste the alkaloid by diverting it from more effective and practical uses. More disturbingly and presciently, Fermi also worried that wholesale administration of quinine would lead to the emergence of resistant strains of plasmodia.[31]

Having rejected Celli's original approach from an early date, the campaign even moved slowly away from the pure doctrine propounded by Grassi. In provinces where the burden of disease was overwhelming, the Italian antimalarial program adopted de facto an aim far less ambitious than radical cure.

Physicians sought instead to achieve the limited goal of making quinine available to everyone who was seriously ill. Saving lives, not eradicating disease, became their mission. Clinicians in the field quietly modified the impractical goal proposed by experimental scientists.

A variety of factors reinforced such redefinition of the campaign's intentions. One set of factors was biological. Unknown to the founders of the state-quinine initiative, the complex life cycle of plasmodia limited the effectiveness of quinine as the key to malaria control. When first injected into the bloodstream, the parasites—then known as sporozoites—do not linger in the blood plasma, where they are vulnerable to the alkaloid. Instead, the sporozoites migrate to the safety of the liver tissues, beyond the reach both of quinine and of the body's immune system. There they multiply during the weeklong incubation period of the disease. Only then do they emerge as merozoites—a new and morphologically different stage in the evolving life cycle of the plasmodium. The merozoites return to the bloodstream and invade erythrocytes. At this stage, however, a complication with major epidemiological consequences arises from the fact that malaria is not a single disease but a complex of three different illnesses caused by distinct species of plasmodia. In vivax malaria, sporozoites continue to take shelter in the liver indefinitely, ready to reemerge at distant intervals and to reestablish disease long after the full recovery of the patient from the primary infection. Here was the mystery of relapses that puzzled physicians until Giulio Raffaele solved the enigma in the 1930s by careful examination of what he termed the "tissue phase" of plasmodia. Decades before Raffaele's discovery, however, Italian clinicians learned by trial and error that quinine—curative and prophylactic alike—was often powerless to prevent relapses and therefore to eradicate disease.

If sporozoites, then, sheltered beyond the reach of quinine, a later phase in the evolution of the plasmodium was simply unaffected by the drug. After successfully multiplying asexually in red blood cells, plasmodia eventually produce male and female cells known as gametes—the strange shapes that had thoroughly baffled Laveran. For the transmission of disease, gametes are vital. During her blood meal, the female anopheles mosquito sucks gametes into her own body, where they initiate the sexual phase of the parasite's reproduction, enabling it to complete its life cycle. But unlike sporozoites and merozoites, gametes, especially in falciparum malaria, are not susceptible to quinine. Thus the power of the alkaloid as a stand-alone instrument of eradication was further seriously weakened by the complex biology of plasmodia.

A further biological difficulty affecting quinine's efficacy was that a significant proportion of malaria victims proved unable to tolerate it. Developing painful and sometimes serious side effects, they dropped out of the program, together with many of those who witnessed their distress. This problem was exacerbated when physicians attempted to simplify the lengthy curative regimen, replacing daily tablets with high-dosage weekly and fortnightly injections. Administered in such concentrated doses, quinine produced more-frequent and more-severe side effects.[32]

Confusion among physicians led more patients to abandon the program. The antimalarial crusade began well before the Italian medical profession had fully absorbed the fundamentals of the new science of parasitology. As late as 1910, some of the eminent physicians on the Superior Health Council, such as Badaloni and Baccelli, were still unconvinced that mosquitoes were the sole means for the transmission of malaria. They clung instead to miasmatic notions that "malaria germs" could nestle in swamps, in the earth, and perhaps elsewhere in the environment and could find conduits other than mosquitoes by which to enter the human body. Frequently, too, clinicians did not understand the proper use for quinine. Mistakenly, they believed it to be an all-purpose febrifuge or even a panacea rather than the specific remedy for malaria. In 1927 the American malariologist L. W. Hackett made a visit to Calabria, where he noted that "in all these towns the doctors continue to prescribe quinine for every headache, fever, cold, or pain which they discover. . . . The peasants have been instructed, badgered, and cajoled for twenty years to take quinine whenever they feel badly, and also to take it as a preventive when they feel well."[33] Other doctors incorrectly assumed that quinine conferred immunity in a manner analogous to the smallpox vaccine. In all such cases, precious supplies of quinine were wasted, while the disappointing results of inappropriate therapy undermined public confidence.[34]

Bitter and highly public disputes among physicians and pharmacists further compromised public trust. There were rifts between those who believed wholeheartedly in quinine and those who regarded it either as entirely useless or as ineffective unless administered with arsenic and iron; between believers in oral administration and partisans of injection; between adherents of Celli's prophylaxis and followers of Grassi's radical cure; between elite academic malariologists and clinicians in the field; and between jealous rivals for preeminence, such as Grassi and Celli. Indeed, the quinine program got under way before the medical profession had assessed the best mode for administering the remedy, before there was any understanding of the long-term effects of prolonged use, before possible counterindications had been evaluated, and before it was known whether there should be different therapeutic regimens for different species of plasmodium. Difficulties arose in part because malaria control had begun hastily on the basis of several leaps of blind faith.

If blind faith created some problems, bad faith gave rise to many more.

Vested interests obstructed the progress of the campaign at every step. Landlords and farmers resented the quinine tax they were required to pay on behalf of their tenants and employees. Indeed, the tax lent itself easily to the criticism that it was arbitrary and unfair. Rates varied widely from township to township, and they took no account either of a landlord's income or of the number of his employees.[35] Frequently, cadastral surveys were out of date, generating tax assessments that were anomalous and unintended by the framers of the legislation. It was also unclear where migrant laborers had contracted their disease, with the result that taxpayers often suspected that they were subsidizing their neighbors by paying to treat cases they believed to be imported. Furthermore, proprietors abhorred the radical message of workers' rights emanating from health stations and schools for peasants. They opposed the new regime of health inspections and restrictive regulations, and they resented the involvement of labor organizers. Many landlords, Grassi noted, preferred to suffer fever in silence rather than purchase quinine for themselves. Imagine, he wrote, their enthusiasm for medicating their employees! For all of these reasons, property owners everywhere resolutely opposed the quinine campaign. Organizers of the program wrote unanimously of the landowners' "hostility," "neglect," and "obstinate refusal" to comply with the objectives of the legislation. Their opposition was so intransigent that Grassi, disabused of his early optimism, suggested that a hundred years would be needed to overcome it.[36]

Landlords, however, were not alone in their opposition to the antimalarial effort. Pharmacists resented state quinine because it entailed the loss of one of their most important sources of income, and they feared that it would establish a precedent for the state to control the prices of all medicines. Members of the middle class—lawyers, notaries, and shopkeepers—often owned small plots of land where they cultivated market gardens, which were now subject to the new levy. Public health doctors often earned inadequate salaries, and they resented a campaign that imposed arduous work for no additional reward. Sometimes physicians had family or marriage ties to pharmacists and therefore faced serious conflicts of interest. In some regions, municipalities outsourced the responsibility for collecting the tax and purchasing the alkaloid. In such cases the contractors had an interest only in minimizing the purchase of medicine.[37]

Townships (*comuni*) were the instruments for the "passive resistance" of the landed classes and pharmaceutical interests to the eradication campaign. Throughout malarial Italy, landlords dominated town halls, serving as mayors, aldermen, and municipal councilors. A salient contradiction of the state-quinine program, therefore, was that its implementation required the cooperation of precisely those people who most adamantly opposed it. Public health officials regularly complained of the "obstructionism," "indifference," "deficient energy," "indolence," and "apathy" of local government.[38] In defiance of their obligations under the law, townships persistently failed to collect the quinine tax, they purchased derisory quantities of the drug, or they delayed purchase until it was too late in the season to carry out the course of medication demanded by Grassi. In many provinces, it took unrelenting pressure from prefects and officers of health to secure even halfhearted compliance. In Trapani (Sicily) and Sassari (Sardinia), for instance, campaigners reported in 1908 and 1909 that hardly a single township purchased quinine in the quantities and at the dates stipulated by the health authorities.[39] At Trinitapoli (Apulia), one of the most malarial townships in the nation, the municipal officer of health was unable to convince the town council to furnish him with a microscope, filing cabinets, pens, or even an office from which to conduct the offensive against the disease.[40]

Under the terms of the quinine legislation, vested interests even had an incentive to practice obstruction. The intention of parliament was that all profits from the state monopoly should be used to encourage the program, chiefly in the form of subsidies to overburdened municipalities. Local authorities rapidly discovered, however, that these very subsidies from the central government could be used to subvert the law. The technique was simple. All town halls had to do was to delay collection of the quinine tax as long as possible. When the subsidies finally arrived — normally at the end of the year — it would be too late to purchase quinine for the purposes envisaged by the state. Councils could then divert the outside funds from their intended objective, using them retroactively to cover antimalarial expenses without the necessity of ever collecting the local quinine tax. The two great negative results were, first, the interruption in the availability of quinine to those who needed it and, second, the draining of campaign funds. Alberto Lutrario, the director-general of public health, termed this corrupt procedure the "posthumous distribution of subsidies" — a procedure that "greatly attenuated the efficiency of the antimalarial campaign" and "exonerated landlords from their legal obligations."[41]

Having experienced the inertia of local government in matters of public health, many commissioners and provincial officers of health, as well as Angelo Celli himself, suggested that it had been a major strategic error to entrust the purchase of quinine to townships.[42] They urged instead that the campaign be reformed by having it provincialized or nationalized. From the outset Grassi had insisted that the eradication program depended entirely upon the abundant supply of quinine to all who needed it, for several epidemic seasons. The only way to achieve that result, he predicted, was for the state to provide it free to local authorities. He claimed that placing quinine as an item on the state budget would cost only three million lire a year—a negligible amount in comparison with many military or public-works programs that provided much smaller benefits to the nation. Indeed, he believed that the savings in medical expenses and productivity would offset the outlay. The decision to make the program dependent instead on a local government tax inevitably diminished the resources available to the malaria campaign, thereby transforming its objective from eradication to emergency intervention. Thus, Grassi wrote in retrospect, the original all-out war on malaria was unofficially but dramatically changed into a guerrilla campaign against mortality.[43]

Natural Disasters as Obstacles to the Campaign

The course of the campaign against malaria was not a smooth and steady advance. On the contrary, sharp, unexpected spikes in mortality and morbidity periodically interrupted progress. Yielding to the temptation to personify the epidemic, contemporary physicians sometimes explained these imponderable vicissitudes as the result of the capricious will of the disease. This was known as its *genio epidemico,* the apparently intelligent strategy by which the disease besieged its human hosts. Nevertheless, these sudden upsurges of disease had simple, naturalistic explanations. One, of course, was the weather. Heavy spring and summer rain, flooding, and intense heat could create ideal conditions for mosquitoes to breed, thus prolonging the malarial season. In years when such weather patterns occurred, Italians experienced violent surges in death and suffering. A typical instance was the sudden increase in malaria cases and deaths in Sicily in 1910, which interrupted several years of hard-won progress. The reason, explained the physician in charge of the campaign at Messina, was the arrival of "heavy rains in August and September." He continued, "Collecting in puddles, the water, together with high temperatures, created ideal environmental conditions—just right for the development of anopheles mosquitoes" and the transmission of disease.[44] Under the right circumstances, flooding alone could set off an epidemic, as the province of Sondrio (Lombardy) learned in 1911. On the night of 21 August, as the malarial season peaked, torrential downpours caused the Adda River to overflow its banks, flooding the fields, blocking drainage ditches with debris, creating limitless breeding sites for mosquitoes, and unleashing a fierce epidemic.[45] Conversely, a prolonged drought and the early arrival of cool weather could create an illusion of progress by lowering the prevalence of malaria even when the campaign itself had stalled or quinine had been unavailable. Thus variations from year to year were often serendipitous and bore little relation to long-term trends in public health.

Because malaria is a disease that thrives on human misfortune, it was also common for sharp upturns in prevalence and mortality to follow in the wake of large-scale public disasters. The mechanisms involved are vividly illustrated by four examples that struck Italy during the early years of the quinine offensive: the earthquakes of 1905 and 1908 in Calabria and Sicily; the cholera epidemic of 1910–1911; and the local fungal catastrophe of downy mildew that destroyed the vineyards at San Ferdinando di Puglia (Apulia).

Reggio Calabria and Messina provinces lie at the heart of a great seismic area in southern Italy where two major quakes struck during the course of the antimalarial campaign—on 8 September 1905 and 28 December 1908. The first, with its epicenter in Calabria, was reported as one of the worst seismic catastrophes of modern history, ranking with the terrible Lisbon earthquake of 1755 (which Voltaire made justly famous) and the fearful Italian earthquake of 1788.[46] "Never," wrote the Socialist newspaper *Avanti!*, "has a disaster stricken a country so inexorably and so pitilessly. . . . It is the most chilling drama that has ever occurred."[47] In retrospect, however, 1905 proved to be only the prelude to the far deadlier earthquake of 1908. By all accounts, the quake of 1908 was one of the most violent ever recorded until that time, greatly exceeding the more famous San Francisco earthquake of 1906 in its destructive power. This quake, along with the tidal wave and the uncontrolled fires that followed in its train, entirely demolished both coastal cities of Messina and Reggio Calabria, together with numerous smaller towns and villages in their hinterland. Even more than the quake of 1905, this event attracted worldwide attention and dismay, and it caused enormous loss of life and property. A city of 150,000 before the disaster, Messina alone suffered 100,000 victims according to the press, and virtually the entire surviving population became homeless overnight.[48]

On both occasions, to the misfortune of the survivors, fearsome local epidemics of malaria followed rapidly in the wake of the quakes. The earthquake of 1905 struck just as the annual malaria epidemic was reaching its peak. Tens of thousands of refugees were forced to flee the centers of cities and villages and to sleep in the open countryside under improvised tents or in hastily constructed sheds that provided little shelter from flying insects. In addition, a change in the weather added immeasurably to the misery of the population, as powerful thunderstorms and unusual heat vastly increased the number of mosquitoes and lengthened the season of transmission. Inadequate food and clothing further lowered resistance and exposed the populace to additional risk. In the terse words of the provincial officer of health for Cosenza (Calabria), "The antimalarial campaign of 1905 was proceeding vigorously when the September earthquake occurred and created a disastrous situation in which vast masses of people were compelled to camp out of doors in the midst of intense foci of malaria while new and most virulent foci were formed."[49]

In 1908 the link between the disaster and the onset of malaria was less immediately apparent. The sole merciful aspect of the 1908 earthquake was that it took place just at the start of the interepidemic malarial period, when cool weather had brought transmission nearly to an end. Unfortunately, however, victims on both sides of the Strait of Messina were still without housing by the summer of 1909 or even by 1910. On the contrary, in 1910 the newly homeless—many of them women and children—were still bivouacking in open fields without adequate sanitation, diet, or clothing. At the same time, the expense of dealing with the crisis and the collapse of revenue that resulted from the destruction of the local economy paralyzed local governments and the antimalarial campaign they directed. Supplies of quinine were interrupted; physicians faced an impossible workload, with patients scattered across the countryside and unreachable; and the international swell of goodwill and commitment to assistance petered out a year after the disaster. As always, displaced populations, poverty, the collapse of medical services, and societal neglect provided ideal conditions for anopheline mosquitoes.[50]

A different type of natural disaster was the epidemic of Asiatic cholera that struck Italy as a limited outbreak in 1910 and then erupted in full force in the summer of 1911. Whereas earthquakes and storms led to *local* upsurges in malaria, the cholera epidemic was of national importance to the antimalarial campaign and led to a spike in mortality and morbidity throughout Italy. Unfortunately, the Italian state orchestrated a campaign to suppress all knowledge of the cholera epidemic by means of official denials, censorship of the press, intimidation of the medical profession, and falsification of public health statistics. As a result, this event has not received historical attention, with the exception of my own book *Naples in the Time of Cholera, 1884–1911*.[51] Reports of the antimalarial campaign reveal, however, that the impact of the disease was so widespread and intense that it caused the antimalarial campaign to stall and mortality and morbidity from fever to soar. Mortality from malaria spiked in 1911, when deaths per million inhabitants in Italy rose from an average of 104 to 127, falling again to 90 in 1912 and 75 in 1913 (see Table 4.1). Significantly, the records of the public health campaign against malaria—from places as distant from one another as Sicily, Sardinia, Basilicata, Tuscany, and Emilia—suggest that the "secret" epidemic of cholera was the reason for this upsurge in death and suffering.

Cholera affected the prevalence of malaria in a variety of ways. In some places, the relationship was dramatically direct. The arrival of cholera, always a source of terror, in some southern towns in the late summer of 1911 caused absolute panic. Sudden in its onset, excruciating in its symptoms, and lethal in the majority of cases that it affected, cholera caused many a local exodus as the inhabitants sought safety in escape. Fleeing for their lives from cholera, physicians reported, anxious peasants slept in the open countryside, where they exposed themselves to high risks of malaria at the height of the season. Unfortunately, the refugees in Sicily, obsessed with the fear that cholera was spread by poisoners, lost all trust in medication and physicians and refused to take the quinine tablets that they thought would hasten their demise.[52]

More generally, cholera affected malaria by diverting the medical and public health resources essential to the campaign. In order to deal with the cholera emergency, physicians and their assistants abandoned the work of locating and attending fever victims. At the same time, local governments, compelled to spend scarce resources on the sanitary measures needed to halt the spread of the cholera bacillus, failed to budget money for the purchase of quinine. Therefore, in many provinces, the precious alkaloid was suddenly unavailable to the poor for the first time since 1900. In a common lament, the provincial officer of health for Siracusa (Sicily) explained that in 1911 quinine was not distributed in the province "because of the struggle against cholera, which absorbed the entire medical attention of the townships."[53] In provinces throughout Italy physicians made identical observations. At Caltanissetta (Sicily), medical officials informed Rome that the antimalarial campaign had ground entirely to a halt because dealing with cholera took priority.[54] In Avellino (Campania), the Department of Health learned, antimalarial activity "was almost totally canceled by the fight against cholera and by the necessity of ensuring the sanitary defense of our towns."[55] In Basilicata, health officials had "less time and less freedom in their control work in the war against malaria" as a result of "the existence of the cholera epidemic."[56] From Emilia, in the North, the medical officer of health in Ferrara noted that the "simultaneity of the campaign against cholera with that against malaria in 1911 . . . absorbed all the energy of the provincial health department."[57] Finally, at Grosseto, in central Italy, the antimalarial commissioner Alfonso Di Vestea wrote, "The worries occasioned by cholera, in addition to damaging the budget, halted the campaign in various localities because the medical personnel that had been hired were no longer available and it was not easy to replace them. These concerns also diverted a significant part of the work of management and vigilance. The result was that the campaign was contained within limits that were much more modest than had been planned."[58] The fight against cholera trumped the campaign against malaria, preempting its resources and allowing fever to strike unimpeded. Only in 1912, when cholera had departed, did the antimalarial struggle resume on a full-time basis.

The cholera epidemic demonstrates the capacity of a medical emergency to promote a national upsurge in malaria. By contrast, the town of San Ferdinando di Puglia illustrates the potential of a plant disease and the economic disruption it creates to promote a local fever epidemic. Although located on the southern border of Foggia province, one of the most malarial provinces in the kingdom, San Ferdinando remained an oasis of health, free of endemic malaria until 1899. It was the good fortune of the eight thousand peasants of San Ferdinando to inhabit a hill town located high above the dangerous plain known as the Tavoliere. They benefited also from the intensive cultivation of vineyards on the slopes of the neighboring hills — vineyards that provided full and remunerative employment and created no environmental conditions that favored the breeding of mosquitoes. Of the nine hundred hectares of the township, eight hundred were devoted to the cultivation of grapes, and the remaining hundred hectares to intensively cultivated market gardens. In striking contrast to the sickly and impoverished day laborers who worked the nearby wheat fields of the Apulian latifundia, the grape growers of San Ferdinando enjoyed economic well-being, stable employment, and freedom from malaria.[59]

In 1899, however, conditions of public health at San Ferdinando began plummeting disastrously when the fungal vine disease of *Peronospora destructor,* or "downy mildew," laid waste to the vineyards. Progressively and rapidly destroying the vines that were the basis of the local economy, this devastating plant affliction impoverished the population. Facing unemployment and hunger, the men and women of San Ferdinando were forced in growing numbers every summer from 1900 on to migrate in search of work as day laborers on the great estates of Foggia province. In a final sign of desperate conditions, many even stayed on after the harvest to eke out a subsistence as gleaners. The former grape growers, lacking any immunity to malaria, fell ill en masse on the wheat fields. By 1906 fully a third of the population of the township was estimated to be ill with malaria, and by the outbreak of the First World War, the disease had become a pandemic that afflicted the whole adult population. By then poverty and a poor diet had formed enduring conditions that predisposed them to disease. Only the children remained healthy because they remained behind in the town while their parents and relatives made the long trek to the plain below.[60]

Political Consequences of the Campaign

Malaria breeds apathy, illiteracy, and inaction. Fever, therefore, had long been a major factor inhibiting the development of a flourishing civil and political society in much of Italy. Conversely, the attenuation of the disease and the national mobilization to combat it stimulated participation, awareness, and organization in fields beyond public health. Indeed, the war on malaria made a major contribution to the expansion of civil liberties and democracy that was such a marked feature of the Giolittian period—before world war and then Fascism led to major setbacks. The great campaign to control malaria with quinine played a substantial part in the rise of the Italian labor movement, the formation of a Socialist awareness among farmworkers, and the establishment of a collective consciousness among women. Particularly important in this regard was the fact that malaria was conceptualized, or "framed," by the campaign not as a poison arising from the environment but rather as an occupational disease that was the product of human agency and all-too-human negligence. This understanding of malaria transformed the abolition campaign into a major social and political force in its own right. Leaders in the quinine campaign such as Angelo Celli and spokesmen for the South such as Giuseppe Tropeano had long insisted that progress in the war on malaria and victory in the establishment of workers' rights were interdependent. Events rapidly confirmed their assessment.[61]

Nowhere was the link between the quinine program and the mobilization of labor clearer than in the case of the famously malarial rice fields in the Po Valley and of the weeders (*mondine*) who worked them. Throughout the "rice belt," weeders were overwhelmingly women under twenty-one years of age. They constituted between 70 percent and 80 percent of the workforce in the three leading rice-producing provinces—Novara, Pavia, and Milan, as exemplified in the crucial district of Mortara in 1904 (Table 4.6).

The reasons underlying the growers' preference for young women were economic, physical, and disciplinary. The Ministry of the Interior estimated in 1905 that the average cost of labor per hectare of rice was 280 lire—double that of any other grain crop in Italy. In this context, weeding was crucial because this single operation contributed disproportionately to the operational cost of rice production, ranging from 96 to 168 lire per hectare. For this reason, growers sought weeders who were cheap, and women in Giolittian Italy earned half the pay of adult males. In Novara province, for example, daily wages averaged 3.7 lire for male rice workers and 2 lire for women and children. Financial constraints became especially compelling after 1880, when the price of rice declined on the newly global market, from nearly forty lire per kilogram in 1873 to just over thirty lire in 1900.[62] As the steamship, the Suez Canal, and the railroad exposed Italian producers to stern international competition, they redoubled their efforts to cut costs.

In addition to considerations of economy, the physical task of weeding favored the bodies of the young female and the child. Weeding, which was

Table 4.6 Age and Sex of Rice Weeders in Mortara, 1904

Sex	Under 13 years of age	13 to 21 years of age	Over 21 years of age	Total
Male	66	2,985	1,639	4,690
Female	80	7,084	3,485	10,649

Source: Data from Prefetto di Pavia, "Relazione sulla campagna antimalarica attuata col chinino di Stato nelle squadre fisse dei mondarisi dell'agro pavese," 30 Aug. 1904, ACS, MI, DGS (1882–1915), b. 120, fasc. "Pavia: Applicazione della legge sulla malaria," 13–14.

performed with the back bent double throughout a twelve-hour day, required elasticity of the spinal column, sufficient flexibility of the limbs to maintain the posture for an extended period, and short stature. Furthermore, muscular strength was no advantage. These qualities suggested the hiring of young women.[63]

Finally, contractors preferred migrant females, whom they deemed more readily subject to labor discipline than adult males. The youth and sex of the migrants; their ignorance of conditions in the provinces to which they were imported; their dependence on employers for meals, shelter, and return transportation to their homes; and the payment of wages only at the end of the season—all of these factors strengthened the hand of the overseers, known as corporals, who recruited and drove the work gangs. Experience demonstrated that locals, who could go home if their demands were not met, were more likely to strike at critical moments when the crop was at risk.[64]

Working from dawn to dusk in water up to their knees, these women were at great risk of infection because they toiled in the midst of virtual swamps just as the epidemic season peaked. Investigators probing the health of weeders noted other factors as well. First among their concerns was the workers' inadequate diet, which normally consisted of five hundred grams of bread and two rations of either polenta or rice soup that they received as partial payment for their work. Other causes for anxiety were the lack of safe drinking water, low wages, overwork, and the absence of health care or basic sanitation. Recruited from the highlands of the Apennines, rice weeders typically also lacked all immunity to fever.

With regard to malaria, however, the most dangerous condition they experienced was their accommodation at night. Perilously substandard workers' dormitories were ubiquitous in the rice belt. Landlords made no costly outlays on healthy quarters for a transient workforce whose long-term welfare was of no concern. Instead, the weeders sheltered at night in haylofts, in stables, or beneath the porticos of farm buildings. There they slept on straw matting—entire work gangs together with no separation by age, gender, or family groupings.[65] English malariologist Sydney James and Dutch malariologist Nicholas Swellengrebel explained the central role of housing in the epidemiology of malaria. Fever, they noted, was not equably distributed among the population. A classic focal disease, malaria spread in clusters, choosing its victims disproportionately among the poor who slept in dark, crowded, and unsanitary dwellings with open windows and porous walls. Overcrowded buildings attracted large numbers of mosquitoes—including *Anopheles labranchiae,* the principal Italian vector—which were drawn by the warmth and by the carbon dioxide emanating from such places. Once inside, anophelines did not content themselves with a single blood meal before taking flight to lay their eggs. Instead, they took up residence for several days and feasted repeatedly, assisted by the fact that sleeping bodies are ideal, motionless targets. In this way numerous human bodies crowded together not only attracted mosquitoes but also posed a direct threat to one another as infected insects transmitted parasites from the blood of sufferers into the veins of their neighbors. The poorly lighted rooms; filthy, unpainted walls; unprotected windows; open rafters; and lack of ceilings, all characteristic of northern farms, also afforded mosquitoes unlimited access and innumerable crevices where they could shelter, unseen and undisturbed, to digest between one meal and the next. Housing, James concluded, was a critical factor that made malaria a focal disease, a social disease, a "house disease," and a classic disease of poverty. A densely populated, unsanitary, and poorly constructed dormitory was the perfect habitat for adult mosquitoes, just as a rice field covered in stagnant water was an ideal nursery for larvae.[66]

Since most weeders were women of childbearing age, pregnant rice workers and their children suffered and died in terrifying numbers from the ravages of intermittent fever. Malaria causes severe complications in pregnancy, leading to high rates of maternal death from anemia and hemorrhage, as well as to disproportionate numbers of miscarriages and of neonatal deaths following premature birth. Of every thousand children born to malarious weeders, six hundred died before completing their first year of life.[67] Furthermore, the infants and small children who accompanied their mothers on the seasonal trek sickened with alarming frequency. Commenting on the severe impact of malaria on pregnancy and neonatal death, the World Health Organization has noted that "pregnant women suffer decreased immunity to malaria, quadrupling their chance of contracting malaria and doubling their risk of death. Pregnant women with malaria are at increased risk of anemia. Maternal malaria increases the risk of stillbirth, premature delivery, low birth weight babies, and intrauterine growth retardation. Low birth weight babies are much less likely to survive their first year of life."[68] Malaria was thus a fearful scourge of rice workers and their families. Conditions were so harsh that the deputy police commissioner at Vercelli testified that the life of the rice workers was "truly sad"—"so sad that I was moved to pity. Although I did my duty, out of common humanity I felt unable to enforce the full rigor of the law against them."[69]

The sole positive factor was the climate of the North. Relatively cool temperatures inhibited the transmission of the most virulent Italian species of malarial parasite—*Plasmodium falciparum,* which is intolerant of cold. In comparison with the rest of the peninsula, therefore, northern malaria was widely prevalent but low in mortality. It caused chronic debility, but it seldom led directly to death. In addition, shorter summers abbreviated the transmission season, mitigating the impact of fever.

To reach nomadic and often inaccessible rice workers, physicians made use of the standard institutions of the Italian campaign—health stations and rural schools. In addition, they appealed to the emerging Italian labor movement. Physicians and educators encouraged trade unionists and Socialist Party leaders to organize farmworkers and to instruct them in the doctrine of malariology. Most dramatically of all, the state itself turned to the unions for help. Here was a sea change in Italian political life. Until the turn of the century, strikes had been illegal. As recently as the early 1890s, Prime Minister Francesco Crispi declared martial law in Sicily and deployed the army to destroy the peasants' union movement known as the Fasci Siciliani. Similarly, in 1898, the army had employed artillery fire to quell workers' demonstrations in Milan. Now, under Prime Minister Giovanni Giolitti, the government encouraged labor organizers to take an active part in persuading workers and peasants of the virtues of quinine. Trade unions, the government reasoned, were often the best channels available to reach the masses with the gospel of quinine. In 1902, the minister of finance, Paolo Carcano, explained this development, in which he took a direct hand:

> It is necessary to note and make use of every means that can be of assistance in overcoming distrust and ignorance. To that end I have involved the Ministry of Agriculture, Industry, and Commerce in order that it might invite agricultural extension lecturers and labor organizations to take a part in convincing the individual peasants they approach, or the workers' associations with which they are in contact, that the most effective, economical, and certain way to treat and prevent malaria is the continuous and rational use of state quinine.[70]

The Socialist movement responded enthusiastically to the call. In infected zones the Socialist press endorsed the war on malaria and made it a prominent theme of its propaganda. *Avanti!*, the party's daily newspaper, noted that socialism and quinine advanced step by step together in the Italian countryside.

Federterra, the national federation of farmworkers' unions and peasant leagues, declared malaria the great occupational disease of its members. Socialist unions therefore adopted the quinine campaign as an official part of their program and their demands against landlords. They also educated their members in its use, organizing lecture tours by physicians, distributing pamphlets, and taking the message of the campaign directly to the workplace. Where distrust was most firmly entrenched, union leaders even organized those therapeutic ceremonies that became a feature of the Italian campaign against malaria, in which league officials, sympathetic teachers, and Socialist municipal councilors gathered in the central piazzas of villages to swallow their tablets and encourage emulation. Under the leadership of its general secretary — Argentina Altobelli, a former weeder and an early organizer of rice workers — Federterra even took the unusual step of taking a stand in the medical debate between Celli and Grassi, calling for the prophylactic rather than the curative use of the alkaloid. It officially endorsed Celli's position as Socialist public health. The fact that Celli, not Grassi, was a leader of the left facilitated this decision.[71]

Rice fields experienced a sudden surge of national attention, as the weeders became symbols of the oppression of women. A variety of anxieties converged to suggest the need for action. Concern about malaria was sharpened by panic about the inevitability of national decline if so many women gave birth to new generations that were unfit for agricultural work, reproduction, or military service. There was a dark Darwinian fear of a eugenic dystopia. A moral panic also erupted concerning the sexuality of tens of thousands of young females removed for long periods from their watchful guardians — fathers, brothers, husbands, and priests. Giovanni Lorenzoni, a leading expert, worried deeply about the ethics of the rice fields. There, he wrote, "anything goes," and the evenings were filled with singing and dancing. Lorenzoni warned of "sexual license" and illegitimate births.[72]

In this highly charged context, the rice belt was perceived as a place in such urgent need of reform that the national legislation on quinine needed to be supplemented in order to safeguard the physical and moral health of female workers. Pressure for additional measures was exerted both from above and from below. From below, the Socialist lawyer and trade-union activist Modesto Cugnolio launched an ambitious initiative to secure the rigorous enforcement of the lapsed law of 1866 and the related provincial regulations that attempted to regulate rice cultivation in order to protect the health of workers. Cugnolio's strategy was to use a strict construction of existing regulations not only to achieve improved health for the rice workers but also to gain such long-term Socialist goals as the eight-hour day and union recognition.

Meanwhile, from above, the state conducted a series of inquiries and then enacted the law of 1907 to defend weeders and their children. The law banned night work in the fields, prohibited all work in the last month of pregnancy, mandated two half-hour breaks in the working day to allow mothers to breastfeed their infants, limited the working day to nine hours, and enjoined that the water used to irrigate rice fields be flowing rather than stagnant. In addition, it required employers to equip workers' quarters with metal screening, to provide gender segregation, to whitewash interior walls, and to face the external walls with impermeable materials that would prevent access by mosquitoes. Finally, the legislation established mediation committees chosen by election, and stipulated that female workers be both enfranchised and made eligible for office.[73]

Thus, in the rice belt, the social question, the "woman question," and the malaria question were joined into a single movement. The Socialist feminists Anna Kuliscioff, Angelica Balabanoff, Maria Cabrini, and Argentina Altobelli lectured tirelessly, and for the first time they found a mass audience. Kuliscioff in particular regarded the public debate that preceded the passage of the 1907 law as an opportunity both to politicize working women and to press the Socialist Party into taking a firmer stance on the issue of women's rights. Change was occurring rapidly in a nation that Kuliscioff, the most prominent feminist of the period, described as surpassed (in Europe) only by Turkey and Spain in its lack of attention to women's emancipation. Italy, she had written in a famous phrase, had long been the "monopoly of men."[74]

In this context, the campaign against malaria played a major role in the politicization of farm laborers in general and of women in particular. The laws on state quinine profoundly altered power relationships. They did so, first, by placing landlords morally, legally, and politically on the defensive. In addition, the quinine legislation provided workers with a sense of injustice and a vocabulary of rights, it placed two professions — doctors and teachers — on the side of social reform, and it established channels by which the twin messages of socialism and women's emancipation reached a large population. Most simply, by reducing the burden of illness, the campaign also enhanced the capacity of laborers to defend their own interests.

The argument here is not one of malaria determinism. The antimalarial campaign was such a powerful catalyst in the emergence of socialism and women's consciousness because it operated in an environment where its message struck a resonant chord at an opportune moment. A variety of other factors were also at work. Among these were Giolitti's proclamation of state neutrality in labor disputes, the concentration of labor on the rice fields and latifundia, the practice of gang working that multiplied horizontal bonds of solidarity, the absenteeism of landlords that negated the possibility of paternalism, the concurrent struggle over common land and use rights that bound communities together in opposition to proprietors, transoceanic emigration that thinned out the labor market and brought growing numbers of women into agricultural labor to replace absent men, and sheer economic distress. The intransigent opposition of landlords to the demands of farmworkers and to the state-quinine campaign also radicalized farm laborers.

In this process the antimalarial crusade was an important force. It was no coincidence that the campaign against malaria in the rice fields was rapidly followed by an upsurge of Socialist organizations and by an outburst of demonstrations in which women played a prominent role. From the 1890s to the First World War there were waves of strikes by rice workers. By 1905 the movement had assumed a thick organizational structure of leagues, cooperatives, and Socialist Party branches. The Ministry of the Interior reported the transformation and sounded a note of alarm. The rice workers' movement, it worried, "has taken on a serious quality that it never had in the past — serious both because of the imposing number of organized workers in leagues and because of the marked character of class struggle that the leagues have assumed."[75] More than merely a local phenomenon, the weeders' movement served as an important step in the establishment of Federterra as a powerful national organization.

At the first Federterra congress at Bologna in 1901, *Avanti!* reported that one of the salient features was a series of speeches by women from the rice fields, all of whom were greeted with thunderous applause. The Socialist newspaper also noted that women weeders played an influential role in establishing the national federation.[76] Indeed, from 1893 until Mussolini's consolidation of power and the destruction of democracy, the league of rice workers at Molinella remained, as the paper already noted in 1901, the "moral center, the vanguard" of the Socialist movement in the Po Valley.[77] Furthermore, a striking and unique feature of Federterra, the largest Italian union federation, was that its leader, from 1906 until its demolition by Fascism, was a woman — Argentina Altobelli, who represented the rice fields. An additional important feature of union politics in some regions was that workers also began to strike in defense of health measures against malaria, refusing to work, for instance, unless estates provided adequate and well-screened accommodation.[78]

Thus the antimalarial campaigners who took the approach that malaria was a multifaceted social problem played a major role in transforming politics. Clinicians, teachers, and trade unionists who staffed health stations and peasant schools or organized farmworkers argued that health depends not only on quinine but also on a series of simple but vital prerequisites. These more humble antimalarials included a sound diet, sanitary housing, safe motherhood, humane working conditions, the right to organize, and knowledge made accessible to all. In pressing these conditions as essential attributes of the campaign, the activists raised issues that contributed not only to the recession of fever but also to the extension of civil liberties that was such a major feature of the period. Malaria and the campaign against it contributed significantly as catalysts in the development of Italian socialism, trade unionism, feminism, and the medical and teaching professions.

5

The First World War and Epidemic Disease

Over and over the old man prayed as he walked in solitude
to king Apollo . . . : "Hear me, lord of the silver bow, . . .
bring to pass this wish I pray for:
let your arrows make the Danaans pay for my tears shed."

So he spoke in prayer, and Phoibos Apollo heard him,
and strode down along the pinnacles of Olympos, angered
in his heart, carrying across his shoulders the bow and the hooded
quiver; and the shafts clashed on the shoulders of the god walking
angrily. He came as night comes down and knelt then
apart and opposite the ships and let go an arrow.
Terrible was the clash that rose from the bow of silver.
First he went after the mules and the circling hounds, then let go
a tearing arrow against the men themselves and struck them.
The corpse fires burned everywhere and did not stop burning.

—*Homer,* The Iliad, *trans. Richmond Lattimore, 1.33–52*

Italy's decision in 1915 to join England, France, and Russia in their conflict with the Central powers of Germany and Austria-Hungary followed fifteen years of unprecedented progress toward control of malaria. From 1900 on, new scientific understandings of the disease were effectively applied to create a rural health infrastructure. Health stations and sanatoriums took medical care to the most remote areas of the nation. Peasant schools educated those at risk about the mechanisms of malaria and the best means of self-defense. Teachers, physicians, and trade unionists mobilized public opinion in favor of workers' rights, improved sanitary conditions, and promoted universal literacy. Parliament passed legislation protecting women and children from forms of exploitation that exposed them to unacceptably high risks of infection. At the same time, central and local governments were charged with making the specific remedy freely available to all who needed it. By 1915 the ultimate objective of eradication remained distant, but a well-organized movement to alleviate the epidemic and to reduce mortality was gathering momentum.

At this moment of hope for Italy's rural poor, the outbreak of war signaled catastrophe. In recent years, the World Health Organization (WHO) has declared war a "complex emergency" that creates ideal conditions for mosquitoes and plasmodia. Warfare, the WHO analysis suggests, is incompatible with progress toward the control of malaria. The Italian experience in the First World War fully confirms this interpretation. As a result of the war, the hard-won gains of fifteen years were reversed, and Italy returned to levels of morbidity and mortality that had prevailed in 1900. Instead of continuing to advance, Italy experienced a great upsurge of sickness and death. A furious outburst of malaria began in 1915 and overran the nation in 1917 and 1918. Only in 1923 did the disease return to the painfully won level of 1914. Tens of thousands—civilians and soldiers alike—perished of malaria, and millions sickened.

The antimalarial campaign became a casualty of war. As the state systematically mobilized resources for total war, it starved the campaign of resources—personnel, funds, medicine, and public attention. At the same time, the voluntary associations that played so large a role in galvanizing the assault on disease—the Society for the Study of Malaria, the National League against Malaria, and the trade unions—ceased activity as their leaders and members were conscripted. Finally, when the campaign resumed full functioning after peace returned in 1918, it did so on the basis of new priorities that were foreign to its founders. The campaign was militarized, and its original goal to redeem suffering humanity was subordinated to the political needs of the state.

Malaria and the Fighting Front

Italy entered the First World War in May 1915, when Prime Minister Antonio Salandra and his minister of foreign affairs, Sidney Sonnino, signed the secretly negotiated Treaty of London and declared war on Austria-Hungary. This decision by Salandra and Sonnino was above all an operation of domestic politics. It constituted a virtual antiparliamentary coup d'état that defied the expressed wishes of the overwhelming majority of Italians. The Liberal majority in parliament, the Catholic Church, the Socialist Party, the trade unions, and leading sectors of Italian industry and finance all opposed joining the fray. The Italian leaders, however, calculated that a short and glorious war would strengthen the authority of the state, stimulate a flagging economy, and put an end to the reforms initiated by Giovanni Giolitti.

For conservatives and reactionaries, Giolitti had perilously undermined law and order by his many concessions to the political left. In their view, he had presided over the rise of a mass Socialist-Party and trade-union movement. To the distress of the political right, Giolitti had also insisted on the neutrality of the state while workers, peasants, and women struck, organized, and challenged the prerogatives of property and patriarchy. It seemed all too possible to conservatives that Giolittian Liberalism would prepare the way for Red revolution. Already in 1908 the right-wing landlord Lino Carrara, who led the establishment of armed self-defense by property owners and advocated the recourse to "extreme measures," had written, "There has been too much reformism. No conflict has ever had greater importance for Italy."[1] His political associate, the landowning deputy Faelli, argued more laconically, "This is the battle of civilization against barbarism."[2] Such fears became especially vivid in the so-called Red Week—a moment of political crisis in the summer of 1914 when the state, under pressure from mass demonstrations across the peninsula, had seemed on the verge of collapse.

Salandra and Sonnino intended, therefore, to buttress hierarchy through wartime discipline and to isolate the Socialists amid an upsurge of patriotism and national feeling. War against the national enemy—Austria-Hungary—would also enable Italy to complete what some regarded as the unfinished work of Italian unification. Italy would extend her boundaries to her "natural frontiers" and incorporate the "unredeemed" territories still under Habsburg rule. A rapid victory, meanwhile, would avenge the military humiliations suffered by Italians at Custoza during unification and at Adowa during Italy's failed imperial adventure in Africa. Finally, the advocates of war expected the conflict to stimulate a faltering economy, slash unemployment, and generate profits. Since the high command under General Luigi Cadorna insisted that hostilities would last only weeks, intervention on the side of the Entente powers seemed an ideal opportunity. Indeed, it was deemed unwise to delay. Italy should not miss the opportunity that Cadorna predicted would be a mere "walk to Vienna."

All such calculations, however, rapidly proved mistaken when the conflict

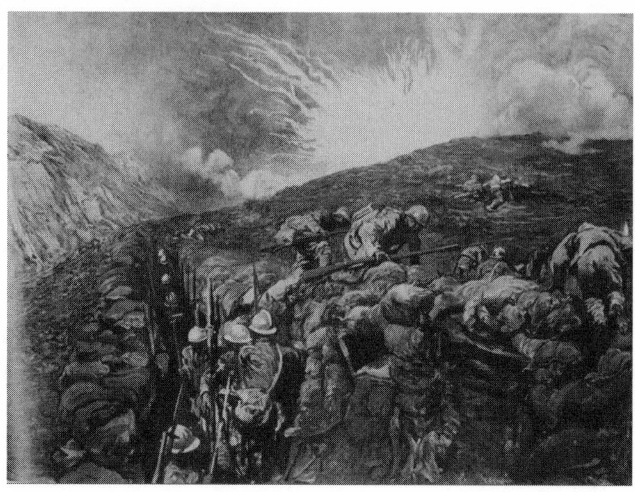

Giulio Aristide Sartorio, *Infantrymen Go over the Top at Santa Caterina* (1917)

settled into a prolonged war of attrition. Instead of tipping the military balance decisively in favor of the Entente as Salandra, Sonnino, and Cadorna had predicted, Italian intervention merely added a great arc of 700 additional kilometers to a line of trenches that soon stretched from the North Sea to the Adriatic. After the Battle of the Marne in September 1914, the western front froze into a war of position as the defensive capabilities of industrial societies overwhelmed all offensive strategies. Entrenchment, barbed wire, the machine gun, and the science of modern engineering perfected the art of "defenses in depth" and halted all strategic advances. At the same time, the ability of the modern state to transport, arm, deploy, and feed almost unlimited troops permitted defenders to fill rapidly any breaches in its outer lines of fortification. Under such conditions, warfare was transformed into a reciprocal state of siege in which each side attempted to bleed the opposing forces to death. The Italian front, which became as violent as any sector of the western front, emerged as yet another killing field where the opposing coalitions sought to deplete one another of men and matériel. For most of the period from May 1915 to the armistice in November 1918, the lines separating Italy and Austria-Hungary remained immobile amid terrifying casualties. Even the names of the battles remained the same, as the two clashing armies fought no fewer than twelve Battles of the Isonzo.

In terms of malaria, the result of such carnage was catastrophic. Of all high-impact infectious diseases, malaria is the most sensitive to the relationship of human populations to their environment, and no activity is more destructive of this relationship than war. From the outset, the conflict led to a steep spike in both mortality and morbidity from fever. Indeed, the longer and more intense the fighting, the higher the numbers of malaria deaths and cases. Already in 1915 and 1916 there was a significant recrudescence, with more cases, more deaths, more pernicious infections, and more zones brought under the sway of disease. Then, as the war reached a climax of violence in 1917 and 1918, ferocious epidemics broke out, ebbing only slowly after the armistice. As the provincial officer of health for Caltanissetta explained, this great outburst of malaria affected "the whole of Italy."[3]

As always, malaria mortality statistics for this time are far more accurate than those for morbidity. In the prewar period there was a consensus that official data for the incidence of malaria were unreliable. The main reason was systemic: because of the gulf between the rural population and the medical profession, physicians saw only a fraction of the people who fell ill. In addition, with a disease as protean as malaria and in an era when many doctors had no access to microscopes, diagnosis was highly uncertain. The state, therefore, had no dependable means of accurately quantifying cases. During the First World War this chronic structural weakness was exacerbated by the near collapse of the antimalarial campaign. Having mobilized the physicians responsible for the rural poor, the state lost contact with most of those who suffered from fever. The doctors who remained were overwhelmed. Claudio Fermi, who attempted to combat the epidemic in Sardinia, noted that wartime statistics were highly dubious for the simple reason that "many health officials do not keep clinical records."[4]

Dead bodies received attention from the authorities more reliably than feverish ones. Mortality statistics, therefore, provide a more accurate gauge of the progress of malaria. These figures demonstrate that between 1915 and 1918 there was a sharp reversal of the steady decline in mortality that marked the Giolittian era (1900–1914). After declining from 490 deaths per million inhabitants in 1900 to 57 in 1914, malaria mortality rose sixfold to 325 deaths per million in 1918, thereby erasing one of the signal achievements of Italian public health (Table 5.1).

Aggregate national figures, however, understate the depth of the setback because of differences between the "two Italies"—North and South. Death resulting directly from malaria continued to be associated overwhelmingly with falciparum malaria, which prevailed in the South (plus the provinces of Rome and Grosseto in the Center). Southern Italians were therefore far more at risk than aggregated totals suggest. In 1900 a national rate of 490 deaths per million inhabitants from malaria corresponded to a rate of 1,056 per

Table 5.1 Deaths from Malaria in Italy, 1914–1923

Year	Deaths	Deaths per million inhabitants
1914	2,045	57
1915	3,835	105
1916	5,060	137
1917	8,407	237
1918	11,487	325
1919	5,163	138
1920	3,443	91
1921	3,456	91
1922	3,188	86
1923	2,274	61

Source: Data from Ministero dell'Interno, Direzione Generale della Sanità Pubblica, *La malaria in Italia ed i risultati della lotta antimalarica* (Rome, 1924), p. 21.

million in the South. Similarly, in 1917 and 1918, national rates of, respectively, 237 and 325 malaria deaths per million inhabitants masked rates of 523 and 718 deaths per million in the South. Malaria, which had begun to lose its place as a major killer of southern Italians by 1914, again reaped a fearful harvest during and after the war.[5]

Official data understate the disaster because mortality figures indicate only deaths caused directly by malaria. Such statistics ignore those more numerous cases in which malaria produced death indirectly through its complications and sequelae—tuberculosis, influenza, and pneumonia. At the turn of the century, Giovanni Battista Grassi argued that an accurate estimate of deaths caused by malaria—directly and indirectly—could be obtained by multiplying the official figure by five. If his suggestion is followed with regard to wartime tallies, then in 1918 malaria probably killed nearly sixty thousand Italians. The most disturbing increase in mortality occurred in Apulia. In 1912, Apulia suffered an already high mortality rate with 199 malaria deaths per million inhabitants, but in 1918, this number climbed to 1,195 deaths per million. In that calamitous year, this single region endured more deaths from malaria than the whole of Italy in 1914.[6]

To focus solely on mortality, however, is to overlook the burden of suffering, debility, and poverty that the wartime upsurge occasioned. In 1917 and 1918, just as in 1900, the ten thousand recorded deaths from malaria were accompanied by a morbidity of millions. Unfortunately, since the war paralyzed the public health campaign, it is difficult to understand fully the cost that war-generated malaria imposed on the most vulnerable Italians. The military emergency itself hid the malarial consequences from sight. For example, until the conflict began, the antimalarial campaign generated an immense documentary record compiled by the commissioners and physicians in the field. During the war, the campaign stalled. Physicians, too few and too burdened, no longer filed detailed reports. At the same time, such private associations as the Society for the Study of Malaria and the National League against Malaria closed shop, while their journals ceased publication. The labor movement and the Socialist press, which had taken up the antimalarial cause as their own, also went into near hibernation. Their publications halted as their members were conscripted and their newspapers were subjected to rigorous censorship. For these reasons, the documentary record of the wartime malarial emergency is limited.

Nevertheless, the officials still staffing the campaign agreed that the epidemic began to assume an unfamiliar gravity very early in the war. Beginning in 1915, malaria became more widespread, the burden of cases progressively increased, and the clinical forms became exceptionally virulent and refractory to treatment. Officers of health all over Italy employed such descriptions as "notable recrudescence of the epidemic," "extraordinary virulence assumed by malaria," "exaltation of the virus," "massive diffusion of malaria," "enhanced severity," "extreme gravity both of intensity and spread," "striking upsurge," "worryingly widespread outburst," and "some new condition that is sudden, violent, and [has] never existed here before."[7] In 1925, Alberto Lutrario, the director-general of public health, surveyed the Italian experience of malaria on behalf of the League of Nations. His account of the war years is somber, portraying a nation subject to recurrent "epidemic waves" that enabled the disease to reclaim areas from which it had previously receded. These waves, moreover, overwhelmed all attempts to control them. His explanation was that "the ordinary methods of combating the disease appear sometimes to be practically ineffective when new factors supervene to provoke epidemic outbreaks—especially new social factors."[8]

An intriguing indication of what was involved emerges from the figures for both morbidity and mortality in the strategically important province of Sassari in Sardinia (Table 5.2). However approximate the statistics, they at least suggest the intensity of the malarial resurgence in a highly affected southern province. According to the data, in the terrible years 1917 and 1918, nearly the entire population of Sardinia fell ill. Claudio Fermi, an expert malariologist, confirmed this conclusion. He reported of the island that "the townships of the two provinces of Sardinia are malarial to the extent of 100 percent. . . . These places, as I constantly repeat, are literally hospitals for malaria patients, except that, unlike true hospitals, 60 percent of the patients receive no treatment at all and the rest receive inadequate therapy."[9] Sardinia was an extreme

Table 5.2 Malaria in Sassari Province, 1914–1918

Year	Cases	Deaths	Deaths per 1,000 inhabitants
1914	15,561	92	5.9
1915	27,982	183	6.5
1916	20,030	174	8.6
1917	41,922	640	15.2
1918	39,330	763	19.3

Source: Data from Medico Provinciale di Sassari, "Lotta antimalarica 1918," ACS, MI, DGS (1910–1920), b. 116, fasc. "Sassari: Relazione sulla lotta contro la malaria."

case, but its experience corroborates a vital conclusion that all the available evidence suggests. As a result of the First World War, tens of thousands of Italians perished of malaria and millions were infected, many severely and repeatedly, and often with parasites of more than one species concurrently.[10] Italians, in other words, paid a savage tribute not only to the god of war but also to the goddess of fever.

Giovanni Battista Grassi's personal career illustrates the gravity of the medical crisis. After being passed over for the Nobel Prize in favor of his nemesis Ronald Ross, Grassi retired in disillusion from malariology. He withdrew soon after parliament passed the legislation launching the antimalarial campaign that was based so largely on his discoveries and his doctrine. Witnessing the terrible wartime epidemic of malaria, however, Grassi experienced a change of heart. Moved to patriotic duty by the disaster of Caporetto, when the Italian army was routed in the fall of 1917, and to pity by the suffering of the peasants of the Roman Campagna, he returned to the fight against the disease. From late 1917 until his death in April 1925, Grassi rededicated himself to the cause, running a research station and dispensary at Fiumicino near the mouth of the Tiber. In his words,

> When the first reports of the disaster of Caporetto arrived, my friend Dr. Cotronei, who had just, and at long last, obtained a leave, . . . did not hesitate for an instant to give up his leave, return to his post, and take his part in saving the men of his unit. This truly noble gesture made a great impression on me, and I thought to myself that I would do well to abandon theoretical laboratory research in order to contribute somehow in a direct and practical manner. Since I lacked the strength for work at the front, I decided to serve the poor country people in their fight against malaria. This disease remains a scourge for our nation, which will never be redeemed until it is removed from our midst.[11]

Why was the First World War in Italy so conducive to an explosion of malaria? Part of the reason was geographical. The border between Austria-Hungary and Italy consisted of three sectors. In the center stood the nearly unassailable barrier of the Dolomite Mountains. Here small tactical engagements between highly trained Alpine units punctuated the conflict, but neither side could hope to effect a strategic advance with large units and heavy equipment in mountainous terrain. The second sector—the great salient of the Trentino—was also unsuitable as the main theater of war. A difficult terrain with hills and mountains interspersed with ample valleys and passes complicated the deployment and supply of large armies.

Inevitably, the main battleground was the lowland coastal sector stretching south from the Austrian border, where the Isonzo, Tagliamento, and Piave rivers completed their journey to the Adriatic Sea. Here a level topography permitted the rapid movement of whole armies and their equipment and allowed the use of roads and railway lines to supply and reinforce the troops. Thus for the first two and a half years of the conflict—from May 1915 to October 1917—the Isonzo front witnessed the headlong clash of the Austro-Hungarian and Italian forces. The fighting cost Italy 1.1 million casualties and Austria-Hungary 650,000—for negligible territorial or strategic gain.[12] Only in October 1917 did the front move appreciably. On 24 October, a combined Austrian and German offensive beginning at Caporetto caught Italy unprepared, overwhelming the Italian troops and hurling them back first to the line of the Tagliamento River and finally to the Piave River, where by January 1918 they regrouped and held their position.

Unfortunately, the coastal zones of the Veneto, where the war was chiefly fought, were notoriously unhealthy. The whole littoral extending northeast from the Po Delta to the Austrian border was intensely malarial. It contained great expanses of wetlands where anopheline mosquitoes flourished. These included swamps and areas that were flooded annually in the spring when the great northern rivers overflowed their banks. The rice fields, drainage canals for land reclamation projects, and unfilled excavation ditches for the construction of roads and railroads added further collections of surface water. Here, in an environment where vivax malaria already prevailed, Cadorna deployed his army of peasant soldiers. As the health officials of the high command observed, the Third Army, stationed in the theater of operations between the Isonzo and the Piave, created "a great concentration of men in a zone that is eminently swampy and malarial."[13]

The potential for a major upsurge in malaria was inherent in such a deployment, especially since the military campaigning season—from early spring until autumn—coincided, like agricultural work, with the seasonal epidemic.

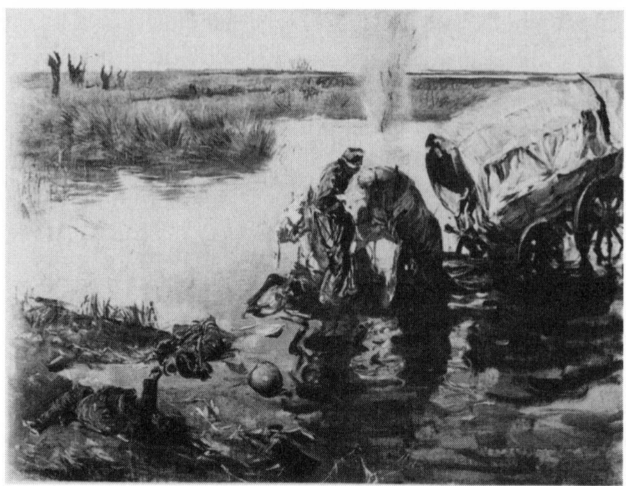

Giulio Aristide Sartorio, *Roundup of Prisoners in the Piave Delta* (n.d.)

Unlike agricultural work, however, trench warfare permitted no restrictions on working hours to permit soldiers to avoid those most dangerous times for the transmission of malaria—dawn and dusk. At the same time, modern, industrial warfare compounded the risk factors to which troops were exposed. In order to escape the fire of machine guns and heavy artillery, soldiers burrowed underground in deep trenches that filled with water and became breeding grounds for mosquito larvae. Trenches were the antithesis of the sturdy, screened housing that the prewar campaign had found to be one of the most effective antimalarial tools. Conditions in the trenches were so bad that the Third Army was known as the "malarial army."[14]

Deep craters gouged into the earth by the explosion of artillery shells and mortars also collected rainwater, giving rise to further larval opportunities. In addition, to the rear of the trenches that made up the front line, military engineers built roads, railway lines, and bridges—all projects involving excavations where stagnant water collected and anophelines multiplied.[15] Those working behind the front line—including soldiers and civilian construction workers—faced an additional risk by sleeping in hastily built and crowded barracks or simply under canvas. Finally, the fact that conscripts arrived on the Isonzo from all over Italy had dire medical implications. Many soldiers from nonmalarial districts possessed neither acquired immunity nor sufficient understanding of the disease to practice self-defense. In addition, the horror of battle on the Isonzo and Piave fronts was so great that some soldiers purposefully avoided taking their quinine. They hoped to contract infection in order to be evacuated and sent home on convalescent leave. Malaria, inten-

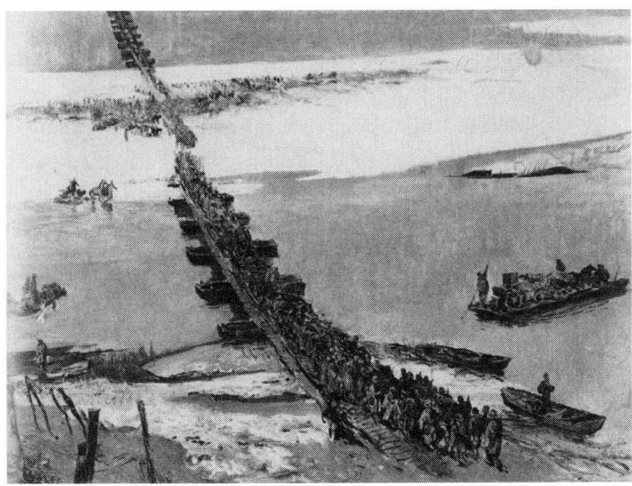

Giulio Aristide Sartorio, *Austrian Troops Return across the Piave* (n.d.)

tionally contracted, provided a desperate means of escape. Doctors described such actions as "malarial defeatism."[16]

In the Veneto, the great Italian war zone, the health of civilians was affected along with that of the army. Some of the hundreds of thousands of soldiers stationed in the region brought infection with them. But the chief danger to civilians arose from the effects of the conflict on the local environment. Malaria in the prewar Veneto had receded in part because of major projects of land drainage and reclamation (*bonifica*). Reversing these arduous gains, the army deliberately destroyed drainage canals, flooding the fields in order to prevent enemy advances. The area of swampland expanded, multiplying the numbers of mosquitoes, and land that had been redeemed from fever once again succumbed to its dominion. At the same time, under war conditions, landlords were unable to clear and maintain irrigation works, so that ditches became clogged with vegetation, creating an ideal habitat for insects. Close to the front, artillery fire and air raids destroyed houses, forcing their inhabitants to seek shelter in unprotected stables or to bivouac in the fields. In the province of Udine, the townships of Latisana and Marano Lagunara became symbols of the horrors inflicted by war on noncombatants. Civilians were forced by military action to abandon their heavily damaged houses en masse.[17]

For civilians in the Veneto, the most devastating period of all followed the defeat at Caporetto. After driving the Italian army back 150 kilometers, from the Isonzo River to the Piave, Austria-Hungary occupied the whole of Udine and Belluno provinces, as well as parts of the provinces of Treviso, Venice, and Vicenza. For an entire year from October 1917 to October 1918, a total of

12,500 square kilometers and 1.2 million people fell under Habsburg military occupation. Furthermore, as the Italian soldiers retreated in headlong flight, some four hundred thousand civilians—men, women, and children—sought to escape with them. The Italian authorities made insufficient provision for these refugees, leaving them to suffer the ravages of inadequate shelter, food, and clothing. They also failed to provide medical care and quinine.[18]

Worst of all was the fate of the 1 million Italians who remained under Austrian occupation. The occupying forces, numbering from 1 million to 1.5 million, were subject to the same insalubrious conditions as their Italian counterparts. In frequent rotation between the front lines and the rear, Austrian soldiers formed an excellent conduit for spreading malaria to the civilians around them. Specific Austrian policies increased the risk. The Austrians requisitioned livestock and food, and they imposed a ration of two hundred grams of flour per person per day and one hundred grams of meat per week. Such rations not only led to hunger but also lowered resistance to disease. Large numbers of Italians in the occupied zone were reduced to begging and eating weeds. At the same time, the Austrians requisitioned all Italian hospitals and pharmacies, and they made no effort to replace the infrastructure of health stations and public clinics that had played so prominent a role in the prewar antimalarial advances. For a six-kilometer stretch along the Piave River, they confiscated—and sometimes demolished—all houses, evacuating forty thousand residents, who were forced to sleep in farm buildings or in the open.[19]

Of all Austrian policies, however, the most savage was the prophylactic strategy known as relegation. Knowing that the territory they had invaded was highly malarial, the Austro-Hungarian command instituted draconian measures to protect its troops. To that end, the army decided to remove the threatening human reservoir of infection. At the onset of the epidemic season in June 1918, Field Marshal Svetozar Boroevic von Bojna systematically evacuated Italians, "relegating" them to an infamous "closed zone." This was a virtual concentration camp, where Italians were confined without economic resources or medical attention, without adequate housing, and without reliable supplies of food or quinine. The medical results, the official postwar Italian investigation concluded, were "real horrors" and "the literal destruction of our population."[20]

Malaria and the Home Front

Even with two warring armies on its soil, the Veneto was not hit as hard by the upsurge of malaria as some other regions. In war, just as in peace, the

North of Italy was shielded by its climate. Cool temperatures ensured that malaria there remained predominantly vivax malaria, which was relatively mild and generated a low rate of mortality. Ironically, the civilian population of the South experienced the worst effects of malaria during the First World War, despite their distance from the front. In 1918 as the epidemic reached its peak, 11,477 Italians died from malaria, of whom 9,547 were southerners.[21] Why was the outbreak so severe at such a distance from the battlefields?

A major factor was the link between the war zones and the rear through the constant large-scale movement of people. Frontline soldiers regularly returned home on leave to recuperate or to help with the harvest, along with Austrian prisoners of war. Inevitably, soldiers who had plasmodia in their bloodstreams brought the disease home. A representative case was Caltanissetta province in Sicily. There in 1917 the prefect reported an epidemic that he described as "very serious," even though an unusually dry spring had greatly reduced the mosquito population. Unhappily, the countervailing factor was the presence of

> a great number of soldiers suffering from chronic malaria who were sent to their homes to complete their treatment. When one takes account of the clinical course of the disease, which was unlike the common experience of these localities . . . , and when one recalls that many physicians insisted that . . . they were dealing with new strains of malaria, then it is appropriate to suspect that the upsurge was chiefly the result of individuals who had been infected elsewhere.
>
> This theory is confirmed by the fact that the disease was especially virulent wherever there were especially large numbers of malarial soldiers returning from the fighting front. . . . The number of sufferers and of deaths was highest in those townships where the soldiers were most numerous, and where Austrian prisoners . . . were sent to perform agricultural labor.[22]

Similarly, in the severely afflicted provinces of Foggia, in Apulia, and Sassari, in Sardinia, the director-general of public health noted that the "most severe health problems" were created by the employment of prisoners of war in the local agricultural cycle, because the number of prisoners stricken with malaria was "notable."[23]

Returnees from the Veneto and Austrians captured in combat between the Isonzo and the Piave, however, would have contributed principally to the spread of vivax malaria, the species that prevailed in the North. In the province of Milan, for instance, officials reported a flood of cases in 1917 and 1918, but these were mild and responsive to treatment. Fatalities were rare. One army medical officer reported, "In the lower Isonzo Valley, and later in the lower Piave Valley, malaria caused serious damage to the army. . . . But an important point to stress is that it was almost exclusively a question of springtime tertian infections with very few of the quartan or estivo-autumnal fevers which always prevailed in Albania and Macedonia."[24]

By stark contrast, the war-related malaria epidemic in central and southern Italy produced a pandemic of pernicious infections—that is, cases of falciparum malaria that were frequently described as violent and resistant to quinine. For instance, the medical officer of health at Potenza, in Basilicata, reported in 1918 that "the course of the epidemic was much more serious than in previous years, with notable increases in morbidity and mortality and with an upsurge of severe and pernicious infections."[25] A disproportionate source of such falciparum infections was a secondary front in the war—the Balkans. In October 1915, Britain, France, and Italy sent troops to Macedonia and to Albania. Their purpose was to save Serbia from being overrun and to strengthen the inclination of Greece and Romania to intervene on the side of the Entente. Unfortunately, the Balkans, like the South of Italy, were a hyperendemic area where falciparum malaria prevailed. Deployed at the height of the epidemic season, all three armies suffered fearfully. They succumbed so rapidly to infection that, in the words of the American malariologist L. W. Hackett, "the three armies were paralyzed before they could strike a blow."[26]

The danger to Italians of warfare in the Balkans was immediate. Fearful of German submarine warfare, troops from all three allied powers traveled overland as far as possible rather than by sea. They journeyed by train to southern Italy, using Apulian ports to embark on their final short passage to Salonika or to the Albanian coast. Later, when they had succumbed to malaria, these soldiers were evacuated back to Apulian hospitals, bearing their plasmodia with them. The Italians among them then returned to their native towns and villages for convalescence, all the while "heaping new fuel on the fire" of the epidemic.[27] Malaria, Hackett commented, "dogged the footsteps of returning soldiers to their homes and infected countrysides whose inhabitants had never known the bitter taste of quinine."[28] Between the spring of 1916 and the armistice, the Italian army alone repatriated 49,701 soldiers who had contracted malaria in Albania and Macedonia.[29] Along with the Italian veterans, there was also a trickle of Austro-Hungarian prisoners of war captured in the Balkan conflict. Thus, allied strategy opened a regular epidemic highway linking the Balkans and southern Italy.

This Balkan connection stoked the epidemic that ravaged the South. As far away as Sicily and Campania, prefects and officers of health reported that falciparum malaria erupted with full force in 1917 and 1918, when Italy suffered the worst malaria epidemic of the twentieth century. Local physicians noted that the key foci of the disease were those townships with the largest numbers of soldiers on leave, especially veterans of the Balkans. More troubling than the sheer number of cases, however, was their severe clinical profile, and the fact that they were often unresponsive to quinine. The consensus was that the veterans had imported strains of falciparum malaria that were new to Italy and to which the local population had no immunity.[30]

While veterans and prisoners from the war zones thus contributed to the recrudescence of malaria, war-related developments on the home front also played an important role. A significant consideration was the effect of war on Italian agriculture and on the men and women who worked the fields. From the outset, agriculture suffered severe hardship as the state systematically diverted resources and manpower from the countryside to industry and the army. Such diversions had epidemiological consequences. Conscription was the most obvious mechanism for the redistribution of resources, as hundreds of thousands of peasants and farmworkers were drafted and sent to the front. The inevitable result was a severe shortage of labor in the countryside and a steep fall in agricultural output. In an effort to sustain their yields, landlords and farmers turned to women, children, and elderly men, whom they employed in ever-greater numbers to replace absent conscripts. In those areas of central and southern Italy where a rigid sexual division of labor prevailed, women and children had traditionally been spared outdoor labor in the fields during the malaria season. Now recruited to harvest and to thresh, these replacement workers, who had no immunity, succumbed to fever at alarming rates. With labor in such short supply, farmers paid scant attention to such vital antimalarial measures as the maintenance of drainage ditches, the cautious irrigation of market gardens, the vigilant removal of small expanses of stagnant water, and the intensification of production, which entailed such benefits as the replacement of workers in the fields by machines, the elimination of fallow in favor of moisture-absorbing crops, and the introduction of animal husbandry (which provided mosquitoes with alternative mammals to feast upon in lieu of humans). There was a consensus among public health authorities that the war thus provided a powerful stimulus to the resurgence of malaria in the countryside. Indeed, in the opinion of one prefect in Apulia, the war was the single most important factor. Summarizing conditions, he wrote in 1918 that "the grave resurgence of malaria, which spread in a worrying manner in recent years, [was] caused above all by the neglect of works that facilitate natural drainage in malarial zones or prevent the development of malaria-carrying mosquitoes in stagnant water."[31]

In addition to its effects on agriculture, conscription promoted malaria through its impact on light industry located in malarial zones. For example, at the brick and tile works at Lucera, in Apulia, the wartime shortage of labor caused the closure of the plants, enabling rainwater to collect in the unused clay pits and basins. As a result, mosquitoes bred in unlimited profusion in immediate proximity to the town. The direct and unhappy consequence was that Lucera took its place at the head of the list of localities where fever raged most intensely.[32]

While conscription diverted men to the front, the state also requisitioned animals. Again, there were immediate medical consequences. Most obviously, in the absence of horses, cattle, and pigs, there was no possibility for "animal deviation" — the redirection of anophelines from man to beast. The development of animal husbandry had played a substantial part throughout Europe in the spontaneous recession of malaria. In Italy during the First World War, however, mosquitoes were left with only humans on whom to prey. Such requisitioning also produced a vicious downward spiral. The disappearance of farm animals greatly diminished the intensity of cultivation, leading to the omission of fodder from crop rotations and therefore to even fewer animals.

Another means to divert resources from agriculture to the military and to war-related industries was the price mechanism. In the rampant inflation that marked the war years, industrial prices far outstripped those for agricultural goods. In the words of the agricultural expert Arrigo Serpieri, "The rural classes during the war experienced an agricultural income whose buying power was lower than before the war. The monetary income, as an average for the four years, rose from 100 to 221; the general wholesale price index from 100 to 287. . . . Comparing the two indexes, we must conclude that in the four years of the war the effective total buying power of agricultural income declined by about one-fourth."[33] The same mechanism affected soldiers — those peasants in uniform whose wages stagnated relative to the general price index.

The results were multiple. At the base of the rural social pyramid, peasants and farm laborers found that their real wages declined from year to year. Many went hungry and resorted to impoverished diets that lowered their resistance to disease. Meanwhile, farmers discovered that industrial products — machinery, parts, and chemical fertilizer — became either unavailable or prohibitively expensive. Harvesters and threshers, for example, began to disappear from the fields. Agricultural machines, however, were an important coefficient of health. They minimized the number of people required in the fields during the malarial season, and they reduced the number of hours necessary to accomplish a task. As machines retired to their sheds, human beings were compelled once more to undertake dangerous tasks and lengthy workdays that exposed them to mosquitoes. At the same time, farmers simplified their crop rotation systems, moving in the direction of extensive wheat cultivation. Unfortunately, the reversion to extensive farming led to poorly cultivated fields with greater moisture and more numerous mosquitoes.

Inevitably, the result was a steep fall in agricultural output. In order to counteract this tendency and to maintain food supplies for the army, the state intervened. One important strategy was to encourage producers by removing legal restrictions and obligations that had been imposed to protect workers from occupational diseases, especially malaria. An important instance of such relaxation of protection concerned the rice fields. In 1916, in an effort to stimulate higher yields of the cereal, the authorities suspended the 1907 law that had protected rice workers from malaria by requiring screening, limiting the workday, and mandating minimal standards of hygiene. From 1916 until 1923 there was a return to the free market and to the neglect that had prevailed before the weeders had begun to strike during the Giolittian era.[34]

Finally, the diversion of resources away from the countryside severely undermined the antimalarial campaign itself. In 1915, combating disease among civilians lost its standing as a national priority. The onset of hostilities entailed severe cuts to the budget available to the quinine program. Thus in Sardinia, the most malarial region, the medical officers of health reported in 1916 that the funds available to run the antimalarial service had become wholly inadequate and needed to be increased fivefold—from 63.65 lire to 318.25 lire.[35] At the same time, the state stripped the rural health stations of their personnel—physicians, nurses, and attendants—to provide care for soldiers at the front. In the Roman Campagna, for example, the health stations faced such an acute shortage of doctors that they were no longer able to offer a comprehensive service. In the province of Verona, the shortage of personnel caused sixteen of the thirty-two functioning health stations to close their doors.[36] In Sardinia, a third of the experienced and committed doctors who knew the region and its people were replaced by teachers, university students, police officers, and priests—people with no medical training who simply distributed quinine.[37] Once regarded by its physicians as an apostolic mission, the antimalarial campaign now suffered a sharp decline in morale and élan as inexperienced, temporary placeholders assumed the responsibility of caring for patient populations whose economic and medical conditions were progressively deteriorating.

At the same time, the action of municipalities in support of the campaign was reported to have slowed as a result of the shortages of personnel.[38] Bartolommeo Gosio, the commissioner for the regions of Basilicata and Calabria, wrote of the actual "suspension" of antimalarial activity.[39] The simplest summary was that of the prefect of Caserta in Campania, who wrote in 1919, "Thousands of ill patients were given limited medical attention because of the shortage of physicians. Confronting an enormous workload, they were unable to devote the necessary diligence to the war against malaria."[40]

A clear sign of the times was the collapse of the campaign's moral driving force—the Society for the Study of Malaria. Following the death of Angelo Celli in 1914 and the mobilization of many of its leading medical figures, and with an ever-growing shortage of funds, the society disbanded and closed its journal of record, the *Atti della Società per gli Studi della Malaria* (Proceedings of the Society for the Study of Malaria). The society remained in suspension until 1926. Although the campaign itself officially continued to operate, it lost its sense of direction. Roberto Villetti, director of Rome's municipal department of health, noted in 1922 that the "wartime upheaval . . . has destroyed all of our previous advances."[41]

To a large and nearly paralyzing degree, the antimalarial campaign also lost its foremost weapon—quinine. Part of the reason, monopoly pricing, was coincidental to the war rather than a direct result of the conflict. By 1914, nine-tenths of the world production of quinine were securely in the hands of a Dutch trust that began to adopt classic monopoly practices by restricting supply of the alkaloid while tripling, and then quadrupling, its price.[42] Thus the cost of quinine rose rapidly—to "fantastic levels," in the words of a report for the Department of Health—just as Italian funds to purchase it declined steeply.[43] At the same time the war itself severely complicated matters. Trade was disrupted as German submarines sank ships bearing consignments of quinine to Italy. Here was a medical effect of Germany's decision to conduct economic warfare against the Entente powers through an unrestricted submarine assault. Inevitably, the combined effects of monopoly prices and U-boat activity were quinine shortages and interruptions. Since the effectiveness of quinine depended on a rigorous and lengthy regimen, such interruptions were severely prejudicial to health.

In order to stretch failing supplies, authorities reduced the dosages that were known to be effective. This was, in effect, a form of medical rationing. The recommended daily dose in 1914 was 0.4 gram, totaling 2.8 grams a week. Under the press of the emergency, public health officials authorized experiments with weekly doses consisting of only 1.0 gram administered in just two installments—0.6 gram on Saturday evening and 0.4 gram on Sunday morning.[44] From an administrative standpoint, such reduced doses spared quinine and eased the strain on overworked physicians. Medically, however, quinine administered in insufficient doses compromised the recovery of patients and negated Grassi's vision of radical cure. Leading authorities argued that it also promoted a new problem—the emergence of drug-resistant strains of plasmodia that were first reported during the conflict. As the malariologist Giuseppe Sanarelli wrote, one of the unpleasant observations of physicians was that the prolonged and inadequate use of quinine led to "the appearance of quinine resistance in parasites" which "rendered patients refractory to treatment."[45] Such rationing diluted not only the medication but also the relationship between sufferers and physicians. Weekly rather than daily doses inevitably reduced contact and, therefore, opportunities for health education.

Quinine did not, of course, suddenly lose its therapeutic value in 1915. Indeed, nearly a century later, it remains one of the drugs of choice for treating malaria. To be effective, however, quinine needs to be administered in strict conformity to a regular and prolonged regimen. Wartime conditions of high cost, limited supply, and diminished dosages meant that quinine, inappropriately consumed, lost much of its effectiveness. Psychological and educational factors also compromised the efficacy of the alkaloid. Villetti made this point with regard to the Roman Campagna. After 1915, families lost their principal breadwinners to the army, experienced rapidly declining standards of living, and often suffered bereavement. Under such severe economic and emotional strain, their enthusiasm for antimalarial activity waned. In Villetti's words, a major problem faced by the antimalarial health stations was "the indifference of populations distracted by the worries of war."[46] In any case, the quinine distributors confronted a patient population that was significantly different from the one that attended the stations before 1915. As malaria expanded into new areas and as inexperienced villagers with little familiarity with quinine were recruited into agricultural work, the campaign once again found itself confronting the distrust and superstition it had encountered at the turn of the century. Educationally, health stations often found themselves returning to the starting point of their activities a generation before.

But there was a further dimension to the problem. In 1900, the leading antimalarial warriors had begun their work of redemption with confidence that they possessed in quinine a weapon equal to the task of eradicating or at least controlling malaria. During the First World War, the medical profession lost its trust in the "divine medicine." The most dramatic case was that of Antonio Dionisi, an eminent malariologist and founding member of the Society for the Study of Malaria. After Celli himself, Dionisi had been the leading Italian advocate of prophylactic quinine to control the disease. Recruited by the army to protect the soldiers of the Third Army on the Isonzo front, he had at first confidently taken the precious tablets himself and administered them to the troops. The result, despite careful adherence to the prescribed regimen, was that both he and the soldiers under his care contracted malaria. Profoundly disillusioned, Dionisi concluded that quinine was unequal to the task. Dionisi's apostasy was widespread, and Ettore Marchiafava reported in 1917 that a "veil of skepticism" surrounded the alkaloid.[47] Both the Austro-Hungarian and the Italian armies had relied on quinine but in doing so had encountered problems that led to universal loss of faith. Without faith to motivate its physicians, the campaign lost much of its dynamism.

Lecce province, in Apulia, illustrated nearly all of the factors that underlay the great wartime malaria epidemic. Beginning in 1916, the medical officer of health at Lecce pointed to a gathering crisis. In 1914, he estimated that, in a population of 725,839 people, 374,021 of whom lived in malarial zones, there were 19,638 cases. By 1917 these had nearly doubled—to 38,046 cases, with 348 deaths. Malaria even erupted in townships from which it had once been banished by the efforts of the prewar quinine campaign. The reasons produced by the Lecce official to explain the sudden upsurge were partly contingent, such as the unusually heavy rainfall for three years in succession, from 1914 to 1917. But the health officer also cited factors that linked the sufferings in the province to the war—the presence of veterans from Albania and Macedonia who had returned to Lecce for treatment; the newly impoverished diet of the people, which compromised their resistance to infection; the demechanization of agriculture; the neglect of drainage and reclamation ditches; a shortage of doctors and health-care personnel; earthmoving projects associated with military efforts to fortify the naval bases at Taranto and Brindisi; and the ignorance regarding quinine that was typical of the inhabitants of localities that had not previously known the disease.

By 1917, therefore, the consensus of opinion was that the war had unleashed a measureless and ever-deepening malaria problem, reversing the gains of twenty years of unceasing toil. In 1918, however, a further calamity compounded the emergency. This factor was the arrival in Italy of the great pandemic of Spanish influenza that swept the globe as the war reached its climax. The "Spanish lady" produced perhaps the most deadly pandemic ever to afflict the earth and the first severe outbreak of influenza to strike Europe since 1889–1890. In the view of the Department of Health, the war itself was the great predisposing factor: "It is useless to pretend otherwise: the pandemic struck the various nations after a long period of fighting. By then all the public services that would otherwise have taken the leading role in prevention were overwhelmed and overstretched. The general disruption resulting from the war effort was important. But even more significant was the fact that the war fully absorbed the energy of the personnel and equipment that were required to defend higher interests."[48]

In Italy there were two waves of flu in 1918—a mild and "almost unnoticed" ripple between late April and June, followed by a great flood that first gathered force in Calabria in July. It then swept the whole nation, reaching its greatest intensity in September and October and then receding through January 1919.[49] There were smaller outbursts in 1920, 1922, and 1923, with each upsurge less devastating than the one before (Table 5.3).

Wartime conditions in Italy created perfect opportunities for an airborne virus to spread widely—the mass movement of soldiers and refugees, over-

Table 5.3 Deaths from Influenza in Italy, 1914–1923

1914	3,559
1915	4,174
1916	5,919
1917	3,814
1918	274,041
1919	31,781
1920	24,428
1921	4,162
1922	13,199
1923	8,806

Source: Data from Mortara, *La salute pubblica,* 213.

crowding, widespread malnutrition, and the preexisting epidemic of malaria, which is immunosuppressive and therefore made Italians particularly vulnerable. Indeed, the vast prevalence of malaria was one of the reasons that Italy was among the nations most severely afflicted by the Spanish flu. The prefect of Caserta, in Campania, made the correct connection when he observed that "influenza was most severe in those townships where malaria raged most virulently."[50]

Although malaria greatly predisposed Italy to influenza, the causal links also operated in reverse: the arrival of a virulent strain of influenza greatly exacerbated the malaria epidemic that was already under way. The reason was biological. Respiratory diseases such as influenza, pneumonia, and tuberculosis are serious "opportunistic infections" that afflict the victims of malaria. In other words, a large but unknown number of those whose death in 1918 was officially diagnosed as influenza really died because they were already ill from malaria. As the prefect of Cosenza observed, it was common for the most serious cases of malaria—those that involved severe respiratory tract complications leading to bronchial pneumonia—to be misdiagnosed as influenza.[51] It was no accident that influenza struck hardest in the South, where the malaria epidemic was most virulent, and that influenza was most severe in those townships where malaria was also most serious.[52]

Influenza also exacerbated the malaria epidemic because it effectively brought the antimalarial campaign, which was already in crisis, to a standstill even more dramatically than the cholera epidemic of 1911. Influenza struck the health-care personnel of the antimalarial campaign, and it diverted the attention of the remaining staff from malaria patients to the victims of influenza. A further problem was that quinine was still widely thought to be a generic febrifuge rather than an antimalarial specific. Therefore, it was given to flu victims in preference to malaria sufferers. A misleading clinical observation led to this unfortunate diversion of already scarce quinine, the prefect of Cosenza in Calabria explained. It had long been observed, he wrote, that "in all those malarial localities where the treatment and prophylaxis of malaria were carried out with the greatest diligence, influenza had always struck most mildly."[53] In the midst of a deadly global pandemic of influenza, it was tempting, if not logical, to conclude that the mildness of influenza in such localities resulted from the fact that quinine was an effective medication against influenza as well as against malaria. Tragically, therefore, an effective medication was systematically withheld from patients it could have helped and administered instead to sufferers of an unrelated disease against which it was useless. Indeed, since it was used in the attempt to contain an epidemic as terrible as the "Spanish lady," quinine soon became entirely unavailable for malaria patients. The Department of Health called for its "parsimonious use" for all patients as the demand "exceeded all reasonable proportions."[54]

Malaria after the Armistice

If war was the direct cause of the vast upsurge in malaria, why did the epidemic not abate until 1923—long after the armistice, which brought hostilities to an end in November 1918? Indeed, in certain localities the process of normalization was even more extended. As the malariologist Alberto Missiroli observed of the Roman Campagna, "After the war, ten years were required to reduce malaria to its former level."[55] Malaria persisted at nineteenth-century levels partly because the immediate effect of the return to peace was to reinforce the plasmodial link between the fighting front and the home front. Peacetime entailed the demobilization of hundreds of thousands of veterans of the Piave and Balkan theaters, many of whom were infected. Upon their return to civilian life, they transmitted plasmodial infection to their families, neighbors, and fellow workers. In the Roman Campagna, public health authorities explained, the first effect of peace was the return of veterans who established new and virulent foci of malaria. Instead of ending the "returned soldier problem," peace intensified the role of the soldier as a conduit for disease.[56]

Even sadder than the lot of ordinary soldiers was the fate of those who had been held as prisoners of war. In the two months following the disaster at Caporetto in October 1917, the Habsburg army captured twice the number of Italian prisoners that it had taken in the whole of the preceding twenty-nine months of war (Table 5.4). The medical consequences of the prisoner-of-war problem were especially severe because Austria-Hungary made no effort to

Table 5.4 Prisoners Captured per 1,000 Italian Soldiers, 1915–1918

1915	25
1916	56
1917	193
1918	31

Source: Data from Mortara, *La salute pubblica,* 34–35, 37.

provide humane treatment for the Italian soldiers it captured. On the contrary, the Habsburg authorities systematically subjected them to the overwork, overcrowding, and filth of concentration camps, where they were starved and denied medical attention. A measure of the inhumane conditions of their detention was that, of six hundred thousand Italians taken as prisoners, ten thousand perished from wounds but approximately ninety thousand died of diseases. In the words of the official report on the health of the Italian army, "This number is strikingly high. . . . In less than a year of detention, on average, our prisoners died at nearly the same rate as infantrymen as a result of combat during three and a half years of bitter fighting."[57] In addition, a large number of these detainees returned home "in a pitiful state" of health and perished soon after their return — of tuberculosis and other respiratory infections, of gastrointestinal diseases, and of wounds received during their captivity. Many of these soldiers also infected others after they reached their destination, and malaria was one of the infectious diseases they frequently bore in their bloodstreams.[58]

In addition to the return of soldiers and prisoners of war bearing disease, another cause for the delay in the return to prewar levels of malaria was the persistence of wartime environmental degradation. In the war zone itself, large-scale investments and years of labor were required to drain fields flooded by both armies, to repair damaged or neglected irrigation ditches, to restore buildings, and to house refugees. More generally, Italy underwent a protracted period of reconversion to peacetime economic conditions. Only gradually did landlords renew their livestock, repair farm machinery, clear drainage canals, improve workers' accommodations, and restore more-intensive crop-rotation systems — measures that slowly created an environment less favorable to the breeding of anopheline mosquitoes. Inevitably, since landlords and farmers began the postwar period with severe profitability constraints, the restoration of prewar levels of investment proved to be a prolonged and painful process. In the meantime, in a period of persistent inflation, agricultural wages lagged behind the general price index. Thus a compromised diet, inadequate clothing, and unsanitary housing continued to undermine the resistance of farmworkers to disease.

Finally, it took years to restore the antimalarial campaign itself because recurrent waves of Spanish influenza continued to drain it of funds, personnel, and quinine—just when the return of so many ill veterans further taxed the available resources. Only after a protracted hiatus did physicians, nurses, and attendants take up their former duties at rural health stations, and only slowly did the quinine market recover sufficiently to make adequate supplies of the alkaloid available.

Significantly, however, the reestablishment of the antimalarial campaign after the war did not entail a simple return to prewar strategies of control and eradication. On the contrary, the great upsurge in malaria that lasted for nearly a decade after 1915 introduced a major transformation by permanently undermining the previously unbounded confidence in quinine. A hallmark of the campaign at its inception by Celli and Grassi had been the belief that quinine alone could free the nation from its bondage to malaria. Experience had taught the necessity of health stations and peasant schools as well, but these had been conceived primarily as means to remove the barriers of ignorance and distance that hindered the adequate distribution of the alkaloid. Quinine was the cornerstone of the program.

The First World War destroyed this overweening optimism. By the end of the conflict, as the British malariologist Sydney James wrote, "Faith in the efficacy of every prophylactic and therapeutic measure had fallen almost to zero."[59] First, the war demonstrated that quinine's inability to lower morbidity effectively—a weakness already apparent before 1915—was a source of permanent danger. In a crisis, a merely attenuated malaria could rebound, sweeping away all that had been gained by years of unrelenting effort. Second, the war revealed that it was dangerous to rely so heavily on a medication that was supplied exclusively by a foreign monopoly. Just when the need for quinine became acute, the Dutch trust made it unavailable either in adequate quantities or at accessible prices.

Most disillusioning of all, however, were the attempts at quinine prophylaxis by armies on both sides of the conflict. The results were uniformly discouraging, as Giuseppe Sanarelli explained. Military doctors, he reported, encountered strains of malaria that were resistant to quinine. They also found that the alkaloid conferred protection for only a limited period, that it altered the symptoms of the disease and thereby seriously complicated diagnosis, that it reduced the number of cases but made them more refractory to treatment, and that it predisposed patients to suffer relapses.[60] Sanarelli, like the Italian medical profession as a whole, concluded that the scientific knowledge of malaria and the weapons available to combat it were inadequate to the task. "New paths" would have to be discovered if the goal of eradication was to be achieved.[61]

By 1917, as the epidemic erupted in full force and the state found itself unable to contain it, quinine remained the sheet anchor of therapy, but it no longer held out the promise of leading Italy to eradication. For this reason, the Department of Health appointed three technical committees on malaria to explore weapons other than quinine to combat the disease. Composed of such luminaries in malariology as Grassi, Sanarelli, Gosio, Vittorio Ascoli, and Pietro Canalis, the committees investigated new means to destroy mosquitoes and their larvae, studied the irradiation of the spleen by X-rays as a means to stimulate the production of white cells (hematopoiesis) and thereby enhance resistance to malaria, and considered the radical cure of malaria patients by compounds of mercury rather than quinine. Already the concept was emerging that, in the postwar period, the approach to the war on malaria should be multifaceted and eclectic.[62]

Most attention was given to the idea of destroying mosquitoes and their larvae instead of attacking plasmodia. Ronald Ross had originally suggested this alternative approach at the turn of the century, and his follower Claudio Fermi had advocated it in Italy. With the ascendancy of the Rome School and its doctrine, however, the "Italian road to eradication" from 1900 until the First World War adopted quinine as its mainstay. With the wartime emergency, the resulting shortage of quinine, and the growing disillusionment with quinine's potential to uproot malaria, health authorities turned their attention from plamosdia to vectors. Fermi dubbed this methodology "de-anophelization," and between 1915 and 1918 he undertook a series of experiments to demonstrate its usefulness. His aim was not to eradicate mosquitoes but to reduce their numbers sufficiently to break the cycle of transmission.

From an early date Fermi had rejected the nineteenth-century theory of "swamp fever," which linked malaria with marshes and vast expanses of stagnant water. He started with the premise that in southern Italy the disease was most directly associated with the microenvironment. Fermi implicated small breeding grounds such as wells, water troughs, drainage gullies, irrigation canals, and excavation ditches. Therefore, after selecting a village to be protected, he began by drawing a detailed map of all such local breeding places within a radius of two kilometers of the inhabited area—the range, he believed, of a mosquito's flight. Then he meticulously eliminated all possible habitats suitable for larvae by closing wells, draining or filling ditches, and clearing canals. Where stagnant water could not be eliminated, he poisoned it with petroleum. This program of microenvironmental sanitation (*piccola bonifica*) demonstrated its capacity to reduce the population of mosquitoes and to lower the burden of malaria in the communities he chose. The Department of Health endorsed Fermi's idea. The plan was to begin the postwar era not by relying on piccola bonifica alone but by employing it as a major adjunct to other means, including quinine therapy.[63]

Beyond the reorientation of the antimalarial campaign away from quinine, the Italian authorities also effected a profound alteration in the campaign's ethos. In Giolittian Italy, the campaign had been associated with democratization and unionization, with universal literacy and women's consciousness, with social reform and the rights of the poor. In the crucible of the First World War, a new antimalarial movement was forged. Angelo Celli and the original medical apostles for the redemption of the nation from fever, the Society for the Study of Malaria and the National League against Malaria, the men and women who had launched the great campaign "from below"—all were gone by the end of conflict, and the state found itself in the position of reconstructing and reconstituting the war on malaria "from above." Malaria remained the great national problem to be addressed, but now it was approached in a more bureaucratized manner and in relation to different objectives.

A revealing contrast is that of the metaphors used by leading antimalarial campaigners before and after the First World War. Before the war, the imagery was largely biblical, stressing liberation and redemption from fever. Alessandro Marcucci, one of the founding fathers of the rural schools, argued that their mission was to bring a "Gospel of truth, liberty, and justice."[64] After 1915, a new set of dominant metaphors emerged that defined the campaign through military vocabulary. The campaigners no longer spoke of a liberating redemption from bondage but of a war conducted by a militia and humble soldiers against an internal enemy. Gosio, who was familiar with the earlier vocabulary, wrote now—in the new lexicon—that "armies fight in peacetime as well for a better tomorrow."[65] In place of the democratic vision of the past, the new language suggested centralization, discipline, obedience, and an emphasis on technique. The First World War, waged in part to contain the democratic impulses that the antimalarial campaign had helped to foment, now enabled the state to redirect the antimalarial effort along more authoritarian lines. War had begun to colonize public health—a process that was destined to accelerate with the rise of Fascism.[66]

The position taken by the Ministry of Agriculture, which turned to the problems of malaria and the postwar world in 1918, indicates how great a transformation was involved. War, the ministry explained, had revealed that Italy was too weak to compete economically and militarily with such Great Power rivals as Germany. The reason was biological: the Italian race was so undermined by malaria and the conditions it imposed that Italians were unequal to northern Europeans either as soldiers or as producers. Therefore, the only solution was genetic—to breed an improved race of Italians whose vitality was neither undermined by disease nor debilitated by urban living. The solution to Italy's economic and military weakness lay in what the Ministry called the "anthropological reclamation" (*bonifica antropologica*) and the "eugenic reclamation" (*bonifica eugenica*) of the population. Victory in the war against malaria was an essential component of this vision. From this perspective, the reestablishment of a national antimalarial campaign had little to do with social reform and everything to do with power politics, eugenics, and the need for Italy to perform better in future wars. In the words of the ministry, "Today war, or the expectation of the consequence of war on the economy of the people, causes a new orientation of eugenic science in relation to . . . the biological improvement of the producer and the worker. In the face of the German peril, present and future, it is impossible to do without an economic and eugenic population policy."[67]

Thus, as the First World War was ending, Italian authorities began systematically to reconceptualize the antimalarial campaign. Disillusioned with quinine, the Department of Health began to evolve a strategy that was multifaceted, making use of all available weapons against malaria instead of relying on a single powerful instrument. At the same time, faced with massive social unrest in the aftermath of the conflict, other officials began to lose faith in the prewar democratic belief that the health and empowerment of the individual patient went hand in hand. For these officials, the urgent necessity was to strengthen the state against the danger of social revolution that seemed so imminent during the time known as the Red Years in Italian history—1919 and 1920. The end result of this process had significant political and public health consequences. Reflecting on the prewar era, Alessandro Marcucci wrote that Angelo Celli had envisaged the conquest of malaria as a means of saving the body, while Giovanni Cena had seen it as a means of redeeming the spirit.[68] By the end of the war both men were dead, while Anna Celli lost her position as director of the rural schools because, as a native of Germany, she fell under suspicion.[69] She was succeeded by a key figure in the enforcement of law and order, Camillo Corradini, the undersecretary of state at the Ministry of the Interior. At the same time, the Ministry of Agriculture envisaged the breeding of an Italian superrace as the solution to Italy's multiple problems—military, economic, and sanitary. In the turmoil of war and the social unrest that followed, a new and authoritarian vision emerged in which health was subordinated to a very different priority—the fashioning of foot soldiers and obedient producers for the fatherland and Il Duce.

6

Fascism, Racism, and Littoria

Too great a sacrifice may be demanded of laborers who do not properly value their own health. It causes me profound sorrow to observe that such a sacrifice can occur, that it can be tolerated, and that it can even be encouraged by a country that, like our own, rightly aspires to a place among the leaders on the road to progress.

— *Giovanni Battista Grassi*

Although this fact is often forgotten, antimalarial campaigning formed a central part of Fascist domestic policy, involving both the substance of the regime and the image it sought to project to the world. Here it is important to recall that Mussolini's movement spent nearly a decade completing its seizure of power after the Blackshirts' famous March on Rome in October 1922. Thereafter the Fascists achieved full political control by a series of incremental measures. Their cumulative effect was to abolish elections, destroy democracy and parliamentary rule, outlaw competing political parties and trade unions, "fascisticize" the state apparatus by placing party members in all key posts, and reach an accommodation with the Roman Catholic Church. Only at the end of this process, in late 1928–1929, did Mussolini and the Fascist Party find themselves in a sufficiently totalitarian position to define the new society that was to replace the Liberal social order. Having finally concluded the negative task of violently destroying parliamentary sovereignty, civil liberties, and political opposition, the regime was free to carry out the "Fascist revolution."[1]

As a pillar of the new order Il Duce enacted the Mussolini Law of December 1928—the only legislation that ever enjoyed such personal endorsement from Mussolini. This law initiated the Fascist campaign to abolish malaria, concentrating on the Pontine Marshes. The Pontine Marshes extended over a vast plain south of Rome that was largely uninhabited because of the extreme prevalence of falciparum malaria. Clearing and settling the region, therefore, offered the opportunity to construct a Fascist society de novo. Here, from the standpoint of the Fascist faithful, were two compelling possibilities. First was the opportunity for Il Duce to demonstrate, in a highly visible manner, the all-powerful, or "totalitarian," will by which he could solve the intractable problem of fever that had thwarted the best efforts of caesars, popes, and Liberals. Second, the Fascists saw in the Pontine Marshes a rare chance to create a Fascist utopia unimpeded by previously existing structures, traditions, and vested interests.

In order to explore the Fascists' attempt at social engineering in the new province they created, we must examine the political and social purposes that motivated the regime to act. What did Mussolini seek to achieve, and what claims did he advance on his own behalf? What do the reclaimed Pontine Marshes reveal about the objectives of Fascism as a movement? Finally, in the supposedly malaria-proof world the Fascists built, how valid was Mussolini's claim that Fascism had solved the ancient problem?

Even before embarking on his plans for the Pontine Marshes, Mussolini had already displayed an interest in malaria and a capacity to intervene in health matters arbitrarily and in defiance of medical opinion. Since a central ideological tenet of Fascism was the cult of the omniscient and omnipotent leader, Mussolini laid claim to godlike attributes, while the party and the public treated him with religious reverence. Unfortunately, Il Duce believed in his own apotheosis. With no medical qualifications, he regarded himself as a healer—the "great physician" of party propaganda. This capacity for sudden and arbitrary intervention was an integral part of the Fascist antimalarial campaign that began in 1928.

For this reason it is important to remember an illuminating intervention by Il Duce in 1925, when he took a first and ruthless stand with regard to malaria. Acting as deus ex machina, he gave personal authorization to a medical experiment that prefigured the work of Nazi doctors. Mussolini allowed two otherwise-obscure Fascist malariologists—Giacomo Peroni and Onofrio Cirillo—to carry out a large-scale experiment at the expense of hundreds of poor and vulnerable subjects. Their work involved two ethically indefensible procedures. First, they withheld quinine, a readily available and effective medication, from a control group of patients suffering from severe and life-threatening malaria. Second, instead of quinine, they experimentally administered mercury as both prophylactic and remedy, and they did so against the consensus of the medical profession and against the specific warnings of the Superior Health Council and its committee of expert malariologists.

By 1925, European doctors had accumulated centuries of experience in using mercury as a therapeutic agent. Most famously, syphilitics had received metallic therapy since the sixteenth century. Because mercury is in fact highly toxic, this therapy was painful and frequently more harmful than the pox itself. It was widely thought, however, that so agonizing a remedy was peculiarly appropriate for a disease that was commonly regarded as the wages of sin. By the nineteenth century, belief in mercury as a healing agent had been profoundly undermined. Indeed, it was a sign of desperation that, in the first half of the nineteenth century, hapless physicians confronting Asiatic cholera widely administered mercury in the form of calomel. In this case, desperate symptoms suggested desperate remedies. Experience rapidly indicated again, however, that this metallic element served only to increase the suffering of patients and to hasten their demise. By the twentieth century, mercury had fallen into terminal disfavor.[2]

Nevertheless, during the First World War, the physician Giacomo Peroni came to the perverse conviction that for malaria, mercury rather than quinine was the therapy of choice. He labeled its use "immuno-metal therapy," and he encouraged his associate Guido Cremonese to package and sell salts of mercury under the trade name Smalarina. Eager to find substitutes for quinine during the wartime crisis, the Superior Health Council appointed a distinguished committee to examine Peroni's claims and arrive at a recommendation for policy. Reporting on behalf of the committee, Ettore Marchiafava and Corrado Tommasi-Crudeli reached an emphatically negative decision on all counts. With regard to the prophylactic use of mercury, they argued that "there are too few data to support the proposal for mercurializing healthy individuals to prevent malaria." Then, with respect to therapy, they insisted that "it would not be appropriate to give state sanction to an effort that may present serious drawbacks."[3]

Denied sanction to prescribe mercury in 1917, Peroni returned to the idea in 1925, when he substituted political influence for the scientific support that he lacked in the medical community. Peroni had been a volunteer in the First World War, he was a Fascist "of the first hour" who had joined the movement in its earliest days in 1919, and he had direct access to Il Duce. Under the new regime, the idea of finding a remedy for malaria that was inexpensive and that reduced Italian dependence on foreign suppliers of quinine fit perfectly with Mussolini's aspirations to Italian self-sufficiency. At Il Duce's personal request, therefore, Peroni gained permission to conduct a mercurial trial on a patient population that was both impoverished and at severe risk from falciparum malaria. The experiment involved over two thousand workers employed on land reclamation projects carried out under the auspices of the veterans' association (Opera Nazionale Combattenti, or ONC) in intensely malarial areas of Apulia and Tuscany.

In these locations (Stornara, Santeramo, and Albarese), the workforce was divided into two groups. The first group was "abandoned to infection" by being set to work at heavy outdoor labor throughout the epidemic season while the Fascist scientists intentionally withheld quinine from them, as well as such protective measures as screening and environmental sanitation. In a manner suggestive of the later Tuskegee experiment in the United States, Peroni and Cirillo wished to observe the impact on the human body of naturally occurring disease when it is allowed to run its course unimpeded. The second group received mercury. Half of this group absorbed the metal as a prophylactic and the other half as a remedy after symptoms developed. In both cases, the strategy involved what Peroni described as the "mercurial saturation of the organism" by intramuscular injection. The "saturation" continued without interruption for four years, until 1929.[4]

Since the data presented by Peroni are incomplete and probably inaccurate, it is impossible to know the extent of the suffering and death that his experiment caused to the thousands of war veterans involved. It is also unclear whether the subjects of the experiment were actually volunteers and whether the risks involved had been clearly explained to them. Peroni merely asserted that his results were "splendid." He claimed that mercury administered prophylactically prevented malaria in 77.4 to 100 percent of his subjects and that when administered therapeutically, it cured 82.9 percent of patients. Peroni concluded, therefore, that mercury was the all-purpose drug of choice for malaria. Far superior to quinine, he argued, mercury was inexpensive, it required just a few injections instead of the lengthy quinine regimen, and it conferred a lasting immunity. Thanks to the metal, he suggested, Italy could achieve both public health and self-sufficiency. Peroni was so optimistic that he wished to "mercurialize" the entire Italian army.

Impartial observers reached far less sanguine conclusions. Once more the Superior Health Council carried out an investigation to verify Peroni's scientific claims. Alberto Missiroli, the eminent malariologist and a member of the council, reported that Peroni's prophylactic method had been repeated in Sardinia with the involvement of 395 subjects. The results were maximally discouraging. Missiroli explained that the disease ran its course among all 395 subjects "as if no immunizing agent had been employed."[5] Mercury, he commented, had no protective value whatever against malaria.[6] With regard to the curative results, the council noted that "the failures that nearly everywhere followed the therapeutic use of Smalarina have caused it to be abandoned in the treatment of malaria, even though its fanatics insist on attributing to it great powers as a prophylactic and remedy."[7]

Under the Fascist dictatorship, it was possible for Il Duce to intervene capriciously in matters of health. Mussolini allowed physicians to whom he was partial and who possessed impeccable political credentials to conduct inhumane experiments involving the poor and generating no new or useful medical knowledge. Totalitarian ideology in this case proved dangerous to health. When Il Duce decided to attempt a much larger experiment in public health and social engineering in the Pontine Marshes, he acted again with arbitrary and peremptory resolve. Here his style of decision making had more lasting repercussions in terms of human suffering.

The Pontine Marshes

Since antiquity the Pontine Marshes had been famously unhealthy. Parliament had labeled them "the largest and most pestiferous swamps that our poor Italy possesses in its midst." A traveler leaving Rome and heading south toward Naples along the famous Roman road known as the Appian Way found the marshes stretching out on both sides for all eighty kilometers between Cisterna and Terracina at the southern border of Lazio. Extending over a width of ten to fifty kilometers, they were bounded to the west by the Tyrrhenian Sea and to the east by the Lepini Mountains. The Pontine Marshes, shunned by settlers for millennia, comprised eighty thousand hectares of lethally inhospitable wasteland that spread across a low rectangular plain. Their poignant history, their natural beauty as unspoiled wetlands, and their affecting contrast with nearby Rome, however, made them an attraction for visiting artists and writers during seasons other than the dangerous summer. In modern times they were famously described by Lord Byron, Johann Wolfgang von Goethe, and Gabriele D'Annunzio, and they were painted by Giovanni Battista Piranesi, Giulio Aristide Sartorio, Duilio Cambellotti, and Ernest Hébert.

So intense was the danger of malaria, and especially of the prevailing falciparum infection, that in 1928 the entire plain possessed a stable population of only 1,637 people and not a single permanent settlement. According to the Italian Red Cross, 80 percent of those who spent even one night in the area during the epidemic season contracted malaria. Population density was only

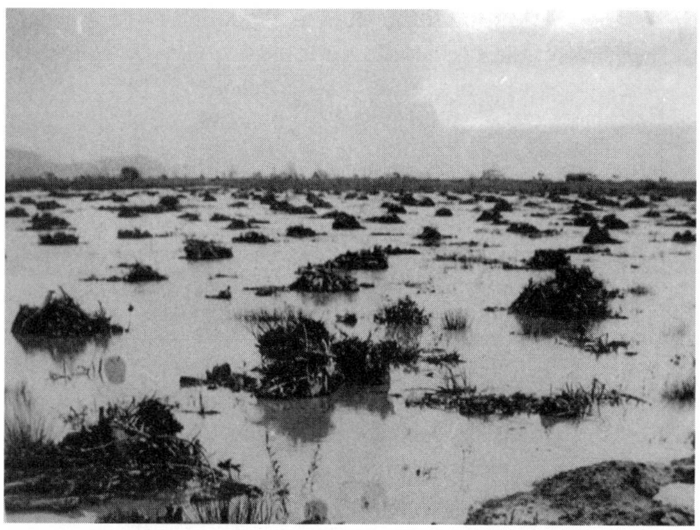

The Pontine Marshes before reclamation

seven people per square kilometer, and of these seven only one practiced agriculture. This forbidding landscape permitted few economic activities—woodcutting, charcoal burning, fishing, shepherding, and buffalo herding, in addition to a strictly limited cultivation of wheat. These ventures were carried out by illiterate, nomadic people who led foreshortened lives in squalor and poverty. Absentee landlords simply abandoned their properties to total neglect, drawing an income primarily from rough pasturage. In the words of the *New York Times,* the area was "inhabited only by a few fever-racked wretches" who lived in straw huts that provided little shelter from the elements and voracious insects. The French racist Count de Gobineau even charged that the unproductive sloth of the Pontine Marshes was an expression of the deficiencies of the Italian race. Even the popular nicknames for localities on the desolate marshland were indicative of ever-present danger: Land of Death, Pool of the Sepulcher, Marshes of Hell, Dead Woman, Land of Bad Advice, and—in a reference to Virgil's boatman over the River Styx—Charon.[8]

Climate, topography, hydrology, and ecological degradation all contributed to the notoriety of the Pontine Marshes for severe malaria. In the wet spring, rainwater rushed off the Lepini Mountains in torrents, causing the rivers to overflow their banks and giving rise to widespread flooding. Because the topsoil consisted of sand and impermeable clay, the water did not readily percolate away. Instead, it collected for long periods on the surface, especially in

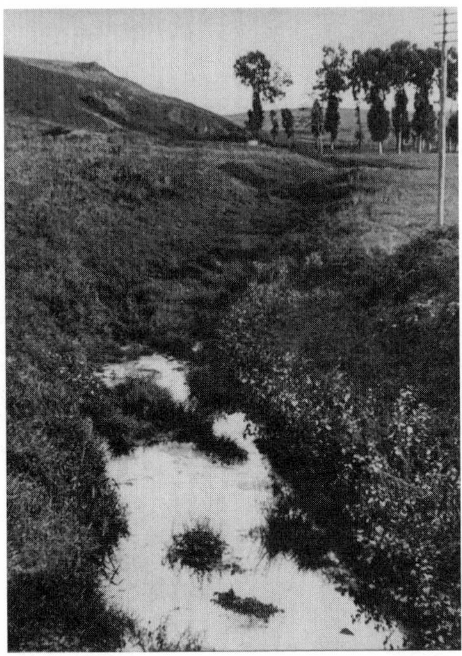

A mosquito breeding site in the Roman Campagna

depressions, where it formed deadly pools. These pools were widely considered the principal source of the epidemics that ravaged the area. Since the plain was broad and the gradient to the sea was slight, the waterways were sluggish. Many rivers even dried up during hot, dry summers, leaving an infinity of stagnant puddles in their beds, where the dreaded vector *Anopheles labranchiae* bred.

In patterns that were typical of malaria south of the Po Valley, these severe hydrological problems were compounded by local environmental damage. Sand dunes along the coast impeded the outflow of water into the sea, the embankments of the Rome-Naples railroad line blocked drainage and collected water on their inland side, and the deforestation of the nearby hills promoted the silting up of riverbeds and encouraged recurrent flooding. Even the great land reclamation attempt of the Papal States in the late eighteenth century only fortified the sway of anopheline mosquitoes over their febrile domain. Through inadequate water flow and poor maintenance, thick vegetation obstructed the ditches that were originally intended for drainage. Ultimately, therefore, the canals commissioned by Pope Pius VI to promote settlement and economic development vividly illustrated the lesson that drainage alone was inadequate as a solution to the problem of malaria. Well into the twentieth century, these eighty thousand hectares remained "the domain of poverty and malaria, of the physical and moral degradation of both the people and the land."[9]

The fact that the Pontine Marshes were so celebrated in art and literature, that they were the site of the great failure of Pius VI, and that they stretched so unacceptably close to Rome made them ideal for a grand display of Fascist power. Mussolini's propagandists designated the campaign to redeem the area a "titanic enterprise" and a "totalitarian land transformation" that demonstrated the political superiority of a single, all-powerful will. Not only would the marshes become habitable, but they would also have a glorious future as the "smiling fields" of "Italy's model agricultural region." The subliminal message was that Fascism itself was the remedy and that Il Duce was Italy's "great physician."[10]

Bonifica Integrale: The Theory

Fascism's great antimalarial effort, established by the Mussolini Law, was a complex reclamation and settlement program known as *bonifica integrale.* The dictatorship proclaimed the program amid great fanfare as "a turning point in history" that rivaled the greatest achievements of ancient Rome. Mussolini himself announced that the law of 1928 was a cornerstone of the Fascist revolution. Bonifica integrale was a "battle" to be waged by the veterans' association, the ONC. This Fascist battle, however, was not conceived as a comprehensive assault on malaria throughout Italy. On the contrary, the main front in the Fascist war on malaria was the Pontine Marshes, which Il Duce had carefully selected as a grandiose pilot project. A comprehensive victory there could then provide lessons for later battles planned for other selected areas in Apulia, Campania, and Tuscany. In the bombast surrounding the project, there was no mention of its first important irony—that the major antimalarial initiative of the regime got under way in an area where almost nobody lived. In the field of medicine, Fascism did not establish its priorities in accordance with need. Here was a major limitation of Mussolini's public health campaign: it was rigidly "top-down" and unresponsive to pressure from below, even when expressed in the eloquent form of human suffering. By unilateral fiat, the Fascist regime proceeded as its first priority to invest massive resources in a landscape devoid of inhabitants.[11]

According to Fascist interpretations, bonifica integrale—loudly proclaimed as the brainchild of Il Duce himself—differed from all previous Italian efforts to combat malaria. Its novelty was that it attempted to deploy all of the weapons known to malariology in a single interlocking campaign. To explain this strategy, Fascist authorities characteristically invoked a military analogy. All earlier efforts, they reasoned, were based on a limited, defensive strategy of containment. Previously, they argued, the objective had been to protect individuals against attack while allowing parasites and mosquitoes to survive. The program of state quinine, for example, provided a chemical quarantine that shielded individuals from infection but allowed the disease to persist, posing a permanent threat to the nation. Inevitably, the Fascists argued, the Liberal campaign had reduced mortality but not morbidity.

By contrast, bonifica integrale, which the regime also termed the "eclectic method," launched an all-out offensive intended to annihilate the enemy within a chosen locality. According to Fascist idolatry, the entire concept was due to Mussolini—to "Him" and "His" will. Contrary to the claims of the cult of personality, however, this strategy was not Il Duce's sudden inspiration but the result of the wartime search for a "rational eclecticism" or "mixed prophylaxis" that would supplement quinine with a full range of other weapons. Giuseppe Tassinari, the agricultural expert who became a leading figure in the Fascist reclamation program, was politically correct but historically inaccurate when he asserted that the first use of the term *bonifica integrale* had occurred in a declaration by Mussolini in 1927. The concept and the term emerged instead within the Department of Health between 1917 and 1923 as it grappled with the dramatic upsurge in malaria unleashed by the First World War.[12]

Already in 1922 the authorities in both the Department of Health and the ONC were using the expression *bonifica integrale.* They defined it as "the effective coordination of three forms of *bonifica*—hydraulic, agricultural, and hygienic—through the cooperation of local official and private bodies under the direction of the state."[13] The first small-scale trial of the new strategy took place without fanfare at Maccarese in the Tiber Delta in 1926—two years before the Mussolini Law and on the basis of a strategy elaborated still earlier. There the regime reclaimed the land and divided up a great estate into forty-five peasant homesteads. Success at Maccarese gave Il Duce the confidence to begin his grandiose experiment.[14] In 1927 Alessandro Messea, the director-general of the Department of Health, drew up a program for extirpating malaria from the Pontine Marshes. His plan contained all of the initiatives Mussolini later proclaimed as his own.[15] More honestly than most Fascist officials, Eliseo Jandolo, the first director-general of bonifica integrale at the Ministry of Agriculture and Forests, argued that Fascist legislation in this field was simply the "codification of experience."[16] Its ambition was to assail malaria on three fronts and on a grand scale. In Fascist parlance, its strength was its "totalitarian vision."[17]

The first front was hydrological, and its purpose was to establish the "preliminary conditions" for a healthy settlement of the land. Called *bonifica idraulica,* this opening stage of the campaign consisted of the elimination of malarial swamps through drainage, flood control, the filling of depressions where stagnant water collected, and the rectification of environmental ravages through reforestation. In Fascist military parlance, this phase of the campaign was also known as the "battle against swamps."[18] Where mosquitoes bred luxuriantly in small collections of surface water as well as swamps, the project also embraced Claudio Fermi's approach of microenvironmental sanitation, or *piccola bonifica.* Collections of standing water were either drained or sprayed with larvicides, such as Paris Green.

Having revolutionized the hydrology of a malarial area, the Fascists intended to attack the disease on a second and more complex front—resettlement and intensive cultivation, or *bonifica agraria* (agricultural reclamation). Merely to drain the land was to repeat the disappointment experienced by Pius VI in the eighteenth century and then by the Italian parliament in the nineteenth century. Applying the paludal, or swamp water, interpretation of malaria, both the Papal States and the Italian Liberal regime approached the struggle against fever as simply an engineering task. Mussolini profited instead from Grassi's doctrine, from the experience of the quinine campaign since 1900, and from the plan that had emerged—unacknowledged—within the Department of Health. He concluded that the only way to succeed against malaria was to supplement the plans devised by engineers. Lasting progress required the settlement of all reclaimed land and the introduction of intensive agriculture and modern animal husbandry. Intensively cultivated crops would absorb moisture and dry the land, a resident peasantry would prevent drainage ditches from clogging and puddles from collecting, and cattle and pigs would divert mosquitoes from humans by providing alternative prey on which to feast. A popular boast was that Fascism would surround every village with sties and place a pig under every peasant's bed.[19] Meanwhile, where there had been only swamps, the ONC would build homesteads, erect fences, construct roads and bridges, and lay power lines. Giving thought to mosquito larvae as well as adults, the planners introduced the voracious freshwater fish *Gambusia affinis* into irrigation canals in order to reduce their larval populations.[20]

After *bonifica idraulica* and *bonifica agraria,* the third front in the Fascist war on malaria was antimalarial hygiene, or *bonifica igienica* (hygienic reclamation).[21] Having settled large numbers of vigilant peasants on the land, the regime intended to protect them from danger. More was involved, however, than humanitarian concern. For the settlers to succumb to infection would destroy the whole reclamation effort, waste the resources dedicated to the program, and discredit Il Duce. To avoid such humiliating failure, the ONC deployed all the defensive measures devised in the Giolittian period. The first such measure was to place mechanical defenses between the peasants and adult anopheline mosquitoes. This step included constructing sturdy and well-screened brick housing that denied entry to flying insects, and whitewashing and illuminating the interior so that the inhabitants could readily see and kill any mosquitoes that penetrated the outer defenses. Second, drawing on Grassi's doctrine, the regime sought the radical cure of all malarial patients by quinine administered through health stations and encouraged by rural schools. Quinine therapy persisted, but it had become simply one weapon among many, rather than the key element of the eradication campaign. Alessandro Messea, the director-general of the Department of Health, explained, "In the antimalarial effort it is of fundamental importance to abandon any exclusive reliance on one method rather than another. By good fortune the weapons of malariology are multiple."[22]

Summarizing the strategy embodied in the Mussolini Law, Antonio Labranca, a leading figure in the Department of Health, wrote,

> In Italy by the term *bonifica* we do not mean the simple draining of swamps. Bonifica has much broader aims. On the one hand, through drainage, it seeks the recovery of land formerly subject to surface water in order to render it suitable for farming. Second, it seeks the gradual transition from extensive to intensive cultivation. Finally, it proposes the sanitation of the territory, complete with an adequate health service and appropriate antimalarial interventions.
>
> These three objectives (hydraulic, agricultural, and hygienic) are closely connected and together constitute what we call bonifica integrale.[23]

A clear shift in emphasis from the prewar campaign was that bonifica integrale treated the control of malaria as primarily an entomological problem—as a matter, that is, of prioritizing the attack on mosquitoes rather than plasmodia.[24]

Bonifica Integrale: The Practice

It was in the threatening landscape of the Pontine Marshes that Mussolini chose to initiate his high-profile "battle for bonifica integrale." Bellicose analogies were foremost in all descriptions of the project. Nallo Alemanni of the veterans' association explained,

> The whole organization had the authentic character of a wartime conquest. The comparison springs to mind in part as a result of the external appearance of the various phases that the battle assumed as it progressed. It also arose from its possession of what is the central character of combat—the fact that it allows no pauses. There could be no rest for those whose task was to ensure the success of the operation or for the immense army of workers on the march who required constant logistical support. But most of all, this battle relied on

> those imponderable qualities of a moral and spiritual nature that are essential to all good soldiers and that are the prerequisites for final victory — discipline, self-sacrifice, and duty. All of these were required in the same measure as they are for a soldier in time of war.
>
> One could continue with the analogy. In this great enterprise it was essential to follow the dictates of wartime strategy and tactics. This was true in all regards — the recruitment of great masses of troops; the assault waves of men uprooting trees, moving earth, and burning wood; the establishment of the supply lines needed to furnish the essentials of life in unhealthy land; the deployment of matériel; and in general all those operations that give such a likeness to war.[25]

This battle, proclaimed in parliament in 1928, commenced in November 1929 with the preparation of the engineering plans for drainage and reclamation and their definitive approval by Mussolini. The project then reached completion — "in record speed," according to its proponents — a decade later. Declaring the battle fought and won, the regime declared victory in December 1939, just in time to celebrate the twentieth anniversary of the founding of the Fascist movement. Three events marked the celebration — the ceremonial incorporation of Pomezia, the last of five cities built on the Pontine Plain; the awarding, in the presence of Il Duce, of land-title deeds to the settlers; and the announcement that, for the first time, mortality from malaria in the area had been reduced to zero. This, the dictatorship announced, was "the first indication of a true and definitive victory."[26]

In the decade between the beginning of the battle in the Pontine Marshes and the victory celebrations of 1939, the regime undertook a program of sweeping proportions. It was, in effect, the most important domestic policy initiative that Mussolini's dictatorship pursued in the 1930s. In the words of a 1999 history of Fascism by Patrizia Dogliani, this project was "the best known, most publicized, and most discussed of the works carried out by Fascism."[27] The goal was to build a model Fascist society and to "solve the age-old problem of malaria fascistically, in the minimum period of time," and on the site of an enormous and lethal wasteland. This program was the last, and one of the largest, efforts made to present to the world a positive vision of Fascist political intentions. It was also the last major initiative of the dictatorship at home before war and the pursuit of a new Roman Empire eclipsed all domestic policies.[28] For these reasons, it is essential to consider the details of Fascist social engineering in Mussolini's model province.

BONIFICA IDRAULICA

In accord with the priorities of bonifica integrale, the first step was hydrological (bonifica idraulica). To prevent the flooding of the coastal plain

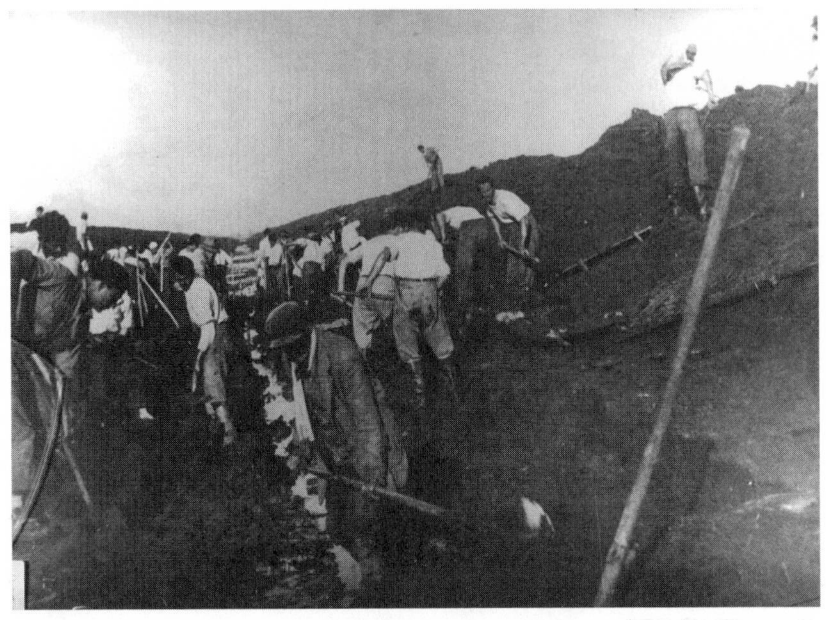

Hydraulic land reclamation (bonifica idraulica) of the Pontine Marshes

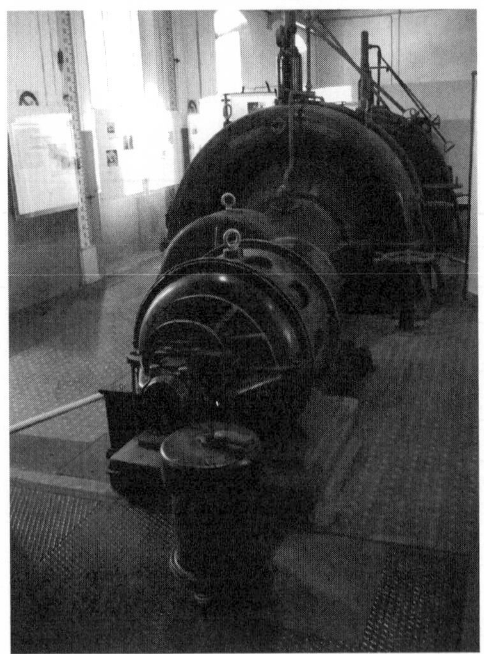

Pumps used for land reclamation at Ostia

entirely, engineers constructed an extensive network of canals. These waterways channeled the annual springtime rush of water from the Lepini Mountains into a final collector known as the Mussolini Canal, which fed the flow harmlessly into the Tyrrhenian Sea. Meanwhile, the planners dug an intricate system of trenches across the plain itself, draining lakes, pools, and marshes. The system of canals, collectors, and trenches ran for a total length of 16,500 kilometers. Engineers also installed eighteen powerful pumps to compensate for insufficient gradient, including the great Mazzocchi Pump (named after the engineer who installed it) with its capacity of thirty-five thousand liters a minute. In addition, they dredged the beds of rivers, shored their banks, and filled all depressions where stagnant water collected.

As this gigantic undertaking got under way, the regime gave no thought to the fate of those few thousand men and women who had eked out a subsistence under the old marshland regime. To realize Mussolini's modernizing fiat, the ONC dispossessed and discarded them—the first casualties of bonifica integrale. Ugo Todaro, the chief engineer for the ONC, made it clear that the sickly woodcutters, herders, fishers, and hunters who inhabited the Pontine Marshes before the Mussolini Law was passed were merely "derelicts of the outdated life on the land" whose health was unimportant. They were obstacles to progress, and their fate was to remain unrecorded in the optimistic statistics by which Mussolini measured his accomplishment. Because the project, in Todaro's words, was "inspired primarily by social purposes," it was not the intention of the regime to allow a few impoverished aborigines to mar the "exemplary, modern, and Fascist life" in the newly constructed society.[29]

BONIFICA AGRARIA

After this transformation in the hydrology and habitation of the Pontine Marshes, the veterans' association turned to the second and more complex front of settlement and intensive cultivation (bonifica agraria). Todaro explained that the intention was to create a sanitary and social utopia embodying the Fascist revolution. In honor of that purpose, the dictatorship declared the area a new Italian province and awarded it the politically correct designation of Littoria in honor of the official emblem of the Fascist Party—the bundled ax known as the *fascio littorio*. The capital city of the new province was to bear the same lofty name, Littoria (which might be rendered into English as Fascistville).

In order to realize the grandiose plan envisioned by Mussolini and implemented by the veterans' association, the ONC imported an army of workers. Their monumental task was to clear and level the newly drained plain, to divide the area into family farms varying in size from four to fifty hectares, and to construct homesteads for the settlers.[30] The workers who carried out this

Table 6.1 Workers Employed in the Pontine Marshes, 1930–1937

1930	41,500
1931	63,260
1932	97,400
1933	124,221
1934	111,117
1935	24,320
1936	22,474
1937	24,420

Source: Data from Oscar Gaspari, "Bonifiche, migrazioni interne, colonizzazioni (1920–1940)," in Bevilacqua, De Clementi, and Franzina, *Storia dell'emigrazione italiana,* vol. 1, 341.

project were manual laborers, employed in the outdoor work of clearing and filling ground, digging canals, laying roads, erecting buildings, and constructing bridges. As the Great Depression swept the nation after 1929, such workers, recruited from the ranks of the unemployed all over Italy, were plentiful. They were also cheap, and in Fascist Italy they enjoyed neither union protection nor political representation. Already in 1929, they began to arrive at the Cisterna railroad station, where they waited in the hope of being hired by the ONC, and set to work in a province that had become one gigantic building and reclamation site. Beginning as a small trickle, their numbers swelled to 41,000 as the first phase of the project—bonifica idraulica—got fully under way in 1930. Then as the battle against malaria broadened into all-out warfare by 1933, the number of workers employed by the ONC and its contractors grew to 124,000 (Table 6.1).

This immense workforce was involved in backbreaking and highly dangerous toil in the marshes. Recruited for deployment in one of Italy's most intensely malarial provinces, many workers arrived at Cisterna without means of self-protection. They often lacked adequate clothing, acquired immunity, the resistance conferred by a sound diet, and the lessons in self-defense imparted by experience with the disease or instruction in rural schools. For such laborers, who were already at risk when they reached Cisterna, well-constructed and sanitary housing was especially important. Unfortunately, sturdy and well-screened accommodation for the laborers involved in reclaiming the land was simply not a Fascist priority. The internal documents of the ONC clearly indicate that the association exposed its workers to a high degree of avoidable risk. Reporting on housing conditions in the first year of bonifica integrale, the ONC leader Enzo Fede wrote, "For workers' accommodations we exploited all available local resources. We used old houses that had been refitted, dormitories that already existed, sheds that were constructed for our needs, and shelters provided by peasants of the surrounding zones and nearby villages. Everything available was used. But, despite inspections, it was impossible not to wish that matters had been better organized."[31] During the second year, as the numbers of workers increased rapidly, conditions deteriorated further. In Fede's words, "It should be noted that housing was not adequate for all of the workers, and one could say that on average it was sufficient for half of them."[32]

The Italian Red Cross also furnished a gloomy assessment of the entrepreneurs' commitment to defending the health of their laborers. In a 1934 report, the Red Cross medical director Nicola Consoli noted that reclamation workers suffered high rates of industrial accidents, tuberculosis, and malaria. With particular reference to the critical issue of housing, Consoli indicated that "the conditions of hygiene are often neglected by the various employers. . . . They are almost invariably reluctant to carry out those hygienic improvements that sanitary professionals recommend to protect the health of their employees. These include the installation of baths and showers, the regular change of the workers' straw mattresses, frequent pest control, . . . and rigorous maintenance of mechanical defenses on doors leading outside."[33] Newly arriving unemployed workers simply slept outdoors near work sites, hoping to replace others who had departed. There they were joined by many who refused to accept the crowded and unsanitary accommodations behind barbed-wire fences that the ONC provided for its dependents.

From the outset, conditions — economic, social, and medical — were severe. Unlike the settlers who followed them, the bonifica workers were temporary and highly expendable. Their role was to sacrifice their own health for the success of the project and then to disappear. Since they were migrants from other regions, their medical fate would never show in official assessments of the Pontine Marshes campaign. Their employment was insecure, their wages were meager, and they received scant medical or sanitary attention. They were also subjected to the rapacious exactions of the contractors who employed them. These entrepreneurs repossessed a portion of the workers' wages by charging them exorbitantly for meals and for the alcohol that flowed abundantly at the close of the workday. Some workers fled, discouraged, before the terms of their contracts had expired; a substantial number contracted malaria; and nearly all experienced sudden dismissal when the first phase of the Fascist project reached completion in 1935.[34]

Unfortunately, there are no known documents that quantify the price paid in death and illness from malaria by the workers who drained and cleared the Pontine Marshes. Various health officials, however, reported a significant burden of disease. Consoli, for instance, described a situation that caused him considerable anxiety. In 1934 he reported that widespread alarm was circulating among the working population of the area. It would be wise, he cautioned, to keep the "many hospitalized patients" out of public view and to conceal the "numerous ambulances making their rounds." "I am learning, perhaps a bit late," he added, "that the truth is not useful in the Pontine Marshes."[35] Similarly, Giulio Alessandrini, the provincial officer of health for Littoria, noted that malaria was sufficiently prevalent in 1933 to cause widespread discontent among the workers. Their grievance was that, when they fell ill, they were transported to hospitals far from their place of employment. After being subsequently discharged, they had to make the return journey on foot, only to find that during their absence, their work tools, clothing, and wage packets had all gone missing.[36] Finally, the minutes of the Provincial Antimalarial Committee meeting of 16 March 1935 contain an expression of serious concern with regard to malaria. Referring to the reclaimed areas of the Pontine Marshes, the committee reported malaria's "special intensity in terms of both the number of victims and the severity of symptoms."[37] Interviewed many decades after the event, Francesco D'Erme, a hydraulic engineer and leading authority on the drainage of the Pontine Marshes, provided a more precise estimate. D'Erme testified in 2003,

> I know as much as anyone alive about the clearing of the waters from the Pontine Marshes. And I know that the workers involved died in large numbers from a variety of causes, especially accidents and disease. If we confine ourselves entirely to deaths from malaria, no fewer than three thousand workers perished from this single cause. Mussolini, however, was supremely indifferent to their fate—at least in private. The reclamation workers, he argued, are like soldiers, and it is the duty of soldiers to die in battle. Publicly, however, Il Duce took care to boast that fewer than one hundred workers died during the project.[38] blatant lie

From the Fascist perspective, such suffering was inevitable and unimportant. The Fascist leader Edmondo Rossoni, for instance, admitted in 1939 that the workers who had been employed on the reclamation and settlement projects had run a serious danger. Like Mussolini, however, he accepted the peril with the nonchalance of a military commander who acknowledges the necessity for casualties during a campaign. "Whoever enters a reclamation project," Rossoni wrote, "can always fall like a soldier going into battle."[39] Contractors were even more cavalier. According to the Italian Red Cross, the contractors "make use of the labor of the humble worker . . . but they abandon him to his own devices as soon as his physical strength has been compromised."[40]

Such results demonstrate the prescience of Giovanni Battista Grassi in his last work. Writing in 1925, just as Fascist plans for the Pontine Marshes were being conceived, he warned that too great a sacrifice would be exacted from laborers "who do not properly value their own health. It causes me profound sorrow to observe that such a sacrifice can occur, that it can be tolerated, and that it can even be encouraged by a country that, like our own, rightly aspires to a place among the leaders on the road to progress."[41] Workers' lives and health were sacrificed to the peremptory timetable set by Il Duce, who wished to demonstrate his power and his ability to sweep aside all obstacles.

After the plain had been cleared and leveled, the ONC and its workforce divided the former marshland into family farms. This phase constituted bonifica agraria (agricultural reclamation). To supervise immigration and settlement, the regime created a new agency in 1931—the Commissariat for Internal Migration and Colonization. The commissariat assumed the task of recruiting healthy peasant families from the Veneto to occupy homesteads as resident sharecroppers in Littoria. The inducement for these families was that the land would become their private property after the successful payment of a series of yearly installments. Between 1932 and the victory celebrations of 1939, approximately sixty thousand peasants immigrated on these terms from northeast Italy. In the words of the president of the ONC, Arnaldo di Crollolanza, "It was not simply a matter of reclaiming land. The goal was to return large numbers of workers to the earth—workers who, from generation to generation, had progressively abandoned the countryside. Through the neglect of the state, this process gave rise to the disastrous phenomenon of urbanization."[42]

Each homestead was equipped in standardized fashion with a sturdy two-story brick farmhouse, stables, a barn, an access road, irrigation ditches, a well, a small vineyard, and fencing. Most important from the standpoint of malaria, the classic "house disease," the ONC placed mechanical barriers—mortar, plaster, and screens—between the settlers and the anopheline mosquitoes that threatened them. The ONC also whitewashed the interiors and equipped the houses with electric lighting so that any mosquitoes that successfully entered the buildings could be seen and killed.[43] In addition, each tenant family received livestock, grain, chemical fertilizer, and a loan to tide the residents over until the property became productive. Furthermore, the Fascist planners built a network of 743 kilometers of public roads and bridges across the province, plus 416 kilometers of access roads to farms; they raised 640 kilometers of high-tension electric lines; they installed 1,080 kilometers of telephone wire; and they planted close to 1.6 million pine trees in rows to break the wind.[44]

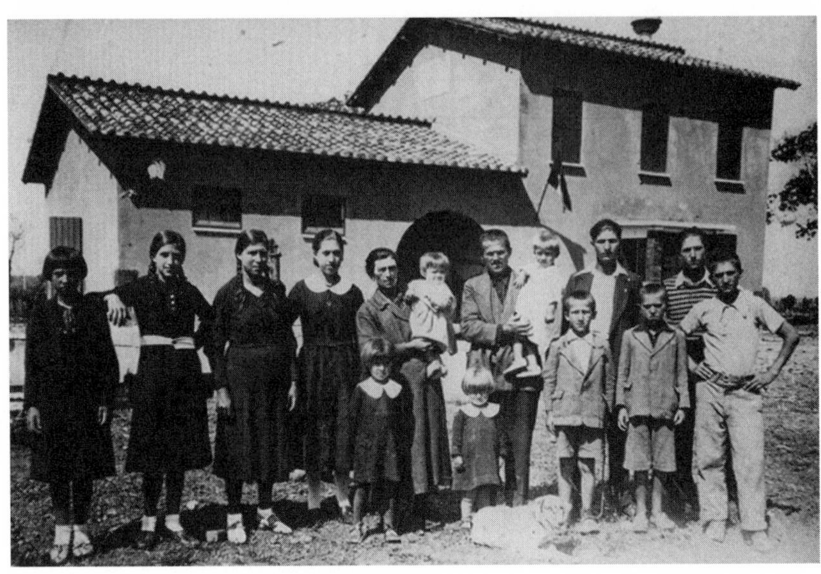

A settler family at their home in Littoria

Then, to cap the rural infrastructure of the new province and to complete bonifica agraria, the ONC built five modernistic cities de novo—Littoria, Pomezia, Sabaudia, Pontinia, and Aprilia, plus eighteen satellite villages (*borgate*). Fascist representatives carefully explained that these urban structures did not contradict the regime's emphasis on "ruralization" and its vision of a Fascist "rural revolution." On the contrary, the cities and villages were centers for "command and control" of the surrounding countryside. Todaro observed that they were just as essential to the agricultural activity of the new province as drainage ditches and roads, and that only a "superficial observer" would regard them as a sign of urbanization. Here, Todaro claimed, was yet another indication of the genius of Il Duce, who invented two new concepts—"rural urban planning" and "cities of bonifica."[45]

The cities of Littoria province served the countryside by housing branches of the Fascist Party and its militia; auxiliary institutions such as the Fascist youth organization Balilla, the leisure association known as Dopolavoro (the "After-Work Association"), and the veterans' association; the police; the church; the tax collector; and local government. There was also provision for such essential services for the rural population as schools, hospitals, and post offices. The satellite villages housed facilities more directly linked with farming—warehouses, grain silos, administrative offices, and lodgings for migrant workers.[46]

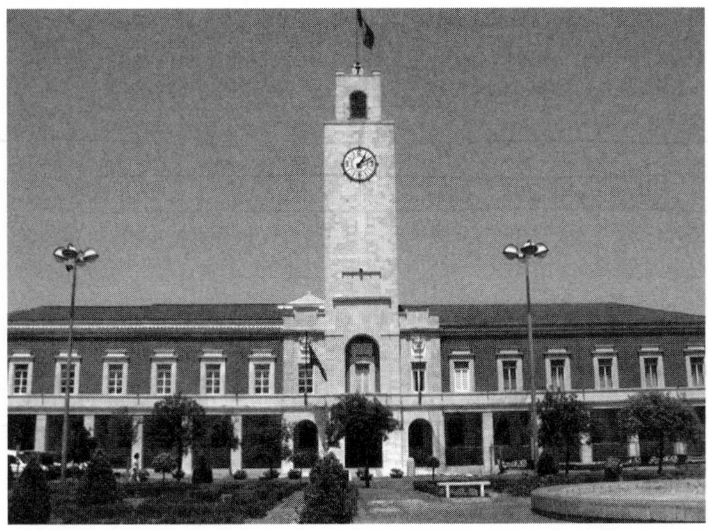

The town hall at Littoria

Todaro further reasoned that the cities and villages of Littoria province would enhance ruralization by making farming a more attractive activity. Through access to well-planned urban centers, peasants could enjoy the benefits of modern life while remaining on the land.[47] Each new municipality would then require its own infrastructure of sewers, cemeteries, piazzas, stadiums, and electric-power-generating stations. To drive home their didactic message, the authorities carefully named the major streets, squares, and buildings of the new cities to honor dates and heroes dear to Fascism. Thus the central squares of Littoria included the Piazza del Littorio and the Largo 28 Ottobre (the date of the Fascist seizure of power in 1922), while the ring road encircling Littoria boasted the name Viale Mussolini (Mussolini Boulevard). Consolidating the regime's selective memory of the battles of the First World War, the satellite villages bore such heroic names as Piave, Isonzo, and Carso.

In the frenzied decade of the 1930s, the ONC and its contractors built all of these structures, raising "centers of healthy rural living" where previously there had been water, bog, and mosquitoes. Measured in terms of cost, the final estimate was that the bonifica agraria of the Pontine Marshes had absorbed 28 million workdays and 549 million lire. But the regime stressed that, in exchange, the entire province had become economically productive. In the late 1930s, the virgin soil of Littoria province provided high yields per hectare and not only fed its constantly growing population but also furnished the markets in Rome with wheat, sugar beet, and hemp, as well as the products of animal husbandry—milk, cheese, and meat.[48]

Controversially, however, bonifica agraria in the Pontine Marshes clearly revealed that the war on malaria was no longer a freestanding objective in its own right, as it had been in the Liberal era. Antimalarial measures instead were conceived as means to further the other political purposes of the Fascist Party. A principal objective, of course, was to provide a dazzling display of power in a highly visible location. Ugo Todaro proudly proclaimed at the outset that the Pontine Marshes would "attract the attention of the whole world" and provide "a grand demonstration of the perfect organization of the Regime when it undertakes the highest tasks demanded by civilization."[49]

For this purpose, Littoria became a showcase for the achievements of Fascism, distracting attention from the comparative neglect of the malarial South, where few initiatives were planned and where fever continued to ravage the population, as Carlo Levi demonstrated in his memoir *Christ Stopped at Eboli*.[50] While the South languished, Littoria became a favorite destination for foreign dignitaries and journalists, as well as for Italian excursionists organized by the Fascist Party, by schools, and by the Dopolavoro. For the edification of those unable to visit Littoria, the regime fulsomely displayed its accomplishments at the grandiose national celebration known as the Decennale, which opened in Rome in 1932 to mark the tenth anniversary of the Fascist seizure of power. The movement also organized a grand exhibition, inaugurated by Il Duce, in the Circus Maximus in 1938 to celebrate the tenth anniversary of the Mussolini Law.[51] In addition, the ONC mounted traveling exhibits devoted to the Pontine Marshes and bonifica integrale, which it presented to the world as the Fascist answer to the Five-Year Plans in the Soviet Union.[52] Within Italy these shows traveled to Rome, Bari, Milan, Turin, Bologna, and Florence. In each of these cities, an exhibit's arrival marked the anniversary of a major event in the Fascist calendar and enjoyed the uncritical adulation of a captive press. The exhibits also journeyed abroad to Munich, Tripoli, New York, and Sophia.[53] The regime also established a newspaper, entitled *Bonifica integrale*, to spread the glad tidings of Fascist accomplishments in the new province. Leading authorities who helped to direct the project, such as Arrigo Serpieri and Giuseppe Tassinari, published annual reports and short popular articles on the Fascists' progress in meeting their ambitious objectives; schools spread news of the regime's victory throughout the peninsula; and the state printed pamphlets in a range of foreign languages to give observers abroad a synthetic overview.[54] On every available occasion, therefore, the Fascist dictatorship announced to the world that the Pontine Marshes were "an achievement that has no comparison in other countries."[55] Postcards and posters bore

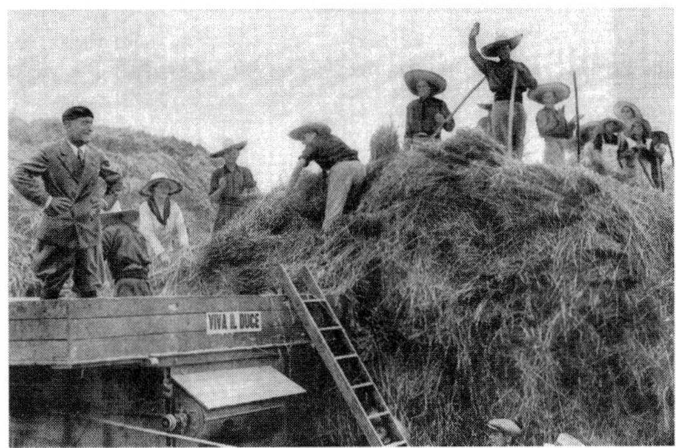

Il Duce visits Littoria

the same message. Most strikingly of all, in his speech inaugurating the new town of Pontinia, Mussolini threw down the challenge that posterity should judge Fascism by the antimalarial policies he had promoted in the Pontine Marshes. Haranguing the faithful from the balcony of the Pontinia city hall, Il Duce announced in 1935, "It is by what we have done in the Pontine Marshes that one must assess the strength of our will, as well as the organizational and creative capacity of the Blackshirt Revolution."[56]

A further important indication of the propaganda possibilities of the newly settled Pontine Marshes was the production of three films devoted to the project. The first was *Camicia Nera* (Black Shirt), a major Fascist propaganda film released in 1933. Made by the official agency Istituto Nazionale LUCE ("L'Unione Cinematografa Educativa" [Educational Cinema Union]) and directed by Giovacchino Forzano, *Camicia Nera* celebrated the first decade of Fascist rule by showing the wonders of Littoria to the world. It portrayed the life of a model worker and wounded hero of the First World War. Revolted by the weakness of the Liberals and the demagoguery of the Socialists, the worker joins the Fascist movement in its violent redemption of the fatherland. After taking part in the March on Rome that brings Mussolini to power, he settles on a farm near Littoria. He and his wife then devote themselves to raising crops and producing sons to become warriors for the future expansion of the fatherland. *Camicia Nera,* therefore, provided an epic depiction of the Fascist revolution, whose culmination was the redemption of the Pontine Marshes and their transformation into healthy peasant farming. In the words of the film historian Elaine Mancini, "The last part of the film concentrates on Fascism's progressive measures. . . . We are shown the draining of the Pontine Marshes, the sample family moving into a better home and buying a tractor, and the country 'returning to order.' A Lexicon of achievements follows: the return of emigrants . . . , construction of homes, public buildings, roads, artificial lakes, train tracks, and 436 kilometers of highways."[57] The message of the film was that Fascism had transformed the "fever of the marshes into the sun of Littoria."[58]

Indeed, the sun figured as a memorable and disturbing trope in the second film—the 1935 documentary *Dall'acquitrino alle giornate di Littoria* (From the Marsh to the Days of Littoria), which was also produced by LUCE. Tracing the history of bonifica, this documentary reached its denouement as the Fascist Party emblem, superimposed on the sun, rose in the east to greet Il Duce. Making his state visit to inaugurate Littoria, Mussolini, as always, spoke from the balcony of the new city hall, which he described as "the symbol of Fascist power."[59]

Appropriately, therefore, the final film was entitled *Sole* (Sun), and it was directed by the famous Fascist cinematographer Alessandro Blasetti. Shot on location in the Pontine Marshes, it bore a heavy weight of political allegory. Blasetti used bonifica integrale as a metaphor for Mussolini's great design to "make Italians." Here the regime claimed to answer at last the famous challenge issued by the Liberal leader and protagonist of Italian unification, Massimo D'Azeglio. D'Azeglio remarked, "We have made Italy. Now we must make Italians." *Sole*'s message was that, by redeeming the swamps, Il Duce had also redeemed Italy and made Italians whole.[60]

The very public proclamation that Littoria (present-day Latina) had become Italy's newest province served a profound political purpose. It evoked major unfulfilled aims of the Italian Liberal government in the First World War—the "redemption" of Italian-speaking territories beyond the borders and their annexation to the fatherland. The Fascist message was clear. While Liberals had failed Italy and Socialists had betrayed her, Mussolini instead delivered a new province to the fatherland—a process that the Fascist theorist Paolo Orano termed "imperial expansion at home."[61] Littoria, moreover, was not a final destination but the dynamic first step toward further conquests abroad as well as at home. The settlement of peasants on newly reclaimed marshland in Italy was a dress rehearsal for colonial expansion in Africa, where Italian settlers would apply the lessons learned in Littoria. In the sly words of the ONC planners in 1932, "The ONC is now beginning its project in the Pontine Marshes, and before long it will be the turn of other areas, both near and far." Indeed, the director of the Health Department of Rome explained that the regime had taken so great an interest in the Pontine Marshes because the conditions there were akin to those Italy would face in East Africa.[62]

Even within existing Italian borders, the example of Littoria was expansive. Fascist planners aimed to rectify the long-term maldistribution of the Italian population whereby fertile lowland areas were thinly inhabited while eroded hills and mountains were overcrowded. Directly addressing this problem, the reclamation of Littoria province served as the prototype for a succession of similar projects in various lowland parts of Italy, such as the Tavoliere, in Apulia, and the lower valley of the Volturno River, in Campania. Begun just as Littoria was nearing completion, these additional schemes were interrupted by the Second World War and never completed. But the intention was clear, as Giuseppe Tassinari, the undersecretary of state for bonifica integrale, explained in 1939 as he surveyed a decade of Fascist accomplishments in the Pontine Marshes. By settling wasteland and bringing virgin soil into successful production, Mussolini hoped to employ the campaign against malaria to advance other Fascist goals such as the "battle for wheat," the "defense of the race," the "battle for births," and the "battle for autarky." In this sense, the regime announced that bonifica integrale embodied the essence of the Fascist revolution. Tassinari wrote, "The battle for wheat and bonifica integrale are thus united in the words of Il Duce because both signify the glory of work, the health of the race, and the independence of the fatherland. The battle for bread and the battle against swamps have been linked . . . in the thought of Il Duce as the foundation for the self-sufficiency in food that is the basis of our battle of autarky."[63]

Internationally famous, the victory at Littoria also lent its luster to legitimize a series of sinister policies that borrowed the magic word *reclamation* (bonifica). The campaign to purge bookstores and libraries of antifascist publications became a "reclamation of books." The imposition of ideological conformity and the racial purging of unwanted Jewish influences became the "reclamation of culture." Meanwhile Fascists misappropriated Grassi's peaceful term for antimalarial therapy, *human reclamation* (bonifica umana), to describe their ultimate, violent goal—to forge a people worthy of Fascism in the crucible of battle.[64]

In addition, settlement of underpopulated wasteland provided a means of permanently relieving the political tensions that had exploded into near revolution during 1919 and 1920—the Red Years of Socialist advance after the First World War. The driving force of this upsurge in political mobilization was the rural workforce of farm laborers in the Po Valley. Already organized in the Giolittian era, these workers acquired additional politicial awareness as a result of the First World War, in which they bore a severely unequal burden of suffering. Since Italian soldiers at the front were overwhelmingly of peasant origin, their already well-articulated grievances acquired an explosive charge of injustice. The revolutionary events in Russia in 1917 acted as an important additional catalyst, especially since Italians viewed the February overthrow of tsarist rule as the seizure of power by the Russian peasantry. Most significantly, in the desperate days that followed the rout at Caporetto in 1917, the state itself, frightened by the combination of revolution in Russia and rebelliousness at home, politicized its army of peasant soldiers. Seeking to give them a reason to fight, it promised land reform after the end of the war. To that end, a newly established Propaganda Service circulated the Leninist slogan "Land to the Peasants!" among the troops together with the promise "Save Italy and She's Yours!" Finally, parliament created the ONC with the specific purpose of aiding landless war veterans in acquiring a homestead. The expectations thus aroused helped to fuel the most powerful peasant movement in modern Italian history as waves of land occupations, strikes, and demonstrations swept the countryside when peace returned and the state lost its reforming ardor.[65]

Therefore, by promising farmworkers land in Littoria province, Mussolini seemed to be making good on a commitment on which the Liberal state had reneged. Thus the Fascist project of transforming the "quality" of Italian demographic expansion by "ruralization" and "deproletarianization" had the avowed purpose of appealing to expectations that had been aroused during the war and then dashed. At the same time, the Fascists hoped to uproot socialist and union militancy at their source. Mussolini aimed to create an obedient and grateful new class of yeoman farmers carefully recruited from the patriotic ranks of the nation's war veterans. In addition, public works on the scale required by bonifica integrale would reduce unemployment and alleviate the social pressures resulting from the Great Depression. While the Western democracies languished, Il Duce strengthened his image as a leader capable of acting resolutely, or as he preferred to claim, "fascistically," at a time of crisis.

It was not by chance that, to achieve this objective, the regime turned for settlers to the Veneto, the northeastern region where wartime devastation had been most intense, where unemployment during the depression was severe, and where the issue of land therefore aroused intense sentiment. The Veneto was also the most deeply Catholic region in Italy. Mussolini hoped that peasants from the Veneto would be deferential to authority and committed to having the large families that both he and the pope, his ally since the signing of the Lateran Pact and Concordat in 1929, so strongly advocated. In this way the Fascists intended that Littoria should become a political and eugenic utopia as well as a sanitary one. Sturdy peasants, thankful to the regime and attached to their newly won property, would breed the many soldiers needed by the dictatorship in pursuit of its expansionist objectives. The Fascists announced, moreover, that settlement on this new frontier was a superior and patriotic alternative to the mass emigration of Italians that had been so salient a feature of the Liberal era. Instead of losing its young men to the New World, Fascism claimed at last to exploit their strength for Italy. As the historian Oscar Gaspari explained, emigration under Mussolini

> was not directed abroad but toward destinations that were domestic or located in [colonial] territories that had been officially proclaimed to be Italian. The intention was that emigration should no longer be "spontaneous" and guided by reasons that were primarily economic. Emigration instead was to be promoted and organized by the Fascist state and designed by it for political reasons. Under the Fascist regime, therefore, the intention was that political emigration would no longer demonstrate the rejection of the government in power by those who departed but would instead display their support.
>
> Fascism sought to transform emigration from a sign of social crisis or even of political protest into an indication of strength and success. At least in the eyes of public opinion, it largely succeeded.[66]

Finally, recruitment of colonists from the Veneto presented medical advantages. Since the Veneto was an intensely malarial region, many of the settlers already possessed experience with the disease, familiarity with strategies of self-protection, and some degree of acquired immunity. At the same time, these colonists from the North, who had been exposed only to vivax malaria, would not harbor the lethal falciparum plasmodia in their bloodstreams. Thus it was possible to recruit colonists with resistance at least to vivax malaria while simultaneously avoiding the danger of introducing the dreaded "pernicious" infections into the new province.

BONIFICA IGIENICA

Having drained, cleared, and settled the land, Mussolini's dictatorship turned to the final aspect of the "eclectic method" that it followed—bonifica igienica (antimalarial hygiene). The purpose was to consolidate the progress gained against malaria through bonifica idraulica and bonifica agricola by treating and protecting individuals. Here Fascist officials introduced few novelties, building instead on strategies devised by the quinine campaign of the Liberal era. In matters of ethos and detail, however, they modified Liberal methodologies to satisfy their own very different ideological ambitions.

To achieve bonifica igienica, the Fascists relied on a variety of institutions that followed in the wake of the settlers. The most important of these was the rural health station, which remained at the heart of the antimalarial effort. As waves of colonists spread across Littoria, two authorities—the appointed governor of Rome (who replaced the capital's elected city council) and the newly created Provincial Antimalarial Committee—established and maintained health stations throughout the Pontine area. G. Pecori and Gioacchino Escalar, the chief health officials for the governor, explained that the health station remained the "linchpin of all effective antimalarial activity."[67] In the annual budget for ongoing antimalarial measures in the Pontine Marshes, health stations received the lion's share.[68]

As in the past, health stations continued under Fascism to provide a comprehensive medical service that sought to win the trust of the rural population, distributed quinine, and brought physicians and auxiliary health-care personnel into the countryside to work and live near the patients they treated.[69] After the disillusionment of the First World War, however, the Department of Health abandoned the hope of quinine prophylaxis, advocated by Angelo Celli and Antonio Dionisi, and elected to rely solely on the radical cure, or bonifica umana, associated with Grassi. The goal was now "to provide treatment that [was] not only immediate but also energetic and prolonged" in order to prevent relapses and to eliminate the mass of inadequately treated patients who were major carriers of parasites.[70] To facilitate such extensive care, every physician in the service was required to compile a census of fever victims, who were to be followed up for six months after their first course of medication.

In addition, the antimalarial service in the interwar period created new categories of officials to carry out two supplementary activities. The first new activity was the task of identifying and treating acute sufferers, and taking aid to chronic patients at their workplaces. This work of detection and follow-up was entrusted to a "nurse/scout." The second new function was the destruction of mosquito larvae. This task, assigned to a "scout," involved locating collections of stagnant water and spraying them with larvicide.

Finally, the authorities attempted to unite the various stations throughout Littoria province into a single network operating in close contact with Rome's fever hospitals, Santo Spirito and San Giovanni. The intent was to eliminate a gap in health-care provision that had weakened the antimalarial service in the past. Because of this gap, malaria victims who had been hospitalized for acute infections often lost contact with physicians after being discharged. Relieved of their symptoms but still carrying plasmodia in their blood, these former patients continued to pose a double risk—the risk (to others) of infection and the risk (to themselves) of relapse. In the 1920s and 1930s, therefore, the campaign instituted a system of close telephone communication between the hospitals in Rome and the health stations in the countryside so that the stations would be notified whenever a malaria patient was discharged from a Roman hospital. Thus alerted in a timely manner, the health stations could then ensure continuity of treatment for the remainder of the lengthy quinine regimen. To reinforce this new system in its dealings with migrant laborers, the hospitals issued patients "health passports" to present to the health station nearest their destination. In this way the policing skills of the dictatorship were brought to bear on public health.

After health stations, the second institution inherited from the past that continued to play a vital part in the Fascist antimalarial campaign was the rural school. Indeed, the regime greatly enhanced the numbers of schools serving the peasantry, systematized and standardized their curricula, and strengthened their role in providing antimalarial information. Fascist authorities regarded rural schools as a critical weapon in the war against malaria. This weapon, moreover, became increasingly important at Littoria as a settled population replaced the nomads of the past.[71] Under Fascism, rural schools proliferated everywhere. By 1943 there were nine thousand, and they had largely achieved at least one goal — the abolition of illiteracy among the rural population.[72]

If the emphasis placed on the teacher in the regime's antimalarial efforts represented an element of continuity with the Liberal past, the content of instruction and the ethos of the schools were profoundly different. In opening the first rural schools in the Roman Campagna, Angelo Celli and Giovanni Cena had conceived of them as institutions of democratic empowerment. Farm laborers and their children heard in Cena's classrooms that they were not mute beasts of burden but thinking citizens with rights and a place in political life. Students received instruction in the three Rs and in the essentials of the new doctrine of malaria. But they also learned that malaria was an occupational disease and that their health depended not only on quinine but also on social justice, on sanitary housing, on a shorter workday, on women's rights, and on union organization. Cena's successor, Alessandro Marcucci, wrote explicitly that "it was necessary to give the peasant the consciousness of being a citizen and a worker."[73] The schools were conceived as an integral part of larger processes of social reform and democratization, which were prerequisites for health.

Fascism was the sworn enemy of the social vision that motivated Celli and Cena. The process of "fascisticization" in the schools, therefore, marked a sea change in the curriculum offered to peasants. In accord with Fascism's hierarchical and military system of values, the schools taught obedience and duty, and they eliminated all discussion of workers' and women's rights. Malaria in Fascist Italy was no longer defined as an occupational disease for which employers were to blame. Schools taught instead that it was a self-inflicted wound for which the sufferer was responsible. Fascist reasoning was that the state had long offered instruction in the basic tenets of malariology and in the necessary mechanisms of self-defense. The disease, in the words of Escalar, "strikes . . . those who do not know how to carry out the specific instruction of the antimalarial campaign or who refuse to do so."[74] Fever, in the eyes of the

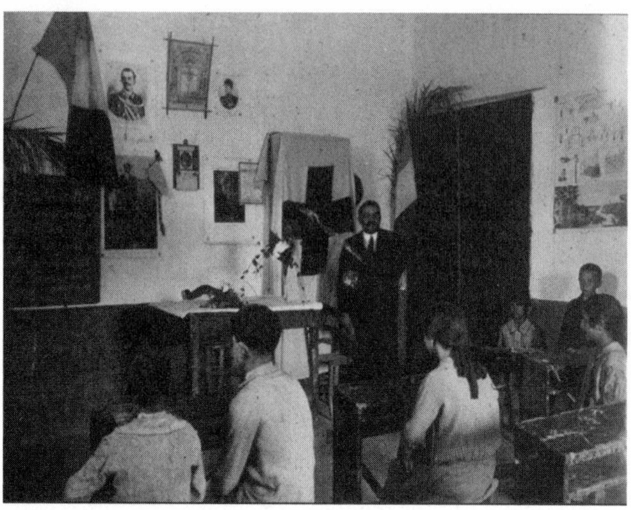

A rural school lesson in Littoria

regime, was the result of ignorance, of negligence, and of the willful desire to shirk personal responsibility. Workers, therefore, no longer had any grounds to call for reforms or to press demands for improvement on farmers and employers.

Explicitly endorsing the military model of imperial Rome, school officials regarded pupils as "young recruits for the great rural army."[75] Accordingly, they were organized into "legions" and "centuries," placed in uniform, and enlisted in the Fascist Party youth organizations — Balilla for boys and Piccole Italiane (Little Italian Women) for girls.[76] Fascist theorist Nicola Pende noted, "It is high time that school in Italy should become the natural breeding ground . . . in which the regime raises its disciplined army of intelligence, of strong arms, and of strong hearts. If it does so, then tomorrow this army will be able to win the triple battle fought by the nation — for economic victory, for political victory, and for victory in the training of the human spirit."[77] In strict adherence to the goals of bonifica integrale, the rural school set out to produce the new "integral man" of Fascism.[78]

As minister of education, the Fascist philosopher Giovanni Gentile had especially favored rural schools in his famous educational reform of 1923. They provided a model of the practical, hands-on, out-of-doors learning that he wished to impart. Marcucci, one of the original founders of the peasant-school initiative, explained that, under Gentile's direction, instruction was bureaucratized and centralized, with the curriculum determined in Rome; the day was rigidly planned and timed; and teachers were encouraged to assume a

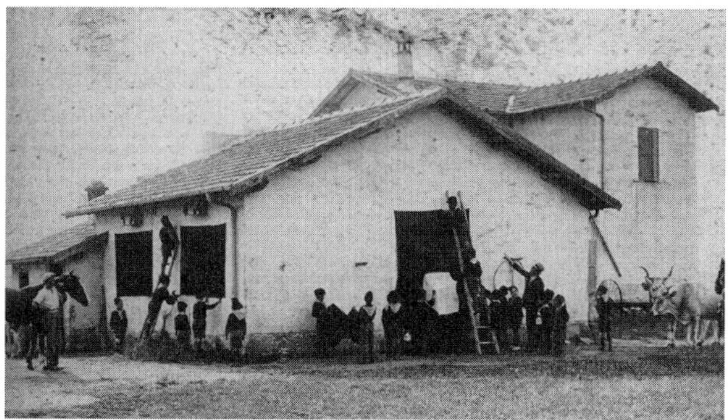

Fascist boy scouts (Balilla) in Littoria learn to use screens

strictly hierarchical relationship with their students, whose role was to be obedient and respectful.[79] Antimalarial instruction in the new curriculum emphasized outdoor activity in the fields, where students learned to locate and treat mosquito-breeding sites, while devoting a minimum of time to classroom activity. Students learned to recognize the symptoms of malaria; to visit workplaces and distribute quinine; to catch imagoes in stables, sties, and homes; to inspect and repair screens; and to appreciate the lengthy regimen of quinine therapy. They were also encouraged to act as informers, reporting to the authorities any family members or classmates who fell ill with suspect symptoms.[80] Finally, students learned the value of Il Duce's agricultural initiatives and how to best support ruralization and the battle for wheat.

In addition to health stations and rural schools, the third important institution inherited from the past by bonifica igienica was the sanatorium. The Sanatorio Antimalarico Ettore Marchiafava (Ettore Marchiafava Antimalarial Sanatorium) brought infected children from the countryside to Rome for a stay averaging two months. There ill children received treatment, a wholesome diet, respite from mosquitoes, and lessons in self-protection from malaria.[81] For the same purpose, the new Littoria province ran a summer camp for children at the seashore—the Lido di Littoria Summer Camp.[82]

The results concerning malaria among settlers were a source of great pride to the regime. In 1939, at the Mostra Nazionale delle Bonifiche, an exhibit on bonifica held in Rome, the Antimalarial Provincial Committee (CPA) of Littoria officially declared "victory over malaria" in the Pontine Marshes.[83] The figures it produced for public display are still on exhibit at the municipal museum at Pontinia (Table 6.2). These statistics, however, make no reference to the plight of the reclamation workers who had preceded the settlers and

Table 6.2 Malaria in Littoria Province, 1930–1939

Year	Population	Cases	Cases per 100 inhabitants	Deaths
1930	5,500	2,625	47.72	4
1931	5,500	1,450	26.63	—
1932	14,106	11,628	82.04	47
1933	41,026	11,507	28.04	14
1934	62,078	10,137	16.32	12
1935	59,877	1,888	3.15	—
1936	51,483	1,263	2.45	1
1937	37,483	435	1.15	1
1938	40,300	228	0.55	0
1939	45,000	33	0.07	0

Source: Reprinted from Gaetano Del Vecchio, "La redenzione igienica," in ONC, *L'Agro Pontino,* table 1, 201.

whose illnesses and deaths were not permitted to mar the official image of constant progress and swift success. In addition, the statistics conflict with the unpublished figures on which the CPA based its annual budgets. Officially, the CPA's figures for malaria in Littoria showed 228 cases in 1938 and 33 in 1939. Off the record, however, the CPA recorded 1,890 cases of malaria in 1938 and 877 in 1939.[84]

The official image was also at odds with an ironic aspect of Mussolini's totalitarian will. According to Fascist propaganda, the regime succeeded in the Pontine Marshes because of the single, all-powerful will of the dictator. Mussolini, his supporters argued, removed with one stroke all of the bureaucratic obstacles that had stymied the parliamentary system. Thus, according to Fascist reasoning, totalitarianism was supremely beneficial to the health of Littoria and its citizens. In reality, however, Mussolini's iron will rapidly found itself mired in bureaucratic tangles and overlapping jurisdictions. Already in the early 1930s the Pontine Marshes witnessed an extravagant proliferation of competing authorities, each with a share of responsibility for public health—the Fascist party and its auxiliary organizations, the schools, the veterans' association, land-drainage consortia, the Ministry of Agriculture with its undersecretary of state for bonifica integrale, the Ministry of Public Works, the Ministry of the Interior with its Department of Health, the Commissariat of Internal Migration, and the provincial and communal officers of health. Instead of cutting the Gordian knot, Fascism created an immense tangle. Indeed, in 1934 it created yet another agency—the CPA—to provide coordination and unity of direction.[85]

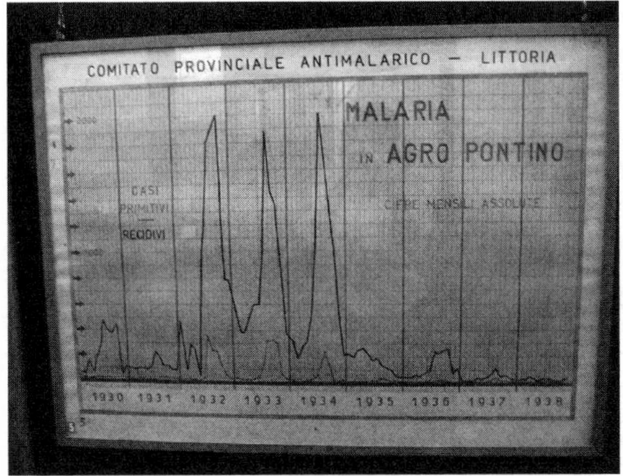

Official graph of the decline of malaria in Littoria, 1930–1938

Even with the CPA in full operation, however, Vincenzo Rossetti, the municipal officer of health for Littoria, reported that unity and coordination were sadly lacking. Neighboring municipalities, for instance, undertook contradictory policies. Furthermore, funds from the ministries "arrived when they arrived," often after long delays, and sometimes only after significant sums had disappeared into mysterious channels of graft and political favoritism. Here in the realm of public health was an Italian manifestation of the phenomenon that under the Nazi dictatorship has been called "institutional Darwinism"—the systematic competition of multiple agencies with overlapping jurisdictions and clashing responsibilities but no public accountability.[86] The effects, Rossetti pointed out, were deleterious to public health. As he explained, "In few sectors is the coordination of all initiatives the fundamental basis of success as it is in the field of malaria. What possible advantages can the officer of health of one township hope to obtain by a well-organized and rationally conducted antimalarial campaign when in a contiguous township little is done, and that little irrationally?"[87]

Racism and Malaria

Perhaps the most sinister aspect of the Fascist antimalarial campaign in the Pontine Marshes was its integration into an overarching scheme to transform Italy into a racial utopia as well as a sanitary one. The newly reclaimed Pontine Marshes became the testing ground for a program to breed an Italian superrace. Ignoring such intractable social problems as the Southern Question, poverty, unemployment, and the ongoing endemic of malaria in great swathes of the nation, racism enabled the regime to mobilize an upsurge of popular delirium by offering biological pseudosolutions. More aggressively, racism legitimized the appetite of the dictatorship for expansion and international violence—an appetite that it whetted in Littoria and attempted to satisfy first in Abyssinia and then in its larger quest for the new Roman Empire, which it promoted by launching Italy on a new round of world war.[88]

To accomplish its purposes, the regime capitalized on a deep-seated current of racial anxiety. Many Italians feared that the poor performance of the military—both in Africa, as demonstrated in the humiliating defeat at Adowa in 1896, and in the First World War—and the relative economic backwardness of the nation in comparison with the more-developed industrial powers were due to an inferior genetic inheritance. Although there was nothing in the teachings of the Rome School or in the doctrine of Grassi and Celli to suggest that malaria led to a tainted heredity, there was a widespread belief that chronic afflictions such as malaria, tuberculosis, and alcoholism led—by biological mechanisms that were never clearly defined—to genetic deterioration and national decline. This idea had a long history in Italy. One of the early anxieties of the Rome municipal council after the city was annexed to the nation was the looming danger of racial degeneration caused by malaria. Fever, the council fretted in 1873, "causes the race to decline by favoring the production of weak and debilitated offspring," who in turn "generate abortive seed for future generations."[89] Half a century later, in 1926, the Sicilian doctor F. Salpietra expressed the same idea—that one of the great perils of malaria is its tendency to produce "progressive deterioration in the development of a race."[90] At nearly the same time, the Red Cross malariologist Franco Genovese, writing in 1924 of his first trip to Calabria, uttered his "dismay" at the sight of "men belonging to a race that has been undermined."[91] Such fears were the essence of the Italian "race problem."[92] It was a sign of anxious times that a leading Fascist cultural journal adopted as its title *La difesa della razza* (The Defense of the Race).[93]

Thus the national campaign against malaria held out the hope of yet another bonifica—the "reclamation of the race." This plan involved two related components. The first was defensive: by reducing the burden of malaria through bonifica integrale, the Fascist regime claimed that it was halting the deterioration of the national gene pool. The second strategy was to improve the national inheritance through eugenics. In this light the regime regarded the Pontine Marshes as the breeding grounds for a great Italian race worthy of empire.[94] The Rome newspaper *Tribuna* (Tribune) clearly understood this objective when its reporter Marco Franzetti toured Littoria and talked to settlers. He reported with pride that he had encountered children who were blond and "of sound race" — "each a future little soldier." At the same time, he admired the adult men for "possessing a serene visage and a body with the strength of Hercules."[95]

To comprehend Fascist eugenics, one needs to appreciate that the dominant racial doctrine in Italy rejected Aryan tenets of racial purity. In the racial cosmology of thinkers like Nicola Pende, Paolo Orano, and Giuseppe Sergi, the world was divided by color into the white, black, yellow, and red races.[96] It was, in their view, a crime against nature to allow miscegenation across any of these color barriers, which also separated Jews from the white race. Only catastrophe and racial suicide could result from such crossings. By introducing laws to restrict interracial breeding, Mirko Ardemagni wrote in the Fascist theoretical journal *Gerarchia* (Hierarchy), the Fascist revolution would save the white race and European civilization.[97] Mussolini explicitly endorsed this rescue mission.

Within the great white race, however, there were various subraces, or *stirpi,* such as Aryans, Latins, Ligurians, Calabrians, and Etruscans. Since these groups shared racial "affinities," the happy result of crossing them would be to produce superior offspring endowed with hybrid vigor. Although racial theorists disagreed about the exact number and identity of the subraces that inhabited the Italian peninsula, they concurred that the historical mission of Fascism was to produce the dynamic Italian "synthesis" or "harmony" of Italy's various related peoples.[98] Indeed, here was the ultimate significance of Fascist plans for the Pontine Marshes. First, bonifica integrale would free the area of disease and hence eliminate the danger of racial degeneration through fever. Then, by settling the new province of Littoria with peasants "carefully selected by anthropometric criteria" from the various Italian racial stocks and allowing  them to intermarry while protecting them from crossings with nonwhites or Jews, the Fascist regime would practice sound "racial eugenics."[99] Acting as the guardian of this racial utopia, the Commissariat of Internal Migration and Colonization screened potential settlers, whom it required to be of "pure Italian race."[100] In Fascist thinking, therefore, the "bonified" Pontine Marshes were the field on which yet another battle was to be fought — the "battle for the race."[101] Littoria province would become the site for "centers for the rational breeding of selected individuals" who should be provided with certificates of racial health entitling them to marry.[102]

In the opinion of Il Duce, a race and its land were inseparable. Thus, in the mystical union of the Italian race with the soil of the Italian peninsula, the reclamation of the land would also improve the biological and spiritual qualities of the people who lived on it.[103] It was as if, by a mysterious inversion of traditional miasmatic teachings, the virtues of a redeemed soil would emanate life-enhancing, healthy effluvia that could penetrate the genes of the fortunate population.

In this heady vision, the Pontine Marshes were "human nurseries" for "crossings among different Italian races"—interbreedings that would yield great rural warriors who would proliferate and build a new Roman Empire. Public health physicians, such as the Littoria provincial officer of health, Giulio Alessandrini, conducted anthropometric measurements to determine the extent to which the children of desirable crossings were yielding the expected results. Alessandrini explained, "In coordination with the Italian Anthropological Society we have begun numerous research projects to determine the influence that immigration into new regions . . . and the crossing of imported and local races can have on the physical and intellectual development of the children."[104]

Indeed, for some of the leading theorists of bonifica integrale, strengthening the race was the primary function of the exercise.[105] For Mussolini himself and for Giuseppe Tassinari, the undersecretary of state for bonifica integrale, the clear and explicit intention was to redeem the race along with the land.[106] A major purpose of their eugenic strategy was to provide a biological solution to some of Italy's most difficult social problems. Fascism claimed, above all, to have solved the Southern Question. According to U. Mellana,

> As a result of centuries of neglect by the governments of the past, there arose in the southern provinces . . . harmful differences between North and South and odious sectionalism. Their roots lie in the different structures of property, of society, and of the economy in the two regions. . . .
>
> Now bonifica causes these differences to disappear, and each region is linked to the other by the unity of a common redeeming direction, by increased wealth and an improved society, and by greater attachment to the fatherland.[107]

The debilitating regionalisms that created such deep fault lines in the nation would be overcome by a deeper biological unity—"a mixing of blood"—brought about by sound racial breeding.[108] The resulting Italian superrace would also be more attached to the soil, more fertile, more creative, and more bellicose. Thus endowed, this master race could resolve the long-term Italian problems of economic backwardness, military defeat, and malaria. Fascism—"the political expression of the Italian race"—needed only to provide the necessary race consciousness.[109]

This rural and racial ideal also had profound implications for the position of women. Littoria province was the Fascist riposte to the feminist advances of the Giolittian era. Mussolini's vision of the Pontine Marshes was of a patriarchal paradise where women performed only their biological and reproductive functions. Here was the subliminal message that lurked behind Fascism's emphasis on superior racial breeding. A world where the function of women was to breed prolifically on behalf of the state was also a world in which women were excluded from public life and assigned a role of dependency in the private sphere. A province where the overriding task was to prepare for war was also a province where the voice of women would not be heard.

A problem with the biological politics of race and antifeminism was that they induced "magic" thinking. For example, the bill authorizing the establishment of Littoria as a municipality presented the reclamation project to parliament as a "miracle."[110] Similarly disquieting was Alessandrini's gushing observation that the city had "risen as if by a magic spell cast by the swift and nimble touch of a fairy's wand."[111] Instead of devising rational solutions to the problems of the South, the economy, and malaria, the dictatorship offered the pseudoscience of race and the utopian vision of traditional family life in an idyllic Fascist community. Still worse, such thinking misled the regime into believing that in the quest for imperial glory, the inherent superiority of the "Italian race" made up for its lack of military, economic, and strategic preparation for modern warfare. This lack of logic contributed in no small measure to the catastrophe that ensued during the Second World War, which resubmerged the Pontine Marshes in water and unleashed a new epidemic of malaria.

Ideology and Malariology

Ideological thinking led to heavy costs in the field of public health, particularly with regard to malariology. Giuseppe Sanarelli, Grassi's colleague at the University of Rome, raised the alarm at an early date. In his 1925 work *Lo stato attuale del problema malarico* (The Present State of the Malaria Problem) he attempted to assess the achievements of science concerning malaria and to indicate the directions in which further basic research was essential if Italy was to solve the greatest of its health problems. While appreciating the worth of the breakthroughs that had been made, from Laveran's microscopic parasites to the more advanced doctrine of the Rome School, Sanarelli believed that there were major areas of darkness that needed to be illuminated before eradication could become a feasible policy. He noted that there was no understanding of such issues as relapses, immunity, the overwintering of mosquitoes, the mechanism of quinine, spontaneous cures, quinine intolerance, and drug resistance. In addition, the speciation of anopheline mosquitoes was only dimly apprehended, and the distinction between clinical cure and radical cure was poorly understood. With such fundamental questions still unanswered, Sanarelli called for a wave of "experimental investigations" to find "new ways" to attack malaria.[112]

Sanarelli was doubtful, however, that such "new ways" would be explored under the regime that had so recently come to power. In the universities, funding for basic scientific research was inadequate because teaching was considered the priority, and there were no major laboratories outside the universities to compensate. Italy lacked institutes comparable to the Pasteur Institute in France, or the Rockefeller Foundation in the United States, and the National Department of Health lacked the facilities for world-class research. Such was the problematic legacy that was apparent even as Mussolini came to power. The problem was that, under Fascism, the needs of malariology and the allied sciences were not appreciated by public opinion or by the political authorities.[113]

Within a few years it became apparent that Sanarelli's warning had fallen on deaf ears and that his proposals had met only "indifference and skepticism."[114] Inherent in the strategy of bonifica integrale was a fundamental anti-intellectualism that was characteristic of Fascism. Bonifica integrale was a policy built on impatience. Mussolini was intolerant of obstacles and delays of any kind. In his view, which gave no importance to the long term, science had already done enough. The "great doctor," who had received no training in science, believed that the time for discussion and research was finished.[115] All that was still needed was the indomitable will that would put what was already known into practice. The search for new knowledge was a wasteful diversion. Alberto Missiroli, the leading Italian malariologist of the interwar period, reflected the thinking of the regime. He announced in 1929, "In the field of malaria I believe, therefore, that the need today is to extend the practical application of the knowledge that we already have rather than to broaden what we know. By that statement I do not mean to imprison learning within the columns of Hercules, but I do intend to stress that our current understanding is already sufficient to prevent this disease, provided that it is well applied."[116] Missiroli was symptomatic of the transformation under way in Italian malariology. An organizer, an administrator, and a willing servant of power more than a pioneering researcher, he did not follow the tradition of Golgi, Celli, Grassi, and Marchiafava.

In this new context, the announcement by the dictatorship, and by a voice as authoritative as that of Missiroli, that the scientific problems of malaria had already been solved created a climate of expectation that was inimical to research and that discouraged young scientists from entering the field. The withering effect of the Fascist regime on basic malariology was well described in the 1930s by the eminent American expert L. W. Hackett, one of the leading scientists of the Rockefeller Foundation. In the 1920s, in recognition of the pioneering role of Italians in the field of malariology, the Rockefeller Foundation chose Italy as a major site for carrying out its program of medical research and philanthropy. It sent Hackett to establish a network of malaria research stations and to encourage the Italian government to adopt a close link between public health and scientific research. The foundation was especially interested in finding new insecticides and larvicides that would allow the state to attack mosquitoes instead of continuing the traditional Italian method of assaulting plasmodia with quinine. The vision of the foundation was that an Institute of Hygiene and Public Health should be founded in Rome to emulate the Pasteur Institute and the Rockefeller Foundation itself.[117] The foundation also hoped that the Italian state would take on its "true function, which is the prevention of disease and the repression of epidemic outbursts"—a function that required a unity of direction that only central government could provide.[118]

These ventures were a disappointment to the foundation, which discovered that the regime lacked enthusiasm and commitment to the cause. Promoting science was not one of its priorities. Hackett found his experience with the Italian authorities to be disillusioning.[119] He wrote in 1932 that the Department of Health was unable to provide effective leadership to the national eradication campaign. Since the department "really lacks credit in the highest political circles," the effect was a system of "mutually independent, inconsistent and often ineffective antimalarial activities scattered over the country."[120] In his diary he also noted paralyzing turf wars between the Department of Health and the Ministry of Public Works, and the lack of commitment to basic scientific research.[121] Despite the monolithic image that it projected, Fascist Italy never operated as a smoothly functioning mechanism of bureaucratic rationality and efficiency under a unitary will.

Thus an Institute of Malariology was established, but it proved to be no rival to the Pasteur Institute or the Rockefeller Foundation. On the contrary, it was dedicated to training public health officials rather than to undertaking basic scientific research.[122] Furthermore, the state, believing that it had found the high road to success against malaria with bonifica integrale, diverted funds from research and provided few incentives for promising young scientists to enter the discipline. Pursuing political objectives rather than public health, the dictatorship cut off funds to the structures that had produced Italian international preeminence in the field, and relied on intellectual capital from the past. The laboratories at the National Department of Health, the Rockefeller Foundation representatives in Italy found, were "inadequate for such a task in space, equipment, personnel, and function." Consequently, "the government lacked an efficient instrument in the Health Department for analytical and research activities, and a health department without an efficient laboratory at its back and unable to undertake . . . field studies and laboratory research is practically inactive except in emergencies, and loses prestige and public support."[123]

At the same time, research in Italian universities stagnated for lack of state funds. R. A. Lambert, another Rockefeller scientist, reported to New York in 1933 that, although there were hardworking and talented Italian investigators, "the difficulty lies largely in the totally inadequate facilities and budgets for research."[124] By 1948, the foundation concluded that "Italian health organization is very inefficient and its reorganization is long overdue."[125] At the same time the *Rivista di malariologia* (Review of Malariology), the journal of record in the field, lamented that the Italian School had lost nearly all of its internationally famous malariologists. Only one—Giuseppe Bastianelli—remained. As a result, Italy was ill prepared either to face the medical crisis that exploded with the Second World War or to resume its role of world leadership in malariology in the postwar era.[126]

7

Creating Disaster: Nazism and Bioterror in the Pontine Marshes

When he broke the fourth seal, I heard the voice of the fourth creature say, "Come!" And there, as I looked, was another horse, sickly pale; and its rider's name was Death, and Hades came close behind. To him was given power over a quarter of the earth, with the right to kill by sword and by famine, by pestilence and wild beasts.

— *Revelation 6:7–8*

With the decision to launch its program of imperial expansion and foreign conquest, Fascism dealt a severe blow to the campaign against malaria. Even before the onset of the Second World War, the shift in political priorities led directly to the erosion of funds for the malaria campaign. Italy, the weakest of the European powers, could not afford both war and public health. Mussolini's belligerent foreign policy signified the end of new state initiatives in the struggle against malaria and a steep decline in support for those already in place. Thus an unspoken corollary of the decision to invade Abyssinia in 1935 was that the period of active Fascist involvement in the war against fever came to an end. Thereafter, preparation for war subverted public health.[1]

When Mussolini entered the Second World War as Hitler's ally in 1940, the effects on the malaria campaign were even more severe. Total war again caused a great upsurge of fever. Indeed, the recrudescence of malaria that

Table 7.1 Malaria in Italy, 1941–1945

Year	Cases	Deaths
1941	118,221	756
1942	164,082	1,075
1943	—	—
1944	373,940	422
1945	471,602	386

Source: Data from G. A. Camperia and T. Patrissi, "La malaria in Italia nel periodo bellico e post-bellico," *Rivista di malariologia,* XVII (1948), 3.

occurred from 1941 to 1945 was a reprise of the upsurge that had prevailed during and just after the First World War, as health authorities noted at the time (Table 7.1).

Just as in the First World War, the disease not only claimed substantial numbers of victims but also reappeared in provinces from which it had been banished, reversing earlier victories. In the words of Felice Jerace, editor of *Rivista di malariologia* (Review of Malariology),

> As everyone now knows, the war left many sad memories, including that of the epidemic upsurge of malaria. For centuries malaria has waxed and waned in accord with the events of history. . . .
>
> Wartime and the consequences connected to it have caused incalculable damage . . . to the bonification facilities, and it has created other environmental conditions favorable to malaria.[2]

The causes that produced the malarial upsurge in the Second World War were similar to those that had so negatively affected public health during the First. Parallels were numerous. Once again, the antimalarial campaign ground almost to a halt as the army drafted physicians and nurses. Just as quinine had become unavailable in the conflict of 1914–1918, so the alkaloid and its synthetic replacements ran short during 1940–1945. Another recurring problem was that warfare reversed the intensification of agriculture, thereby providing mosquitoes with extensive breeding opportunities. Mobilization, which disproportionately affected the peasantry, deprived the countryside of labor. As a result, irrigation ditches, reclamation projects, and environmental sanitation were all abandoned amid general neglect. Inevitably, women, children, and elderly men, all lacking immunity, were forced to the fields to replace absent soldiers, thus exposing themselves to infection. There was also an influx of veterans who had served in the Balkans and who carried disease back to their homes upon their return.

Another similarity to the conditions of the First World War was that standards of living declined severely for the civilian population, lowering resistance, undermining productivity, and greatly increasing exposure to anopheline mosquitoes. Serious disruptions in the economy led to widespread unemployment and wages that lagged far behind the cost of living, which, in turn, led to hunger, rationing, and malnutrition. The requisitioning of animals also led to the collapse of zooprophylaxis—the attempt to divert mosquitoes from humans to other large mammals. At the same time, the passage of warring armies through the peninsula caused widespread destruction of housing and displaced whole populations, who were forced to sleep in open fields or seek shelter in barns and stables. Artillery shells and bombs also produced deep craters that rapidly filled with rainwater and insect larvae.[3] Hospitals, in the words of the United Nations, "were doubly handicapped—first by destruction of buildings and secondly by the systematic looting of beds, equipment, X-Ray facilities, and ambulances by the retreating enemy. They thus had to face the almost insuperable problem of having insufficient space, beds, and equipment with which to deal with an unprecedented flow of patients."[4]

Alberto Missiroli, the Italian physician who collaborated most closely with the Rockefeller Foundation in its antimalarial initiatives in Italy, directed the campaign to combat the upsurge created by the Second World War. He noted the striking similarities between the medical events of both world wars. Indeed, he argued that the only salient difference was the absence of pandemic influenza as a complication of malaria during the second conflict. Missiroli wrote in 1945,

> During the Great War . . . a marked increase in malaria was noted, due in part to the movement of large non-immunized population groups from malaria-free to extremely malarious zones, and in part to the slowing up of preventive measures and to the importation of gametocyte carriers to zones hitherto free from malaria. . . .
>
> Thus during the Great War we observed the re-appearance of malaria in numerous regions in Italy where it had previously ceased to exist and its increase in those regions where it already existed. . . .
>
> If we wish to compare the mortality and morbidity of malaria from 1938 to 1944 with the same data covering the period 1914–1918, we must bear in mind that the rapid rise in the mortality curve during the years 1917–1918 was due to a great extent of malarious persons from pneumonic influenza. Keeping this in mind, it is clear that the mortality curve for malaria during the period 1939–1943 presents the same characteristics as that covering the last war.[5]

Ironically, Littoria (renamed Latina after the fall of Fascism), which Mussolini had intended to make malaria-proof, now became the province of Italy that suffered most severely from the war-induced epidemic. The Littoria epidemic of 1944–1946 dramatically demonstrates the failure of Mussolini's greatest antimalarial program, laying bare the hollowness of the Fascist claim to have solved Italy's ancient problem of fever. Ultimately, Mussolini's foreign policy comprehensively destroyed the great Fascist reclamation project, restoring the province to the conditions that had prevailed in the nineteenth century.

Littoria and the German Retreat

To understand how Mussolini's alliance with Germany destroyed his accomplishments in the Pontine Marshes, we need to note the rapidly deteriorating position of Hitler's army in 1943. By the middle of that year the Axis had fallen apart. Facing military catastrophe, King Victor Emmanuel III ordered Il Duce's arrest on 25 July 1943 and appointed a successor government led by General Pietro Badoglio. Then, on 8 September 1943, in one of the most dramatic moments of the war, Italy changed sides in the conflict. Once Hitler's ally, Italy became a co-belligerent alongside Britain and the United States.[6]

For the German leadership, this betrayal recalled the Italian apostasy of the First World War, when Italy declared war on Germany despite being her ally (in the Triple Alliance of Germany, Italy, and Austria-Hungary). Indeed, Germans now suspected that the Italian presence in the Axis had always been a matter of sheer opportunism. Italy, they believed, had hoped to take advantage of the victories of the Wehrmacht while bearing a minimal share of the burdens of war. Many of the foremost leaders in Hitler's regime saw in Italian behavior a simple proof of what they had always suspected—the racial inferiority of the Latin peoples, who were born to be slaves rather than world conquerors. Nazis also feared that the Italian example of bloodlessly overthrowing Mussolini in July 1943 could set a dangerous precedent for cashiering Fascist leaders—a precedent that, under the pressure of military defeat, could spread across the Alps with destabilizing effects on Hitler's rule. Refusing to accept responsibility for the disaster befalling the Reich, many Nazi leaders also selected Italy as the scapegoat they could blame for the German defeat in the East. The Nazis held the Italians responsible for draining the Wehrmacht of resources at critical moments through their inept campaigns in the Balkans and North Africa. Nazi reaction now was swift and punitive. In a 1993 study, Richard Lamb illustrated the German desire for vengeance by recalling the view of Colonel Eggenreiner, the liaison officer between the Wehrmacht and the Italian army: "Following the events of 8 September, German public opinion was 'exceptionally bitter' toward Italy. . . . [Eggenreiner's] view was that, had it not been for the 'good discipline' of the army, German soldiers in Italy would have committed outrages against the civilian population. Anti-Italian feeling was certainly reflected in atrocities against surrendering Italian soldiers."[7]

In the immediate aftermath of the September betrayal, German troops occupied most of the territory of their former ally (now turned enemy), save for a corner in the southeast controlled by the government of Badoglio and King Victor Emmanuel. The German army also rescued Mussolini from imprisonment and installed him as the head of a puppet regime in northern Italy—the notorious Republic of Salò, which had no independent power base, no army, and no mass following. Tellingly, the ultimate result of Mussolini's arrest in June was that, faced with military defeat, the Fascist Party had simply dissolved, undefended and unmourned. Mussolini's hastily reconstructed neofascist Republic, therefore, served primarily to provide a cover of legitimacy for the harsh reality of German occupation. Now regarding the Italians as treacherous enemies and racial inferiors, Hitler's army began systematically subjecting them to the same brutal policies that had been applied in Eastern Europe. An outburst of partisan activity just behind the fighting front further enraged German commanders, who employed a strategy of terror to deprive the resistance of popular support. Occupation, therefore, rapidly produced a crescendo of violence as the Germans embarked upon the tasks of plundering Italian economic resources, conscripting forced labor, destroying Italian Jews, and terrorizing the population into submission.[8]

A sinister leap in violence occurred in May 1944 when Heinrich Himmler and the commander in chief of the Wehrmacht, General Wilhelm Keitel, reached an agreement on the nature of the occupation and transmitted their conclusions to the German authorities in Italy. As two leading scholars of the German occupation—Michele Battini and Paolo Pezzini—explain, this agreement between Himmler and Keitel, reinforced by a series of orders from the German commander for the Italian theater, General Albert Kesselring, involved three critical determinations affecting the welfare of Italian civilians. The first was that the Wehrmacht under Kesselring should have full authority for directing all aspects of the occupation. The second was that German forces should make no distinction between the treatment of combatants and resistance fighters on the one hand and unarmed civilians on the other. The third was that subordinate commanders would not be held responsible for any excesses they committed in applying the new policy.[9] According to Battini and Pezzini, these decisions and Kesselring's subsequent orders established an "organized, coherent, and planned system" that unleashed a "war against civilians" marked throughout the area under German control by a grim succession of such events as the massacre of unarmed men, women, and children; the destruction of entire villages; the confiscation of farm animals and livestock; and the abduction of able-bodied men to perform slave labor for the Reich. As Battini, Pezzini, and other scholars make clear, such atrocities occurred repeatedly for the remainder of 1944, often without the provocation of partisan activity in the areas where they were committed and without apparent military advantage. As in Eastern Europe, so too in Italy terror against the civilian population became an end in itself. An indication of the extent of German atrocities in Italy is the intention of the British authorities just after the end of the conflict. After carefully gathering evidence, they resolved to conduct a second Nuremberg trial in which the German occupying forces would be systematically prosecuted for war crimes committed between 8 September 1943 and 5 May 1945.[10]

By 1943 the tide of war had turned definitively against the Third Reich. The decisive events were occurring on the eastern front, and the Mediterranean theater of war was secondary. Nevertheless, the diplomatic revolution of 8 September and the subsequent declaration of war on Germany by the Badoglio government greatly weakened Germany's global military position. After losing Sicily to the Allies, the German army took up defensive positions on the Italian mainland along the Gustav Line, which stretched across the peninsula from a point just south of Gaeta on the Tyrrhenian Sea to Ortona on the Adriatic. Already, however, the Germans expected further Allied advances. The German command anticipated that the Allies would outflank the German defenses, anchored at Cassino, by carrying out a landing on the Tyrrhenian coast somewhere between Gaeta and Livorno. Their fears materialized when British and American forces landed at Anzio and Nettuno in January 1944. Since Hitler was unwilling to divert significant resources from his apocalyptic struggle against Bolshevism in the East, the desperate strategy of the Wehrmacht in Italy was to hinder Allied progress for as long as possible in order to delay the final assault on Germany itself and to allow the Führer time at last to deploy his terrible "secret weapons." This strategy implied fiercely defending the Gustav Line and containing the Anzio beachhead to the last possible moment, then slowly retreating farther north while German engineers constructed a new fortified position—the Gothic Line—across the Apennines in central Italy. In this stage of the conflict, the gathering signs of final defeat and the urgent need to shield Germany enhanced the savagery of occupation policy toward the Italians.

It was in this context of impending military crisis and vengeful occupation policy that Germany implemented a violent scheme—a plan of biological warfare carried out in the reclaimed Pontine Marshes. German motives were twofold: to delay final defeat by any means and at any cost, and to exact revenge. In pursuit of these twin ambitions, the Germans carried out the only known example of biological warfare in twentieth-century Europe.

Even before the Germans implemented this plan, warfare had already caused a serious decline in public health in the province of Littoria. As early as 1942, the Provincial Antimalarial Committee (CPA) reported a worrying upsurge in the incidence of fever. The population, the CPA explained, was susceptible to disease because the poverty and inadequate diet resulting from economic collapse had compromised its resistance. Quinine prophylaxis had also ceased because the province lacked both supplies of the alkaloid and the medical personnel necessary to distribute them. At the same time, mechanical protection had become impossible because metal was no longer available to install or repair screening. As a result of the shortage of labor, it had become impossible to maintain the drainage works that had been the pride of Fascism. Finally, returning veterans from Greece and Albania had introduced new and resistant strains of falciparum malaria.[11] Already the health officials of Littoria were alarmed that such a recrudescence of fever in Mussolini's medical showcase would have serious and destabilizing political repercussions, "especially if one thinks of the magnitude and high aims of the reclamation work conceived and carried out by the regime in the Pontine Marshes."[12]

In this already compromised environment, the Germans carefully and scientifically devised a strategy of biological warfare with a dual purpose. By late 1943, the Pontine Marshes occupied a strategic position in the direct path of any further Allied movement up the peninsula. By flooding Littoria province and unleashing a public health crisis, the Germans hoped, first, to buy themselves time and, second, to settle scores with the Italians for their betrayal.

Detailed knowledge of the hydraulic mechanisms that were used to contain malaria in the Pontine Marshes informed German strategy. Although bonifica integrale had dramatically reduced the prevalence of malaria, Mussolini's intervention had not entirely eradicated the disease. Indeed, German scientists knew that malaria was already on the rise in the province. They calculated that, by destroying the hydraulic infrastructure of bonifica integrale, they could create ideal conditions for the most deadly vector in Italy. The result would be an epidemic of extraordinary virulence.

During the period of the Axis alliance, German malariologists had worked closely with their Italian counterparts in a variety of settings—at the University of Rome, at the Superior Institute of Hygiene, and at the School of Malariology in Nettuno. Their Italian hosts had explained with pride the epidemiology of malaria in the Pontine Marshes and the means that controlled the disease. The Germans understood that, as a result of the poor natural drainage of the plain, one could create a flood simply by halting the pumps that lifted water and ensured its flow into the Tyrrhenian Sea. Accordingly, in October 1943, as the rainy season began, the German army ordered that the great water pumps that cleared the plain be stopped. This action was intended to create a watery obstacle that would slow the British and Americans when they broke through the Gustav Line.

In addition, however, German scientists Erich Martini of the University of Hamburg and Ernst Rodenwaldt of the University of Heidelberg were aware of a further lethal detail. One of the major advances in malariology during the 1930s was a growing understanding of the speciation of anopheles mosquitoes. With respect to the Pontine Marshes, the relevant point was that, of the multitude of mosquito species infesting the area, only one—*Anopheles labranchiae*—was capable of breeding in water with a high saline content. A native of North Africa, *Anopheles labranchiae* had originally filled the ecological niche of the Mediterranean coastal zones. After migrating to Italy during the Roman Empire, it had evolved—unlike indigenous Italian mosquitoes—to breed in both fresh and brackish water. In its adopted home, it rapidly became the principal vector of malaria.

Martini and Rodenwaldt devised a plan to take full advantage of the unusual breeding habits of *Anopheles labranchiae*. One of the leading malariologists in Europe, Martini had been a pioneer investigator of the speciation of anopheles mosquitoes. In 1931, contemporaneously with L. W. Hackett and Alberto Missiroli, he had solved the biological riddle of the *Anopheles maculipennis* group to which the species *Anopheles labranchiae* belonged.[13] Thoroughly acquainted, therefore, with the habits of the most deadly Italian vector, he was as well prepared as anyone in Europe to make use of this knowledge for an evil objective. He was also capable morally of using his learning for such a purpose. Martini was a devout member of the Nazi party, a protégé of Heinrich Himmler, and an authority on germ warfare. The ideal Nazi doctor, he was now in a position to misuse medicine by putting it to the purpose not of saving lives and minimizing suffering but of taking lives and maximizing pain.[14] Less illustrious than Martini, Rodenwaldt was a malaria specialist who was fully conversant with his colleague's discoveries and with the intricate public health mechanisms that held malaria in check in Littoria.

In advising German engineers on how best to flood the Pontine Marshes during the rainy season between October 1943 and March 1944, Martini and Rosenwaldt fully understood the consequences of their suggestions for public health. They knew that the German army would create an ideal habitat for *Anopheles labranchiae* so that the upsurge of malaria that had already begun in the Pontine Marshes could erupt into a full-scale epidemic. Indeed, their plan was to put the water pumps into reverse action so that they drew seawater onto the plain and to open the tidal gates at the mouths of the chief waterways. These acts would create a vast swamp of brackish water in which *Anopheles labranchiae* alone would be able to flourish. Missiroli explained, "As is well known, in southern central Italy, malaria is carried chiefly by *A[nopheles] maculipennis elutus* and *A[nopheles] maculipennis labranchiae*, which can tolerate a certain degree of salinity in the water; for this reason, in salty waters the malaria-carrying races have the advantage over their rivals and are responsible for the appearance of malaria."[15]

Indeed, one reason for the success of bonifica idraulica in dramatically reducing the level of malaria transmission in the Pontine Marshes was that it increased the flow of freshwater across the plain and into the sea. This action cleansed the brackish pools along the coast and decreased the population of the leading malaria vector. As a result, with each year that passed after 1932 the population of *Anopheles labranchiae* in Littoria province declined relative to indigenous anophelines.[16] Martini and Rodenwaldt envisaged reversing this process. Not only would there be vast numbers of insects when the malaria season of 1944 began, but also nearly all of these mosquitoes would be members of the species principally responsible for transmitting both falciparum and vivax malaria. Indeed, in some localities investigators reported that in 1944, 100 percent of all adult mosquitoes were *Anopheles labranchiae*, as opposed to less than 30 percent before the German intervention.[17] "Here," wrote Missiroli,

> the Germans have flooded the coastal areas of the Lazio region and of the province of Caserta, in part with fresh water and in part with salt. The presence for a considerable time of fresh water on land composed of alluvial deposits which have as their foundation old marine beds has caused a slight salinification of the water, sufficient to favor the breeding of *A. Maculipennis labranchiae*, which has re-appeared immediately in large numbers, since each species belonging to a given region rapidly becomes predominant when conditions are established which are favorable to its own development, while unfavorable to the development of rival races having the same habitat and the same food habits.[18]

There could be no better way to ensure the highest possible level of transmission and therefore the most intense possible outbreak of fever. Seawater would also cause the greatest environmental damage to agriculture and animal husbandry. Missiroli, aware of the Germans' intentions, feared that in the summer of 1944 the Nazi scheme would unleash in Littoria province the deadliest epidemic of malaria ever recorded. In his estimation, "The enormous increase in marshy areas and particularly of water will facilitate the breeding of a vast number of malaria-carrying anophelines and as a consequence of this situation will produce the greatest epidemic recorded by human history."[19] Italian malariologists therefore pleaded with their German colleagues to confine their activities to the short-term military objective of slowing the oncoming Allied forces by simply halting the pumps and taking no further action. By this means, all legitimate German military objectives would be accomplished, and when the impending battle was over, Italian public health officials could rapidly intervene to repair the damage and save civilian lives. The Italian malariologist Enzo Mosna wrote a poignant report in November 1943:

> We were concerned to determine how it would be possible for the German army to achieve its war aims without causing damage to both public health and to agriculture that would be permanent or would last for a long period after the end of the war.
>
> In its own time the German government sent to Rome, on the fourteenth of the current month, Professor Erich Martini of the University of Hamburg and presently chief of the department of entomology of the Military Medical Academy of Berlin, and Professor [Ernst] Rodenwaldt of the University of Heidelberg and presently director of the department of tropical medicine of the Military Medical Academy of Berlin. Their purpose was to study the possible damage that would result from the flooding of lands that had been previously reclaimed and bonified.
>
> Professors Rodenwaldt and Martini immediately contacted the director of the laboratory of malariology of this institute, and they carried out an on-site inspection at the delta of the Tiber in order to examine on the spot the serious problems that arise from the return of the Roman Campagna and the Pontine Marshes to their ancient swampy condition.
>
> After a careful examination of the situation that is occurring, we took advantage of the long-standing friendship that binds us to those eminent scientists to make the following recommendations: (1) not to divert saltwater onto the bonified fields because the dilution of saltwater with freshwater would create more favorable conditions for the development of malaria-carrying mosquitoes and the appearance of serious epidemics of malaria; (2) to suspend the working of the water pumps, but not to create serious damage to the machinery that would be difficult to repair in the years to come after the end of the war; (3) not to requisition milk-giving cattle in the bonified areas as they produce the milk that allows us to give a half ration of milk to babies and patients; (4) not to divert the civilian and military medical personnel from the tasks to which they are assigned, in view of the severe sanitary conditions that will prevail in the Roman Campagna and in the hinterland of the open city of Rome after the return of the bonified lands to their swampy state.
>
> Professors Rodenwaldt and Martini recognized the importance of the is-

> sues that we raised, and they promised that they would recommend to the German command that it give the most benevolent consideration to our suggestions.
>
> Before leaving, Professor Martini was able to assure us that all flooding with saltwater would be avoided, except for restricted zones along the coast, and that all military and civilian personnel would respect the Geneva Convention.[20]

By invoking the Geneva Convention, Mosna explicitly reminded Martini and Rosenwald that the actions of the German army were bound by a framework of international "Laws and Customs of War." This framework had been established by the Hague Conventions of 1899 and 1907 and the Geneva Protocol of 1925, all three of which Germany had signed. In the "desire to diminish the evils of war," the Hague Conventions boldly declared that "the right of belligerents to adopt means of injuring the enemy is not unlimited."[21] Of specific relevance to events in the Pontine Marshes, the conventions further established that it was forbidden "to employ arms, projectiles or material of a nature to cause superfluous injury."[22] But most applicable of all was the specific ban by the Geneva Protocol on the first use of chemical or biological weapons, "binding alike the conscience and the practice of nations."[23]

Unfortunately, both in the Pontine Marshes and in the Tiber Delta just to their north, the German response to Mosna's invocation of international law was to ignore it. With the evidence now available, it is impossible to determine who in the German chain of command gave the lethal order to implement the plan devised by Martini and Rodenwaldt. It is uncertain whether the responsibility lies with one of Kesselring's subordinate commanders, with Kesselring himself, or even at the very top with Himmler or Hitler. The commission of atrocities at the expense of Italian civilians, however, had been the general thrust of the Wehrmacht occupation policy through the first half of 1944, and in May "war against civilians" became systematic. Kesselring, moreover, was an enthusiastic supporter of harsh measures toward Italians, and he bore direct responsibility for ordering a series of massacres behind the German lines in mid-1944—deeds that prompted his trial and conviction for war crimes in 1947. The plan devised by Martini and Rodenwaldt, therefore, was consistent with the punitive tenor of the Wehrmacht occupation strategy and with Kesselring's well-documented modus operandi.[24]

Regardless of who gave the immediate order, it is undeniable that the Wehrmacht implemented a complicated and inhumane plan that involved not only stopping the pumps and blocking drainage canals but also deliberately diverting seawater onto the fields. Paul Russell, the eminent malariologist and consultant to the surgeon general of the U.S. Army during the Italian campaign, reported in October 1944 that

> one of the tragedies of the war has been the systematic destruction by the German Army of the grand land reclamation projects or so-called bonifiche of Italy. Not only has this smashing of pumps, blocking and mining canals, and deliberate reverse diversion of sea and river water greatly increased the breeding of *Anopheles* malaria mosquitoes. It has also driven from their homes thousands of peasants, has flooded thousands of acres of farm and has set back disastrously the economy of entire provinces. The area of farmland in South Italy flooded by the Germans is estimated at 37,000 hectares or 98,000 acres.[25]

Then, just before withdrawing in May 1944, as the Wehrmacht began systematically to carry out the draconian occupation policy approved by Kesselring, the Germans dynamited some of the pumps and mined the fields and canals surrounding them. In the words of Henry Kumm, a leading American expert on yellow fever and malaria who served on the Allied Control Commission, "Practically all of the pumping stations in the Pontine Marshes were systematically sabotaged."[26] Kumm was also specific about German intentions. He wrote, "As the war advanced that situation changed for the worse. The retreating Germans systematically destroyed the pumping stations of the bonificas, flooding huge tracts of country with the dual purpose of rendering more difficult the advance of the Allied Armies and of magnifying the problems subsequently to be dealt with by the allied civilian administrations."[27]

In addition, the Germans physically removed other pumps and shipped them by train to Germany. Their purpose was clearly to maximize the epidemic and to ensure that reversing the damage would be a lengthy and dangerous process that took the heaviest possible toll on the civilian population.[28] The Germans flagrantly violated both the Geneva Protocol and the Hague Conventions by being the first to use biological weapons and by deliberately causing extensive "superfluous injury" to innocent noncombatants. Thus in a 2003 interview Mario Coluzzi, the recipient of the Ross Prize for malariology in 1998, concluded that "this is certainly a war crime, and a representative of the German government should apologize to the Italian people."[29]

Indeed, the most compelling account of the events surrounding the epidemic at Littoria is the diary of Mario Coluzzi's father, Alberto. A physician and malaria expert like his son, Alberto Coluzzi was responsible for drafting plans to combat malaria first at Cassino (Campania) in 1944 and then in the Pontine Marshes in 1945 and 1946. Knowing the area well, he made on-site inspections in the wake of the German flooding. It rapidly became apparent to Coluzzi that he had become witness to a carefully executed plan that had nothing to do with creating a natural barrier to the advancing Allied armies. After making a tour of inspection, he reported,

> The thing that I was unable to understand at that moment was the flooding created in some sectors where it was not possible either for men or equipment to advance. Nor did I understand the flooding of vast zones that were not useful even for the purpose of stopping a cat. I began to suspect that the Todt organization, which had concerned itself—together with the Fourteenth Armored Division—with defending the lines, had been given the suggestion of causing flooding in some places for other reasons. These suggestions must have been given by someone who knew that malaria can cause losses far greater than those caused by combat, by someone who had a good knowledge of "man-made malaria." . . .
>
> These on-site inspections allowed me to gather information about the damage suffered by the antimalarial structures in these sectors and about the reorganization of services. The province of Littoria had obviously suffered the worst damage because there were many places in which the Germans had put up resistance and because it contained many extensive sectors that could be easily flooded. Here too my attention was drawn by the vast areas that had been inundated, and by the fact that such flooding made no sense if looked at only from the standpoint of creating defensive barriers. I was able to make the same observations in the coastal stretches of the Roman Campagna. It was absolutely clear that the work had been carried out in order to create enormous larval nurseries, and for no other purpose.[30]

Initially based on the topography of the flooded zones, Coluzzi's conclusion was reinforced by the reverse operation of the water pumps by German engineers. "In this respect," he wrote,

> I can add further information. Not all the pumps that were located along the coast were taken away or destroyed. Some of them were still functional, but they had been positioned to function in reverse. A number of people, including specialists who worked to repair the equipment, told me that the Germans had used them in this manner for the purpose of obtaining seawater to increase the flooding. This is not so. A pump so positioned cannot be used to cause flooding. It could be used only in order to give a certain level of salinity to the freshwater that collected in those coastal areas. Clearly there was someone who knew full well that brackish water could favor the development of certain species of mosquitoes, and that those were the best vectors for malaria.[31]

The Germans also took great care to ensure that the disease and the environmental conditions that caused it would be long lasting and difficult to combat. A clear example was the fate of the motorboats that the antimalarial campaign operated in Littoria as means of clearing drainage ditches and canals of vegetation. Their function was to keep the waterways free flowing and clear of mosquito larvae. Coluzzi reasoned,

> Another important fact is this: the Provincial Antimalarial Committee of Littoria had flat-bottomed motorboats that were equipped to remove vegetation for the purpose of controlling mosquito larvae. They pompously called these boats fitted with shovels "the vegetation removal flotilla." The Germans devoted a great deal of time to finding them wherever they had been placed or hidden, and they systematically destroyed them all.
>
> Such actions clearly demonstrate that they intended scientifically to create special swamp conditions that it would be difficult to modify for a long time.[32]

Finally, Coluzzi's suspicions settled into a firm conviction when he learned of German actions at the Department of Health in Rome. In its warehouses the department had stockpiled nine metric tons of quinine for the purpose of containing an outbreak of disease. To prevent the Italian authorities from making use of this precious medication to protect the population, the Germans confiscated the stocks and hid them in the Tuscan town of Volterra. In this manner they ensured that when the epidemic erupted, the specific remedy was in short supply. As Coluzzi argued, "These medicines, if carefully administered and prescribed, would have prevented the substantial shortages that in fact occurred."[33]

What must be added is the frightening reaction of the Italian malariologist Missiroli to the crime committed by the German army as it carried out the plan devised by Martini and Rodenwaldt. Missiroli of course was not responsible for German actions, and he specifically sought to convince Martini to minimize the lasting impact of his strategy. After the Germans flooded the Tiber Delta, however, Missiroli surprisingly and disturbingly withheld quinine from the victims of the malaria outbreak that he knew would follow. His motivations were twofold. In the first place, he regarded treating so large a number of patients as excessively arduous, especially since—in self-exculpation—he wrote that it was a question "only" of vivax malaria, which he regarded as mild. Here Missiroli's argument is self-serving and misleading not only because vivax malaria is itself a serious and sometimes fatal disease but also because the epidemic that erupted produced a profusion of cases of falciparum malaria as well as vivax.

Missiroli's second motivation was even more disturbing. In his view, to medicate those who were ill or at risk would ruin an experiment in which he was passionately interested—the first large-scale trial of DDT as an antimalarial weapon. Here was the long-awaited trial of a technological solution to the problem of malaria in nearly ideal field conditions. In order to observe the effectiveness of the new chemical, therefore, he intentionally stayed his hand and allowed the victims to suffer. In his own unethical words referring to the winter of 1944 and the spring of 1945, Missiroli wrote,

> We had also foreseen the development of numerous cases of malaria in the event that chemical prophylaxis was suspended. These cases in fact did occur late in the months of March, April, May, and June. We could have avoided the development of these cases by administering [the synthetic quinine substitute] Atebrin from late March until the end of June. But since it was a question of benign tertian malaria, which is innocuous for the victim, we thought that it was not worthwhile to resume such an arduous task. This was all the more in our minds because that would have disturbed the experiment of DDT, since at the end of that trial we would not have learned whether success was due to chemical prophylaxis or to DDT.[34]

As a close associate of the Rockefeller Foundation, Missiroli had foreknowledge of the coming use of the new and uniquely potent larvicide, and he wished to observe its effectiveness in a trial when it was used alone. Missiroli also had a detached, "scientific" interest in passively observing the brutal work of his Nazi colleague Martini. He wished to note the effect of the flooding on the relative breeding success of *Anopheles labranchiae*—a mosquito species in which both the Italian and the German shared an abiding entomological interest. By his own admission, therefore, he did nothing to mitigate the epidemic he had foreseen.

With respect to the military outcome of the war in Italy, the consequences of the German strategy of flooding the Pontine Marshes and unleashing *Anopheles labranchiae* were virtually nil. In a decisive thrust northward in May, the Allies simultaneously broke through the German positions at Cassino and at Anzio. Fighting against weakened German defenses, they reached Rome on 4 June 1944. Neither water nor mosquitoes significantly hindered the Allied advance. With regard to malaria, the troops were aided by the timing of military events: the Allies crossed the marshes rapidly and safely before the onset of the malaria season in mid-June. In addition, they benefited from extensive advance preparation that included instruction in the fundamentals of malaria transmission; the carefully supervised distribution of Atebrin; and the use of insect repellent, protective clothing, head netting, and mosquito-proof bivouacs. Well-trained teams of scouts also sprayed insecticide at strategic locations in advance of the troops.[35]

For the civilian population of Littoria, however, the results were dramatic, as both Martini and Missiroli had anticipated. During the hostilities and the flooding, most of the population had fled, seeking refuge on the slopes of the Lepini Mountains or in neighboring provinces. In September 1943 the German army ordered the evacuation of all remaining civilians who lived within a radius of ten kilometers from the shore. This removal of the inhabitants from the war zone ensured that there were no eyewitnesses to German actions affecting the hydrology and fauna of the plain. Their deeds were thus hidden from view at the time, and they have remained shrouded in mystery ever since. It was all too clear, however, that when the German army withdrew and the residents returned to their homes in the summer of 1944, they encountered conditions that rendered them immediately susceptible to disease. Because the standard two-story brick dwellings built by the veterans' association (Opera Nazionale Combattenti, or ONC) under Mussolini's settlement program were ideal for sheltering tanks and snipers, both the German and the Allied armies had systematically leveled homesteads throughout the province, while rising water caused further havoc. In total, 2,298 homes built by the ONC as well as 1,631 public buildings were damaged or destroyed in this manner.[36] As the malarial season got under way, the citizens of Littoria therefore lacked adequate housing, and many were forced to sleep in the open under canvas or in stables, where they lacked all protection from insects. Moreover, with agriculture and the economy in ruins, hunger and malnutrition were widespread, compromising resistance to disease. In addition, in the wake of the wartime disruption, the health services collapsed so that medical attention and hospital care were unavailable. Because of the German sequestration of Italian quinine reserves, effective medicine was also in short supply. Finally, there was extensive environmental degradation. As a result of the war, there were bomb and shell craters in the clay soil that served as breeding grounds for mosquitoes. The network of irrigation and drainage canals that covered the plain had also been neglected and were clogged with vegetation or blocked by German dynamite. It was in these dire circumstances that the inhabitants faced the torment of unprecedented swarms of *Anopheles labranchiae*.[37]

Such a combination of wartime devastation and bioterrorism produced the epidemic that both Martini and Missiroli had envisaged—one of the great upsurges in malaria in modern Italian history. The chairman of the CPA, Leone Leppieri, commented in November 1944 that the situation was "tragic" and that the entire population of the province had fallen ill with fever.[38] So serious was the crisis that the health official Mario Alessandrini considered ordering the evacuation of the entire province.[39] Between 1944 and 1946, the number of officially recorded cases spiked to nearly ten times the number of cases in 1939 and 1940 (Table 7.2). Even these disturbing figures, however, understate the scale of the disaster, as Vincenzo Rossetti, the provincial officer of health for Littoria, stressed. The reason was that the personnel of the anti-malarial campaign were severely overburdened with patients. They failed therefore to carry out the required paperwork that determined the official profile of the epidemic. A more realistic figure for cases in 1944, he argued, was in excess of 100,000 in a population of 245,000.[40] Indeed, nearly half of

Table 7.2 Cases of Malaria in Littoria Province, 1939–1946

1939	614
1940	572
1941	730
1942	1,793
1943	1,217
1944	54,929
1945	42,712
1946	28,952

Source: Data from CPA, "Riunione del CPA del 19 ottobre 1946: Mario Alessandrini, 'Relazione,'" ASL, CPA, b.3/1, fasc. 2/1 ("Anno 1945: Adunanze del Comitato"), 4–5; Henry W. Kumm, "Malaria Control West of Rome during the Summer of 1944," 26 Jan. 1945, RAC, Record Group 1.2, 700 Europe, box 12, folder 102, 1–2.

the patients in many localities carried a double infection of both *Plasmodium falciparum* and *Plasmodium vivax* in their bloodstreams. Alessandrini, reporting to the CPA, described the situation in 1944 and 1945:

> In effect, as soon as the population of the province of Latina descended from the mountains and returned to the fields, the people were stricken with malaria in an unprecedented manner. Because of its rapid spread, malaria assumed an epidemic character in some cities, such as Fondi, where 92 percent of the inhabitants were afflicted.
>
> In the spring of 1945 the situation in the province was simply tragic, and we talked of evacuating the most affected cities.[41]

The medical emergency caused by the German plan lasted for three epidemic seasons and exacted a fierce toll in suffering from unarmed Italian men, women, and children. The Pontine Marshes had been returned to the conditions prevailing before bonification. In Paul Russell's words, "It is probably no exaggeration to say that in some areas, as in the Agro Romano, the appearance of the countryside when the Germans were driven back, was that of 1880 before the earliest advance in land reclamation had been made."[42]

8

Fighting Disaster: DDT and Old Weapons

One unfortunate result of the partial knowledge which has been gained by superficial study of the spontaneous disappearance of malaria was the feeling that if we could only find it there must be some easier way to deal with the disease than any of those laborious methods with which we have been struggling for a quarter of a century — some biological miracle which might banish it by the waving of a wand. Such an attitude is often paralyzing to present action.

— *L. W. Hackett,* Malaria in Europe: An Ecological Study

A new stage in the world history of malaria began in the midst of the emergency that had engulfed the Pontine Marshes. In June 1945 Alberto Missiroli announced in a speech to the Provincial Antimalarial Committee (CPA), over which he presided, the availability of the new and magic weapon of DDT (dichloro-diphenyl-trichloroethane). It was so powerful that he predicted — "to the unanimous skepticism of his audience" — that within five years malaria would be vanquished both locally in Littoria and throughout Italy.[1] In this unexpected declaration, Missiroli had in fact proclaimed the beginning of a new era in malariology that was to last for a generation. It was characterized by American dominance, euphoric optimism, and reliance on DDT to slay the hydra of malaria.

DDT was not a new chemical; it had been discovered in Germany in 1874. In the frenzy to find ways of controlling disease during the world crisis of the 1940s, this long-forgotten product was rediscovered and given its first large-scale trial. The first use of DDT to control disease began on 15 December 1943, when the Americans introduced it to control a ferocious epidemic of typhus that struck Naples and its overcrowded slums.[2] As Fred Soper recalled, the Allies employed the deadly hydrocarbon without regard to its risks and possible side effects. The experiment was, he remarked, "a very hush-hush subject. The toxicology of DDT was relatively unknown, but we did not hesitate to pump it under the clothing of some 3,000,000 people and to assign workers to the pumps in rooms which were unavoidably foggy from the DDT dust in the air."[3] No other means were known that could destroy lice with sufficient rapidity to bring an almost immediate end to a major typhus epidemic. In a stunning display of its killing power, DDT deloused seventy-three thousand people per day, bringing an end to the outbreak in midwinter, despite the most appalling sanitary conditions. As Professor G. Fischer recalled in 1948 in his presentation speech at the ceremony awarding the Nobel Prize in medicine to Paul Müller for discovering the power of DDT as a contact poison, "1,300,000 people were treated in January 1944 and in a period of three weeks the typhus epidemic was completely mastered. Thus, for the first time in history a typhus outbreak was brought under control in winter. DDT had passed its ordeal by fire with flying colours."[4]

Even before the audacious experiment with typhus ended, the American army resolved to make a second trial of the product, using it for the first time against malaria the following summer. This new test took place at Castel Volturno in Campania, where DDT was sprayed inside houses to destroy overwintering mosquitoes.[5] Because the area was a war zone, however, the results were neither clear nor easy to interpret. For that reason, the Americans decided to conduct a further trial, in the delta of the Tiber River and in the Pontine Marshes. This trial was the plan that Missiroli announced to his stunned audience at Littoria.

To wage war against the anophelines of Littoria, the American army converted to public health purposes a technology originally developed for warfare. As the Rockefeller Foundation Health Commission explained,

> The first problem was to work out a method of using standard army equipment for spraying an oil solution from an airplane.... It was found possible to adapt the fog-making tanks of the Chemical Warfare Division to the anti-mosquito tactics. Each tank would hold 33 gallons of the insecticide, a series of tanks were fitted on the bomb racks under the belly of an airplane, and a means was found to discharge their contents at the required rate of two quarts per acre....

> As a further step in this study the unit used an A–20 airplane as a flying laboratory. . . . The upshot of this experiment was a very efficient apparatus for covering a wide area with insecticide under very precise control.[6]

With this means of spraying all extensive areas of standing water, the American army launched its great experiment on 5 June 1944. The effort then continued in successive waves of spraying until 4 September. Clearly impressed, Missiroli concluded his June 1945 speech with a five-year plan for total eradication of malaria.

In this experiment in using DDT against anophelines, far more was at stake than the health of the citizens of Littoria. One consideration was immediate—the protection of Allied soldiers from infection. As Henry Kumm explained, "The flooded areas were a menace not only to the indigenous inhabitants of the region but also to all non-immune allied troops stationed near Ostia-Lido, of which there were at times considerable numbers. For those reasons plans were drawn up to treat the flooded areas . . . with weekly applications of larvicides until such time as the pumps could be put back into operation again."[7] A further consideration was less immediate, yet more important on a global scale. As the Cold War began (with Italy as one of its earliest stakes), the United States and the Soviet Union were involved in a competition for the division of the world into their respective spheres of influence.[8] In this contest, the United States regarded Western medicine and technology as important means of establishing American claims to world leadership. Determined that the postwar world should be based on free-market economic principles, the United States realized that, in what came to be termed the "emerging markets" of the Third World, laborers and consumers needed to be healthy in order to sustain development. There was also a great humanitarian concern to take a dramatic step toward improving world standards of living. From a global as well as an Italian perspective in the immediate aftermath of the Second World War, malaria was the greatest public health challenge. Fresh from the immediate task of defeating the Germans, therefore, the United States had a long-term interest in developing effective methods of exterminating anopheles mosquitoes. If successful, the Italian trial could yield lessons for application in the tropical world, with important implications for the economic and sanitary underpinnings of the postwar era. At the same time, eradication would provide a compelling demonstration of the power of American technology and a lucrative market for the manufacturers of insecticide. After the successful use of DDT against lice in Naples, the DDT lobby was eager to test the insecticide on mosquitoes in a large setting.

To combat the Littoria epidemic that threatened to escape all control, the

Allied Control Commission, in which American influence predominated, enthusiastically accepted the suggestion of the Rockefeller malariologists Fred Soper and Paul Russell to employ DDT over a substantial area. Their idea was that Littoria should become in effect the first testing ground for a new strategy of malaria eradication that would be rapid, effective, and cheap. This was what L. W. Hackett and his Italian disciple Missiroli had termed the "American solution" to the problem of malaria. The disease, reconceptualized as "an entomological rather than a social problem," was to be resolved by a technological "quick fix" rather than a complex program of social reform, agricultural investment, and environmental improvement in the manner of bonifica integrale.[9] If the initiative in Littoria was successful, then the new weapon could be applied to all of Italy.

Just as in Naples, so too in Littoria the Americans took the decision to employ DDT as a daring wartime experiment without knowing its long-term consequences for the environment or its possible toxic side effects for human and animal populations. The results, however, accorded with Missiroli's optimistic forecast: by 1949 *Anopheles labranchiae* had been eradicated in the province, all other anophelines were greatly reduced in numbers, and malaria transmission had ceased.[10] Vincenzo Rossetti, the provincial officer of health for Littoria, observed that the chemical produced a "true miracle."[11]

Results in Littoria seemed to confirm the Rockefeller vision of malaria eradication by means of a single chemical weapon. Indeed, the apparently successful application of DDT in the Pontine Marshes led rapidly to similar campaigns in Sardinia and then in Italy as a whole. There is no doubt that DDT made a significant contribution — first, to combating the emergency created by the retreating Germans and, second, to vanquishing malaria from 1962 until now. But was DDT the miracle weapon that Hackett and the Rockefeller Foundation had been seeking as the shortcut to eradication?

In evaluating what took place in Littoria, one needs to avoid the superficial impression that the final victory against malaria was due solely to DDT. It is all too easy to forget that before DDT was sprayed from the air, the CPA launched an emergency program that was based on hard-won lessons in antimalarial campaigning. It took full advantage of the institutional and cultural accomplishments of the national campaign that had begun in 1900 and had continued almost uninterruptedly for half a century. Not least among these advantages was the fact that public health officials could begin work immediately and effectively because they already possessed a clear strategy and set of priorities for their operations. Among the first initiatives of the CPA were reopening the devastated health stations of the province and distributing quinine. Returning to the province in the summer of 1944, the physicians and nurses of Littoria

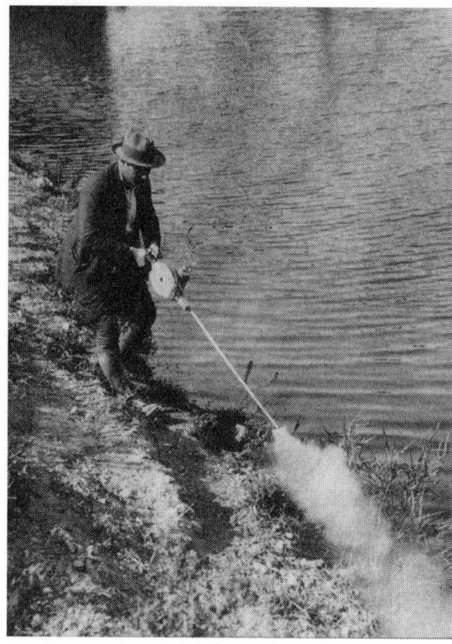

Spraying larvicide in Littoria

succeeded by the end of the year in treating seventy-five thousand fever patients and in providing prophylaxis to an additional fifty thousand people at risk. Such figures indicate that, in its first half-year of reactivation, the campaign reached nearly 50 percent of Littoria's population of 245,000.[12] To achieve such success in the midst of vast wartime devastation, the committee built on the accomplishments of its predecessors, from Angelo Celli and Giovanni Battista Grassi to Giulio Alessandrini and Alberto Missiroli: literacy, the familiarity of the population with quinine, the widespread understanding of the mosquito theory of transmission, the residents' awareness of the danger they faced, and the availability of trained and experienced health personnel. Quininization was an effective strategy because the citizens of Littoria were already "medicalized," educated, and familiar with the priorities of the antimalarial program.

If opening health stations and distributing quinine were the first priorities before the introduction of DDT, two additional measures were the restoration of mechanical protection and local environmental sanitation. Where possible, citizens were encouraged and assisted in the work of repairing their homes, reinstalling metal screens, and planting crops. Campaigners also launched an assault on larvae by clearing ditches and canals and by spraying small collections of stagnant water with the larvicide Paris Green—piccola bonifica, in short. Thus, even before the DDT spraying began, an effective and balanced program to save lives and restore health was well under way. The very low level of mortality in the province in 1944 and 1945 despite the overwhelming prevalence of both falciparum and vivax malaria is a clear indication of its success.

Thus, when converted bombers began to spray DDT across the province, they deployed their deadly new weapon in a context in which malaria was already under attack. Instead of operating in isolation, the DDT spraying proceeded side by side with the traditional initiatives of the CPA. Indeed, as the war ended and funds were made available by the Allies, the CPA devoted great effort to such tasks as rebuilding homes, roads, and the infrastructure of the province; restoring production; improving diet; draining fields; clearing canals; repairing pumps; and distributing quinine and synthetic antimalarials. Here, unstated, was the essence of the multifaceted "eclectic method" that the National Department of Health had devised in the 1920s with a view to deploying all of the available weapons in a combined assault on malaria. Working together, these familiar weapons of the past and the new insecticide achieved an extraordinary outcome that accorded with Missiroli's sanguine prediction.

The experience of Littoria was mirrored in the other mainland case for which extensive archival records are available—the Veneto, where a regional committee known as the Istituto Interprovinciale delle Venezie (Interprovincial Institute of the Veneto) directed the campaign. As in Littoria, a series of war-related factors led to a major upsurge of malaria. These included environmental degradation, the collapse of public health services, the interruption of agriculture and land reclamation schemes, the displacement of populations, poverty, malnutrition, and the importation of infection through the movement of troops. This upsurge in the Veneto began in 1941, accelerated in 1943 with a "notable intensification of the malarial epidemic," and reached alarming proportions in 1944, when there was a "substantial malarial recrudescence in nearly all the provinces of the region."[13]

Just as the CPA directed a broadly based battle in Littoria, so the Istituto Interprovinciale drew up a comprehensive strategy based on Italy's experience since 1900.[14] The Istituto organized the mass distribution of prophylactic and curative quinine; the production of detailed local maps indicating all mosquito breeding sites to be treated with Paris Green; the reestablishment of health stations and of sanatoriums for children; the reinstitution of home visits by nurses and malaria scouts; the repair of environmental hazards through the clearing of canals and ditches; and the establishment of refectories to provide adequately nutritious meals for children.[15] Only in 1946 was DDT adopted as a complement to the campaign that was already under way. In January 1946,

Augusto Giovanardi, the president of the Istituto, announced the decision "to carry out the antimalarial battle in some zones in a grand style with the use of a new chemical, DDT. This has been made possible by the involvement of the High Commissariat and by the understanding and good will of the Allies, who wish to contribute to our campaign by experimenting with the new preparation in our region."[16] DDT was to be sprayed across the whole of the coastal zone between the Po Delta and the Tagliamento River.[17]

As in Littoria, the spraying campaign continued for five successive years, but again it was accompanied by the simultaneous acceleration of the campaign based on the tools of the pre-DDT era. In addition, a decisive factor in the campaign occurred spontaneously — the end of the war. With the war's conclusion, land drainage — "the indispensable premise for the complete sanitary redemption of the lands of the Veneto" — resumed, and there was a corresponding end of flooding. At the same time, there was a resumption of intensive agricultural production, while the crowds of displaced refugees and soldiers who had been such a disturbing feature of the final years of the conflict disappeared.[18]

Massive welfare spending played a vital role as well. Beginning with the invasion of Sicily in July 1943, the Allies invested heavily in health and welfare in an effort to prevent "disease and unrest." Acting until 1945 through the Allied Commission and then through the United Nations Relief and Rehabilitation Administration (UNRRA), the Allies, and especially the United States, distributed food, clothing, and medical supplies; rebuilt and supplied hospitals; and housed refugees and others made homeless by the war. Between 1943 and 1947 they spent a billion dollars on such efforts in Italy, hoping to prevent epidemics, restore the shattered Italian economy, and forestall an outburst of revolutionary activity fueled by social distress. For the year ending in March 1947 an average of more than three ships per day of UNRRA supplies arrived in Italian ports. An aliquot part of the substantial medical resources supplied by UNRRA made their way to the Veneto.[19] Tellingly, the Istituto Interprovinciale concluded that, on the strength of such an array of initiatives, malaria in the Veneto was already under control before the introduction of DDT. In late 1945 in the province of Venice, for example, the Istituto reported,

> a simple glance at the statistics shows that the malaria situation in this province is greatly improved in comparison with the last two years of the war. The drop in the number of cases is undoubtedly favored by the change in local conditions tied to the war itself, such as flooding . . . and the movement of displaced people from damaged centers to malarial locations. A natural tendency toward a definitive improvement in health will be achieved in the coming years with the resumption of drainage and reclamation activity and with the return to the normal maintenance of the canals and ditches.[20]

Thus the Veneto, where eradication was achieved in 1950, presented a situation similar to that of Littoria with regard to DDT. The introduction of the insecticide provided an important new weapon, but it made its contribution in combination with the multifaceted, eclectic methods of the Italian past.

Thus the experiences of both Littoria and the Veneto indicate that success was due to a multifactorial approach. By contrast, the final case for which there is ample documentation — Sardinia — has suggested to many observers the ability of DDT alone to achieve the "miracle." Indeed, partly for this reason, the "Sardinia Project" has enjoyed a disproportionate share of the attention that scholars have devoted to the postwar phase of the Italian eradication campaign.[21] Like Littoria and the Veneto, the island of Sardinia received a comprehensive spraying from 1946 to 1951 under the direction of the Rockefeller Foundation malariologists. Sardinia, however, was a case apart, where eradication occurred under the auspices of a specially created agency — ERLAAS (Ente Regionale per la Lotta Anti-Anofelica in Sardegna [Regional Agency for the Antianopheline Campaign in Sardinia]) — that had the specific objective of testing the power of DDT to annihilate anopheles mosquitoes. Its mission, in the words of Paul Russell, was "to determine whether or not, within the limits of funds available, it would be possible to eradicate *Anopheles labranchiae,* an indigenous vector of malaria, from an area like Sardinia."[22] By systematically spraying the inside of every structure on the island as well as all outdoor breeding sites of mosquitoes, the project achieved a dramatic but qualified success, which was defined not as the elimination of malaria but as the "larval negativism" of the species *Anopheles labranchiae.* The Sardinian campaign failed to eradicate the dreaded vectors entirely, but it so comprehensively reduced their numbers that it broke the transmission cycle and eliminated disease. In terms of its formal objective, the project failed, but in terms of the health of Sardinians, it was a resounding victory. When the campaign concluded its spraying in 1951, the island was malaria-free. As the trustees of the Rockefeller Foundation explained,

> At the end of the effort it was still possible to find an occasional Anopheles labranchiae mosquito — and so one could not say that the campaign for eradication had been successful. The experiment demonstrated that an indigenous insect is more difficult to exterminate than a species that is lately come to the environment. But while the answer to the eradication question was negative, the results of the experiment in terms of public health advancement were rewardingly affirmative. Thus, in 1946, the year the campaign began, there were 75,447 reported cases of malaria in Sardinia; in 1947 they dropped to 39,303; in 1948 to 15,121; in 1949 to 1,314; in 1950 they totaled 40; and in 1951 there were only 9 cases.[23]

In drawing lessons from the Sardinian experience, however, one needs to exercise considerable caution. One reason is that the sources on which scholars have relied are almost solely those of the malariologists attached to the Rockefeller Foundation, which directed the project. This aspect of the documentation means that there is inevitably an institutional and scientific bias. That is, because the Rockefeller Foundation was the dedicated proponent of the "American" technological solution of eradicating malaria with DDT alone, its documents need to be read with circumspection.[24]

Nevertheless, even in the files of the Rockefeller Archive Center there is a suggestive report by the entomologist C. Garrett-Jones of the London School of Hygiene and Tropical Medicine.[25] Garrett-Jones was troubled by what he regarded as the unscientific manner in which the Sardinia Project had been conceived. In his view, it lacked a clearly defined objective, it was carried out in undue haste without regard to the possible consequences of DDT to the flora and fauna of the island, and it made no provision for careful monitoring of the effects of the powerful new insecticide. Everything was conducted according to what some charged was the Rockefeller motto: "If in doubt, spray!" Furthermore, Sardinia witnessed a troubling new development—the emergence through Darwinian selection of DDT-resistant mosquitoes. This development failed to raise due concern at a time when the new chemical was being hailed uncritically as the centerpiece of the DDT era of malariology.

Although the leading DDT enthusiasts of the period—Fred Soper and Paul Russell—regarded the Sardinia Project as a successful application of their strategy, their blindness to historical context is misleading. Even in Sardinia, the "American" appearance of a purely technological victory over malaria by the means of a single weapon is deceptive. In the severely impoverished Sardinian economy, for instance, ERLAAS became the largest single employer on the island, hiring at its height some fourteen thousand peasants as scouts and sprayers. In this manner, the agency inadvertently added a second variable to the equation. By providing mass employment, ERLAAS substantially reduced the hunger and malnutrition that so many considered the essential substrate of malaria on the island. Social questions that the Rockefeller scientists were so eager to exclude stubbornly trespassed on the experiment. Paul Russell himself argued that the Sardinia Project initiated a progressive upward spiral in which mosquito reduction and agricultural improvement mutually reinforced one another. The spraying program, he wrote in 1949 while it was still in progress, had already produced "collateral benefits to Sardinia." Peasants were able to "open up new lands for agriculture" and to "go ahead with bonifica projects formerly impossible because of malaria."[26]

Equally important, ERLAAS and the Rockefeller Foundation did not act alone on the island in matters related to malaria. As on the mainland, UNRRA intervened in a manner that had significant implications for public health. UNRRA established a substantial assistance program that targeted the most vulnerable sectors of the Sardinian population—expectant mothers and small children. During the spring of 1946, 102,732 Sardinian nursing mothers and children received UNRRA food supplies, clothing, and shoes. During July and August thousands of children also received free accommodations and a nutritious diet at a series of summer camps "situated in specially healthful districts in the mountains, at the seaside, [and] in national parks." These measures, which had direct implications for the malaria epidemic afflicting the island, were renewed in 1947. Clearly, DDT was no longer a single, isolated variable but part of a complex interaction involving humans, the environment, and the economy.[27]

Another issue is the legacy of literacy, medicalization, and antimalarial propaganda in the countryside of Sardinia. In the early years of the century such antimalarial campaigners as Alessandro Lustig and Achille Sclavo reported that the greatest obstacle to the successful quininization of the population was its ignorance and suspicion. During the establishment of rural health stations and schools in the early years of the twentieth century, Sardinian peasants and shepherds widely suspected that the physicians who sought to treat them were actually poisoners. Half a century later, however, ERLAAS reported that the descendants of those who had so fiercely resisted quinine now warmly accepted DDT even when it was sprayed in their homes and in the waterways that they depended on for their own survival and that of their flocks. Here one detects the success of the malaria physicians, the rural schools, and the health stations in their fifty-year campaign to create a "sanitary consciousness" and a relationship of trust between doctors and their patients. Sardinian peasants accepted ERLAAS because they understood the significance of its mission and because they were aware of the peril of malaria and of the mosquito theory of transmission. Indeed, ERLAAS itself built on this legacy by carrying out an educational mission of its own. It offered weekly lessons in Grassi's doctrine to its personnel; it provided the schools of Sardinia with a syllabus on which to base lessons for all the children of the island; it broadcast radio programs on malaria and the mission to eradicate it; and it printed leaflets, posters, and bulletins for distribution across the region.[28]

In addition, apart from the general acceptance by Sardinians that ERLAAS describes, there is the question of the peasants it employed as scouts and sprayers. Unless they too had already absorbed the teachings of the Italian School, they would have been of little value to the Rockefeller scientists. Without stating the reason, ERLAAS in fact adopted a policy of hiring "peasants from the districts in which they were to work. . . . ERLAAS needed their thorough knowledge of the terrain and ability to find all the water."[29] The agency, in other words, made extensive use of the peasants' ability to relate their knowledge of the locality to Giovanni Battista Grassi's teaching that standing water breeds anophelines, and anophelines transmit malaria. Again, one suspects that Angelo Celli and Giovanni Cena were right in arguing that education was just as powerful an antimalarial as any chemical. In their haste, the Rockefeller experimenters failed to perceive a vital additional factor that was critical to the success of their mission. Marston Bates, one of the leading Rockefeller scientists, revealed more than he realized when he wrote that "eradication is possible, but requires a tightly organized and smooth functioning administrative machine."[30] Such a machine could emerge and run smoothly only because the island possessed abundant personnel educated in Grassi's doctrine to staff it.

Furthermore, in the furious campaign that they launched against *Anopheles labranchiae* and in their meticulous mapping of its six hundred thousand breeding places, the Rockefeller scientists did not begin de novo. On the contrary, they benefited from the extensive epidemiological and entomological studies that the antimalarial campaign carried out in the Giolittian era and during the interwar period. The American scientists, in other words, depended far more than they realized on the patient, tireless, and unacknowledged labors of Italian doctors during their long decades in obscure and uncomfortable rural postings.

Finally, throughout Italy demographic developments since the First World War assisted the antimalarial warriors in their task. Had Italian women heeded the injunctions of the pope and Il Duce to produce large families, the task of eradicating malaria would have been immensely more complicated because of overcrowding relative to available resources and because of the additional strain on the already overtaxed agencies of the antimalarial campaign. For the whole of the interwar period, however, Italian women silently resisted the intrusion of the authorities into their bedrooms by defiantly practicing birth control, with the result that the birthrate fell significantly. In the words of the volume UNRRA devoted to its activities in Italy, "The rapid decrease of the birthrate after the first world war was not balanced by a similar decrease in the death rate: the result was a decrease of the population surplus." Clearly signaling the importance for health of this noncompliance by women, UNRRA documented the demographic trend prominently on the first page of the chapter devoted to health and welfare (Table 8.1).[31]

Thus in all three regional settings for which there are extensive archival sources—Lazio, the Veneto, and Sardinia—the process of eradication be-

Table 8.1 Average Annual Rates of Birth and Death in Italy per 1,000 Inhabitants, 1881–1936

Years	Births	Deaths
1881–1885	38.0	27.3
1886–1890	37.5	27.2
1891–1895	36.0	25.5
1896–1900	34.0	22.9
1901–1905	32.7	22.0
1906–1910	32.7	21.2
1911–1915	31.5	19.7
1916–1920	23.0	24.4
1921–1925	29.8	17.4
1926–1930	26.8	16.0
1931–1936	23.8	14.1

Source: Data from UNRRA, *Survey of Italy's Economy,* 159.

tween 1944 and 1951 was intricate and complex. In each case, the introduction of potent insecticide was crucial, but the chemical was so effective because it was part of a broad-based campaign. The DDT program built on the experience, the education, and the lessons of a nation that had actively dedicated itself to malaria control since 1900. In no case—even in Sardinia, where DDT was especially important—did the campaign rely on one weapon alone.[32]

In 1945, on the strength of the local success in Littoria, Italy launched its final push for national eradication. As Missiroli explained, "After analyzing the data gathered from the work we carried out in the Pontine Marshes and after considering the area of the malarial zones of Italy, we concluded that it was possible to eradicate malaria from Italian soil in no more than five years."[33] In this plan, a tripartite division of labor emerged among international, national, and local initiatives. At the international level, UNRRA provided DDT and, together with the Rockefeller Foundation, funding for its deployment. Nationally, the High Commission for Hygiene and Public Health, which replaced the Department of Public Health and had Alberto Missiroli as its guiding figure, divided Italy into four zones in which malaria was to be attacked in turn. The commission also furnished financial support. Locally, the various provincial campaign agencies throughout Italy, including the CPA in Latina (formerly Littoria), the Istituto Interprovinciale in the Veneto, and ERLAAS in Sardinia, recruited the necessary personnel, housed the workforce undertaking eradication, and provided transport and logistical support.

With such powerful impetus, and with the background of five decades of

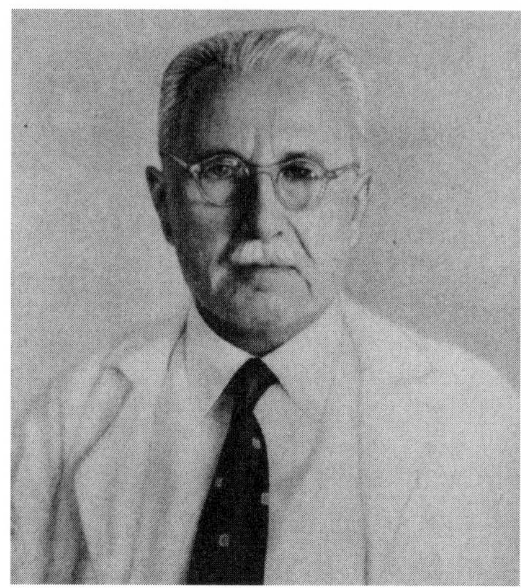

Alberto Missiroli

effort, the five-year eradication program succeeded—not only in Latina, the Veneto, and Sardinia but also throughout the nation. The last substantial outburst of the disease erupted at Palmo di Montechiaro in Sicily in 1956, when seventy-eight people fell ill with *Plasmodium vivax* infections. The last two indigenous cases of malaria occurred in 1962 in Palermo province. Finally, the state lifted the dreaded designation "malarial zone" from the whole territory of Italy in April 1965.[34]

The Italian experience from 1944 to 1962 suggested to many that Italy had pioneered the high road to eradication by means of a single chemical. Here, it seemed, was a solution to the world malaria problem that was quick, cheap, and universally applicable. This proposition—that malaria could be eliminated from the earth by means of DDT—was the chief article of faith for what came to be known as the American School of malariology, in conscious opposition to the slow, incremental, and multipronged strategy of the Rome School. Missiroli, who embraced the Rockefeller enthusiasm for technology, drew this tempting conclusion immediately. In 1946, after witnessing events in Latina, he decided that DDT was a stand-alone panacea that made previous antimalarial weapons redundant. Missiroli even envisaged an insect-free Eden in which all infectious diseases had been eliminated through the extermination by DDT of all noxious pests. According to Missiroli, "We have now achieved the radical aim of preventive medicine, which is not only to avoid disease and prolong life but also to render life itself full and happy."[35]

The most influential proponent of DDT, however, was Paul Russell, who in 1955 published a book entitled, with premature confidence, *Man's Mastery of Malaria*. Russell declared that the world had entered the era of DDT, and he predicted that the new, all-powerful weapon would produce a swift global victory over the ancient scourge.[36] The World Health Organization (WHO), "backed by the optimism of industry and the impatience of politicians," took up Russell's challenge by launching its own worldwide eradication drive with DDT as the major component.[37] The eighth World Health Assembly, which met in Mexico City in May 1955, officially launched the ambitious new campaign after a debate in which Russell himself played a leading role. Reliance on DDT radically simplified the malaria problem by eliminating the need for knowledge of the history, climate, epidemiology, and environment of specific localities; for additional research; for the education of the target populations; and for the establishment of costly health-care infrastructures. Spraying DDT was sufficient everywhere. Emilio Pampana, director of the WHO's Division of Malaria Eradication, even produced the *Textbook of Malaria Eradication* in 1963, confidently outlining what had become the standardized four-step approach to eliminating the disease—"preparation, attack, consolidation, and maintenance."[38] In the same spirit, George Macdonald, one of the founding fathers of "quantitative epidemiology," elaborated a mathematical model for eradication by mosquito reduction to such an extent that "malariometric rates" approached zero. Macdonald also advocated the reigning unified procedure, which he regarded as valid for malaria and probably for all other mosquito-borne tropical diseases as well.[39] In the malariologist Jose Najera's droll observation, Macdonald's model was especially persuasive because few physicians or public health officials understood its mathematical formulas.[40]

Thus inspired, the global drive continued from 1955 until 1969 when, after losing momentum amid mounting difficulties, it collapsed in total disarray. Most discouraging of all were the results of pilot projects in tropical Africa, where failure to interrupt transmission was reported in Cameroon, Ghana, Nigeria, Tanzania, Ethiopia, Zanzibar, and Zimbabwe. Other fully established programs in Afghanistan, Haiti, Indonesia, and Nicaragua failed to secure the expected advances. As a result, newly independent governments with scarce resources were understandably unwilling to invest in malaria eradication programs. Then in 1963 the United States, the major financial contributor to the project, eliminated its funding. Thus the WHO campaign stalled at the outset in the region of the world where it was most needed. Furthermore, outside Africa, "problem areas" rapidly emerged that did not respond to the prescribed "attack phase" even after it had been implemented according to the recommended procedures.

It soon became clear that Soper, Missiroli, Russell, Pampana, Macdonald, the Rockefeller Foundation, and the WHO had drawn misleading lessons from the Italian triumph. Contrary to the expectations of its ardent proponents, DDT—like quinine and Paris Green before it—was not a panacea but a tool with its own uses and limitations. The hydrocarbon failed when confronted with such problems as resistant species of mosquitoes, warfare and population displacement, overwhelming environmental degradation through such practices as the application of slash-and-burn techniques to forest areas, insufficient finances and political will, inadequate or nonexistent educational and health-care infrastructures, the inaccessibility of peripheral populations and regions, lack of attention to the treatment of cases, and the sheer magnitude of the task the WHO had undertaken. Tragically, the belief in a magic panacea also complicated matters by discouraging governments and industry from investing in research to provide additional antimalarial weapons. It also deterred physicians and scientists from entering the field of malariology that, everyone believed, was so soon to be made obsolete.[41]

In 1978, the thirty-first World Health Assembly officially buried the global eradication experiment, replacing it with national programs aiming at the more limited objective of control and making use of a broad array of antimalarial weapons. The era of DDT and the hegemony of the American School, with its unbounded confidence in technology, had come to an end. In Najera's words, "The selection of control methods was to be made following what was defined as the epidemiological approach, i.e. taking into fullest possible consideration the biological, ecological, social and economic determinants of the malaria problem, and those factors which might influence the applicability or effectiveness of individual control methods and their possible combinations."[42] What, then, are the more compelling and useful teachings of the Italian experience, which was the successful prototype for such national programs? What lessons are available for the contemporary world malaria emergency?

Conclusion

The Italian triumph over malaria has enormous importance as an example of the successful eradication of an incapacitating disease that continues to hold much of the world in thrall. Today approximately five hundred million people fall ill of malaria annually, and over one million die, making malaria the most significant tropical disease and, synergistically with HIV/AIDS and tuberculosis, the world's most serious infectious disease.[1] Unfortunately, the number of victims is increasing such that the World Health Organization (WHO) has declared reemerging malaria a "global emergency" and journals such as the *Lancet* have written of a "malaria disaster."[2] This dramatic problem is concentrated above all in the nations of sub-Saharan Africa, which experiences 90 percent of the cases, the vast majority of which affect pregnant women and children under five.[3]

In this somber context, the Italian history of antimalarial victory is especially suggestive. Soon after national unification in 1861, Italians discovered the overwhelming burden of death and disease imposed by malaria. Italian conditions in many respects prefigured the plight of those contemporary nations where malaria is hyperendemic or epidemic. At the close of the nineteenth century, two million Italians were infected or reinfected every year, and nearly every province in the nation paid annually in human suffering and death. Like the nations of the Afrotropic ecoregion today, Italy rapidly learned the truth of Ronald Ross's dictum that an intensely malarial nation can never be prosperous. Even when it fails to kill, malaria destroys the capacity of its victims to work and inflicts such severe neurological damage and cognitive impairment that they remain illiterate and unable to participate in civil society. Malaria also undermines the immune systems of sufferers, leaving them susceptible to a wide array of other diseases, especially the respiratory diseases of pneumonia, influenza, and tuberculosis. Thus in Italy malaria undermined agricultural productivity, decimated the army, destroyed communities, and left families impoverished. Above all, the Southern Question in Italian history —the relative inability of the South to achieve economic development and modernization—had a biological basis in the annual summer epidemic of malaria that debilitated the people of the region.

Facing such an immense problem of public health, Italy resolved in 1900 to create a national campaign—the first of its kind in world history—to control the ancient scourge and perhaps rid the nation of it entirely. In a burst of euphoria, Giovanni Battista Grassi, perhaps the most influential of the founding fathers of the campaign, argued that, properly directed, the eradication effort would require only a few years to accomplish its great task. Inevitably, reality proved to be more complex, and the Italian road to eradication was far from smooth. The campaign struggled amid unanticipated difficulties of every sort, and on more than one occasion it changed direction and strategy. The rural population, far from welcoming the health crusade, initially responded with suspicion and resistance. In addition, the campaign was disrupted by such poorly developed communications and such extensive patterns of migrant labor that large swathes of the population were almost beyond reach. Finally, every advance against the disease was threatened by a series of "complex emergencies" that subverted health, diverted attention, and monopolized scarce resources—two world wars, an economic depression, a series of natural disasters, and a brutally repressive Fascist dictatorship. Nevertheless, the campaign held firm for more than half a century—until final victory in 1965 when the state proclaimed the entire nation free of the disease and abolished the dreaded designation "malarial zone" from the whole of the peninsula.

What are the lessons to be drawn from this signal victory? What were the decisive factors that led to success in humanity's first experiment at creating a national malaria eradication program? In 1998, the WHO established Roll Back Malaria, a global initiative—the first since the failed eradication campaign of 1955–1969—with the aim of halving the world burden of malaria by 2010 and then halving it again by 2015. What can this program hope to learn from the Italian experience of the past?[4]

A first and vital lesson concerns magic thinking—the faith that a new technological weapon can serve as a panacea capable of destroying malaria on its own. At two points in its history—first at the outset, just after 1900, and then again in its concluding years, after 1944—the Italian campaign opted to rely exclusively on just such weapons. The first magic bullet was quinine, which the campaign deployed to destroy plasmodia in the human bloodstream. The second was DDT, which the campaign employed to annihilate insect vectors and their larvae, putting an end to transmission. Technology alone, it was thought, held the key to Italy's liberation. Here was the strategy that Fred Soper and the Rockefeller Foundation later made famous as the "American" strategy to combat malaria by relying solely on chemicals, with no need to tackle complex issues involving living conditions and the relationships of human beings to one another and to their environment. In the words of the malariologist Socrates Litsios, "With the arrival of DDT, the detailed understanding that had been built up in the course of tens of thousands of studies was put aside and a monolithic approach took hold. With victory in sight, there was no need for further studies."[5]

The technological approach, however, was misleading from the outset. Quinine provides a perfect illustration. At the turn of the twentieth century, Giovanni Battista Grassi and Angelo Celli, two of the founders of the Italian antimalarial campaign, wrote of quinine as though its usefulness, distribution, and ingestion were unproblematic. In fact the ability to make quinine available to every Italian at risk presupposed complex institutional, financial, and educational requirements, some of which were unspoken and remain all too conveniently forgotten today.

The first unspoken criterion was one of scale. It was essential to Italian success that it adopted the proper target area for its program. Because mosquitoes and migrant workers are not bound by political and administrative borders, it would have been impossible to eradicate malaria in any single township, province, or even region. Thus a crucial, if seldom mentioned, presupposition for the Italian strategy was that it was national in scope. It aimed at eradication simultaneously throughout the territory of the country, so that success in one area was not undone by inaction in another. The scale of the Italian program perfectly matched the area of transmission.

Similarly, Italy's geographical isolation proved to be a precious asset. Success would have been inconceivable had Italy bordered on other malarial nations, which might have taken no antimalarial action themselves and instead generated a constant supply of infected mosquitoes and feverish migrants. In these senses, Italian unification and Italian geography made essential contributions to the success of the antimalarial campaign. To be a unified territory surrounded by the waters of the Mediterranean Sea rather than by malarial neighbors was of incalculable benefit. Thus in the differently configured context of sub-Saharan Africa, or the rest of the tropical world, programs must assume transnational scope in order to encompass entire areas of transmission.

Unification was a powerful factor in the Italian victory over malaria for the additional reason that it enabled resources to be mobilized and directed appropriately. Camillo Golgi's famous dictum that, in the matter of malaria, there were "two Italies"—North and South—unknowingly prefigured the far larger international North-South divide of the contemporary world. Impoverished and crippled by an overwhelming burden of disease, southern Italy benefited from the financial resources, the trained personnel, and the research institutions of the North (and the capital at Rome) that were deployed to combat the common enemy. Just as such partnership between North and South was a prerequisite of Italian success, so an alliance between the industrial world and developing nations is a precondition for the control of malaria today. In an impoverished nation with hyperendemic malaria, the burden of disease so absorbs resources that establishing an effective control program is impossible without outside assistance. A measure of the crippling strain that malaria imposes on health-care systems is that in many of Africa's poorest nations 50 percent of all hospital admissions are due to this single cause.

In voting for the legislation that created Italy's antimalarial campaign, the Italian parliament demonstrated a clear sense of enlightened self-interest. North and South were linked by a common disease that did not acknowledge regional borders. In the larger contemporary global context such an understanding is urgently needed. One of the powerful causes of malaria is societal neglect. The nations of the industrial North devote pitifully few resources to tackling the malarial catastrophe of the Afrotropic ecoregion. In 1998, the total resources earmarked for malaria control worldwide by the twenty-three wealthiest nations of the world totaled just $60 million—an amount that increased to only $200 million in 2002, even after the WHO initiative. These figures, in the words of David Alnwick of the Roll Back Malaria secretariat, were "extremely low, and incommensurate with the magnitude of the disease."[6] Indeed, the consensus within the public health community and among the most afflicted nations is that the amount of annual aid necessary to accomplish the task set by the WHO is in the region of $1.5 to $2.5 billion. By contrast, as of 2003, allocations compared unfavorably with the budgets of such major Hollywood films as *Titanic.*[7] It is forgotten that, by trapping sub-Saharan Africa in ineradicable poverty, malaria undermines world stability, peace, and the global economy. As a major immunosuppressive disease, malaria also provides a substrate for the two other diseases—HIV/AIDS and tuberculosis—that now hold the potential to undermine world health.

Indeed, in an age of rapid transportation and mass migration, it cannot be confidently assumed that malaria will never reestablish itself in countries from which it has been expelled. In Italy, for example, the great malarial vector *Anopheles labranchiae* is still present in densities little different from those of the past. Furthermore, the accelerating pace of arrivals en masse of African immigrants bearing plasmodia in their bloodstreams has led to a rapidly growing number of imported cases of malaria that are treated in Italian hospitals. Public health authorities are therefore concerned about the possible reestablishment of malarial transmission. To date, it has been Italy's good fortune that the overwhelming majority of cases have been treated and isolated in urban hospitals rather than occurring in the countryside. In addition, although there is no known biological barrier to the transmission of *Plasmodium vivax* in Italian conditions, *Anopheles labranchiae* shows little receptivity to present-day African strains of *Plasmodium falciparum*.[8]

What Grassi and Celli regarded at first as a technological assault on disease in fact involved a prior unspoken development—a great national awakening to the problem so that Italy was prepared in 1900 to tackle two of the greatest preconditions for epidemic malaria—ignorance of the problem and societal apathy. From the outset, a galvanizing influence on the campaign was the partnership of a succession of governmental and nongovernmental institutions that focused attention on the issue, funded research, educated the population, and provided trained personnel to staff antimalarial facilities. These institutions included the Society for the Study of Malaria, the National League against Malaria, the Italian Red Cross, and the Department of Public Health. Equally, at the end of the Second World War when the nation had been devastated by war, economic collapse, and German occupation, the final push for eradication would have been unimaginable without international partnership. In particular, the effort depended on the provision of funds and skilled personnel—largely American—through UNRRA and the Rockefeller Foundation.[9]

Today the Roll Back Malaria program of the WHO relies heavily on a strategy of distributing a technological product—mosquito nets impregnated with insecticide—just as the Italian state once relied on distributing quinine. For this reason it is vital to note a further aspect of the early Italian decision to entrust eradication to technology alone. The physicians who staffed the rural health stations and public clinics where quinine was distributed rapidly reported that education was no less important to success than the alkaloid. Sufferers were not willing to follow the strenuous regimen required for quinine prophylaxis and treatment until they knew and trusted the health personnel who distributed advice and until they understood the impact of malaria on their lives, the mechanisms of transmission, and the logic behind the daily ritual of pill taking. Very quickly, therefore, the idea of distributing quinine led to a recognition that universal education was one of the most effective of all antimalarials. The campaign established rural health stations as the sheet anchor of the program, and the function of these institutions was educational no less than medical. Doctors combating malaria discovered that it was impossible to overcome the superstitions and the resistance of the rural poor unless they gained their trust by providing a comprehensive medical service. The poor could not be brought to the clinic; the clinic had to go out to meet the patients. Only after physicians had gained access to peasant homes and won their confidence by becoming a presence in the community, delivering children, setting bones, binding wounds, and treating influenza and measles could they hope to persuade their patients to swallow an unknown and suspicious chemical even when they felt well. The campaign also set up rural schools as an essential weapon in this struggle for the minds as well as the bodies of patients—a struggle that forged a lasting health education alliance between the doctor and the teacher.

Similarly, in the Afrotropic ecoregion the provision of impregnated mosquito nets alone is merely a gesture rather than an effective policy of control. Successful use of nets presupposes a dedicated and rigorous daily discipline. Studies published in 2003 indicate that, even in African households that possess netting, the vast majority of the population most at risk—pregnant women and small children—does not use them at all, or at least not according to specifications. In intensely malarial regions not even 10 percent of pregnant women and children regularly sleep under netting.[10]

There is no shortcut on the high road to health. The conquest of malaria presupposes that patients have been empowered to act in their own self-defense through knowledge, that they have access to care and regular contact with nurses and physicians, and that they have a sufficient education to understand the nature and essential mechanisms of this complex and dreadful illness. Italy succeeded in eradicating malaria only after the Italian state had saturated the nation with a thick network of rural health stations and rural schools that nearly eradicated illiteracy even before they eradicated the plasmodium.

In addition, it must be stressed that the advances the Italians made with quinine were predicated on the fact that care and the medication itself were furnished to the poor without charge. To recommend a technological product, even of a relatively humble kind, to the impoverished on market principles is in reality to deny them health. The products of Western medical science are useful weapons to combat malaria only to the extent to which they are universally accessible.

Another reason for rejecting an approach relying on a single, high-tech panacea emerges powerfully from the Italian experience. Although it was a potent antimalarial specific, quinine alone proved inadequate to the task of eradication. Physicians running health stations and clinics rapidly reported problems that eroded confidence in quinine's potential to accomplish the vast task with which Celli and Grassi first entrusted it. Quinine, first of all, had biological limits. Some patients were intolerant of it, experiencing such severe or unpleasant side effects that they abandoned the regimen. In addition, the malariologist Giulio Raffaele discovered in the 1930s that *Plasmodium vivax* often nestles at length in the liver tissues of patients, safely beyond the reach of the alkaloid. Here was a physical basis for the relapses that so puzzled physicians and frustrated Grassi's vision of radical cure. Another biological limit, which Italian physicians noted as early as the First World War, was the problem of parasite strains that were resistant to the medication. Human nature also proved to be a nearly insurmountable barrier on the path to eradication because the quinine regimen is so demanding and so lengthy. Populations cannot be expected to follow the requisite disciplined behavior before they have even developed symptoms or after the symptoms have ceased. Thus quinine demonstrated that, while it radically lowered mortality from malaria, it was incapable of lowering morbidity to the same degree or of achieving the ultimate goal of eradication.

In the same manner, DDT made a major contribution to the final push to eradication that began in 1944, but it cannot reasonably be credited with the entire final success in eradicating the disease. In the years since the end of the Second World War, Italy has profited from many interlocking factors affecting the vulnerability of the population to malaria. Italians did benefit immediately after the war from five-year programs of spraying DDT throughout the peninsula. In addition, however, malaria rapidly receded under the press of other circumstances—environmental sanitation, the breakup of latifundia and the introduction of intensive cultivation in crucial malarial zones (such as Apulia), the reestablishment of the antimalarial campaign and the resumption of mass quinine distribution, and greatly improved housing and diet through economic recovery and aid from the Marshall Plan. The nation also made ample use of institutions already long in place—rural health stations and schools, universal literacy, facilities for patient treatment, and the presence of trained and experienced personnel.

The WHO and the international public health community initially drew an inaccurate lesson from the Italian DDT experience, reaching the fallacious conclusion that because eradication followed DDT, it was caused by DDT. The fact that reality is more complex and recalcitrant was indicated in the 1950s and the 1960s, when the attempt to imitate on a global scale the purported success of Italy with the seemingly all-powerful hydrocarbon failed comprehensively. Contrary to legend, DDT was no stand-alone panacea. Indeed, it also gave rise to serious environmental issues. By 1969 the effort was entirely abandoned.[11]

What the Italian experience suggests instead is strikingly different. Technological means are important, and one of the features of the Italian School of malariology was its attempt to transform discoveries in the laboratory and in the field into useful advances in the clinic. The control of malaria requires ongoing scientific research and the practical use of its results. Nevertheless, the antimalarial campaigners who ran the rural health stations learned even before the First World War that the idea of relying on a single scientific and technological weapon was misguided. Malaria, they reported after painstaking epidemiological investigations at health stations throughout the nation, closely reflects the totality of the relations of human beings with their environment and with one another. It is at once a disease of poverty, of environmental degradation, of overpopulation, of poor nutrition, of inadequate housing, of illiteracy, of neglect, of population displacement, and of improper agricultural cultivation. As progress occurred before the First World War, therefore, the campaigners attributed the advances not only to free quinine but also to improved housing and wages (a result of mass emigration and industrial advance), to increased literacy, to better nutrition, and to the moral commitment of the political authorities of the nation. These factors were antimalarials of no less importance than quinine itself. Malaria receded, in other words, with advancing social justice. In the words of the malariologist Jose Najera in 2000, "All the accumulated experience . . . shows that malaria control cannot be undertaken without careful consideration of its socioeconomic and environmental relationships."[12]

It is one of the tragedies of present international responses to the burgeoning crisis of malaria in the tropical world that it focuses instead on two poles of magic thinking, one low tech and one high tech. At the low-tech pole, Roll Back Malaria urges reliance on impregnated mosquito nets and concentrates much of its effort on discovering means to make the nets cheaper, more widely available, and more reliable. The problem, however, is not with the nets. Impregnated nets are likely to be useful, but only if they are combined with a multifactorial approach that includes attention to other major determinants of malaria in the Afrotropic ecoregion. These determinants include malnutrition, illiteracy, migrant labor, warfare, poverty, environmental degradation, displaced persons, and the failure of both local governments and the industrial powers to recognize the magnitude of the public health crisis.

At the other pole, the public health community bases its hopes for the final control of malaria on high-tech research involving the development either of an antiplasmodial vaccine or of genetically reengineered mosquitoes. Waiting for the vaccine while devoting a disproportionate share of scarce resources to the effort is not a valid strategy. There is no precedent for an effective vaccine against a pathogen with a life cycle as complex as that of a plasmodium. Vaccines that demonstrate some effectiveness against one stage of its development have all proved to be useless because they fail to provide immunity against the parasite in all of its forms. It even remains an open question whether an antimalarial vaccine is biologically possible. According to a gloomy 1997 assessment in the journal *Lancet,* "Developing a vaccine against malaria has more in common with developing a vaccine against breast cancer than one against smallpox."[13] Meanwhile resources are drained from simpler but known antimalarials and patients continue to suffer and die. Relying on a future magic bullet will not roll back malaria.

Similar considerations apply to the objective of producing mosquitoes that are resistant to the parasite, oriented to animals (zoophilic) rather than humans as a result of chromosomally altered olfactory systems, or incapable of transmitting disease because of the artificially selected traits of their salivary glands. Such research is important and may indeed ultimately yield new weapons in the war against malaria. An excessive reliance on such potentially illusory hopes, however, avoids the use of those more humble antimalarials that are less dramatic but have already proved their effectiveness, promises results that will be posthumous for the millions now in the vise of this implacable killer, and bypasses the contribution that communities and individuals can make to their own self-defense. There is also a serious question of what possible protocols would induce a nation to allow the mass experimental release on its territory of a notoriously hematophagous mosquito on the strength of laboratory assurances that it had been engineered to be harmless. As in the case of DDT, the possibility of doing unintended but serious harm to the environment is a major cause of concern. Finally, a reasonable conclusion from the history of promised medical miracle weapons is that hope has nearly always exceeded performance. Even in the case of the most powerful antimalarial technologies, the question remains, What is the appropriate context for their deployment? With respect to this issue, Angelo Celli adopted as his own a Latin motto that has enormous contemporary relevance—"Do one thing, but do not omit others" (*Unum facere et alterum non omittere*).[14]

Ultimately, the lesson of the Italian case is that an effective antimalarial program needs to involve a multifaceted strategy. It should include North-South partnership, the moral awakening of affluent powers to the vicious cycle of poverty and disease, education to teach populations how to advance their own health, ready access to care and affordable treatment, environmental sanitation, and social justice along with basic scientific research. Finally, Italian success demonstrates the essential importance of an international framework of activity and large-scale international assistance. Italy realized the final goal of eradication with the scientific assistance and the financial support of the United Nations and the United States, which was given on the basis of an explicit recognition that the disease was an international problem in which the entire world community had a vital stake. It is both morally shortsighted and practically ineffective to expect national governments in states that form part of larger transnational ecosystems to solve a problem of such magnitude. Malaria is a crisis not of nations but of humanity. As Litsios writes in his work *The Tomorrow of Malaria,* "If malaria is not controlled in the twenty-first century, it will no doubt be because we have failed to put a stop to patterns of development which have destroyed natural resources, degraded environments, and uprooted and dehumanized peoples everywhere. . . . Thus the Tomorrow of Malaria represents more than doing battle with malaria-causing parasite species or malaria-carrying mosquito species; it is the Tomorrow of the Human species."[15]

In addition to its relevance for contemporary concerns of public health, the experience of the Italian antimalarial campaign is important for the discipline of medical history. Malaria provides an irrefutable demonstration that epidemic diseases are not a specialized or esoteric subdiscipline. On the contrary, malaria was an integral part of the big picture of modern Italian history. Its impact was deeply felt throughout Italian society, influencing high politics, the labor movement, women's rights, economic development, the Southern Question, military performance, education, and the domestic politics of the Fascist regime. Indeed, these issues cannot be properly understood without carefully considering the burden of this disease and the transforming effect of the campaign to eradicate it. The mobilization of resources to wage war on malaria for over half a century, and the deployment of two professions—physicians and teachers—to conduct the campaign, left a profound imprint on all facets of Italian life. Furthermore, the men and women who carried out the great struggle produced a vast outpouring of reports that constitute one of the best available sources for the social history of the era. The extensive reports by doctors available in archives and medical journals vividly document conditions of life and work throughout the peninsula. Historians for too long have neglected the light such sources can shed on how Italians lived during the century between unification in 1861 and eradication in 1962.

Malaria is also relevant to the understanding of Italian history since the completion of the eradication campaign. Denis Mack Smith, the most prominent English-language historian of modern Italy, wrote, in a striking insight that scholars have too long ignored, that the eradication of malaria was arguably "the most important single fact in the whole of modern Italian history."[16] Oddly for a country where the state had long proclaimed that this overwhelming and devastating illness constituted an insuperable obstacle to economic and social development, studies of postwar Italian history largely ignore the role of eradication in unleashing the resources of the nation. Such phenomena as the "economic miracle," for example, directly presupposed that malaria no longer continued to stunt productivity, limit education, consume resources, and enforce poverty. Most important, then, the Italian triumph over this disease provides a message of hope for a world struggling with the great present-day medical emergency. Contemporary Italy, now among the most healthy nations of the world, is an illustration of the social, economic, and cultural possibilities that become available when malaria is vanquished.[17]

Notes

Abbreviations for archival sources are identified in the Select Bibliography.

Introduction

1. For a brief overview of the history of malaria in Italy, a useful starting point is Gilberto Corbellini and Lorenza Merzagora, *La malaria tra passato e presente* (Rome, 1998). This work is the official guide to an exhibit on the history of malaria in Italy shown at the University of Rome "La Sapienza" in the fall of 1998. Other studies since the Second World War include Arturo Bianchini, *La malaria e la sua incidenza nella storia e nell'economia della regione pontina* (Latina, 1964); F. Bonelli, "La malaria nella storia demografica ed economica d'Italia: Primi lineamenti d'una ricerca," *Studi storici,* VII (1966), 659–687; P. Corti, "La malaria nell'agro romano e potino dell'Ottocento," in A. Pastore and P. Sorcinelli, eds., *Sanità e Società* (Udine, 1987), vol. II, 285–324; Paola Corti, "Malaria e società contadina nel Nezzogiorno," in Franco Della Paruta, ed., *Storia d'Italia, Annali 7: Malattia e medicina* (Turin, 1984), 633–678; Gianfranco Donelli and Enrica Serinaldi, *Dalla lotta alla malaria alla nascita dell'Istituto di Sanità Pubblica: Il ruolo della Rockefeller Foundation in Italia, 1922–1934* (Rome, 2003); Bernardino Fantini, "*Unum facere et alterum non omittere:* Antimalarial Strategies in Italy, 1880–1930," *Parassitologia,* XL (1998), 91–101; J. Farley, "Mosquitoes or Malaria? Rockefeller Campaigns in the American South and Sardinia," *Parassitologia,* XXXVI (1994), 165–173; John A. Logan, *The Sardinia Project: An Experiment in the Eradication of an Indigenous Malarious Vector* (Baltimore, 1953); Elisabetta Novello, *La bonifica in Italia: Legis-*

lazione, credito e lotta alla malaria dall'Unità al Fascismo (Milan, 2003); and E. Tognotti, *La malaria in Sardegna: Per una storia del paludismo nel Mezzogiorno, 1880–1950* (Milan, 1996). A guide to sources on the subject is Archivio Centrale dello Stato, *Fonti per la storia della malaria in Italia* (Rome, 2003).

2. *Naples in the Time of Cholera, 1884–1911* (Cambridge, England, 1995).

3. *Inchiesta sulle condizioni dei contadini in Basilicata e in Calabria (1910)* in *Scritti sulla questione meridionale*, vol. IV (Bari, 1968), 109. See also 20, 26–27, 44, 87–110. All translations are my own unless otherwise indicated.

4. Giuseppe Tropeano, *La malaria nel Mezzogiorno d'Italia* (Naples, 1908), 43.

5. For the papers given at the conference, see the special edition of the journal *Parassitologia,* XLI, nos. 1–3 (Sept. 1999).

Chapter 1. Malaria

1. Corrado Tommasi-Crudeli, *The Climate of Rome and the Roman Malaria,* trans. Charles Cramond Dick (London, 1892), 59–60.

2. *The Birth of Modern Italy: Posthumous Papers of Jessie White Mario,* ed. Duke Litta-Visconti-Arese (London, 1909), 250.

3. For a brief history of malaria in the city of Rome in the nineteenth century, see G. Pecori, "La malaria dell'Urbe nei tempi passati e la sua salubrità attuale," *Capitolium,* I (1925–1926), 505–509. On the experiences of 1849 and 1870, see Anna Celli-Fraentzel [M. L. Heid, pseud.], *Uomini che non scompaiono* (Florence, 1944), 59–75. The misadventure of Daisy Miller is the subject of Henry James, *Daisy Miller* (New York, 1900).

4. *Della periodicità nelle febbri e della sua causa e natura* (Pesaro, 1826), 8.

5. "La legislazione e l'organizzazione sanitaria per la lotta contro la malaria in Italia," *Rivista di malariologia,* VII (1928), 714.

6. For Torelli's bill, see "Senato del Regno. Progetto di legge presentato dal senatore Torelli preso in considerazione nella tornata del 27 gennaio 1883. Bonificamento delle regioni di malaria in Italia," *Atti parlamentari della Camera dei senatori, Discussioni, Legislatura XV, sessione 1882–86, Atti interni,* vol. I, no. 17, 1–11. The weather also played a role in alerting Torelli to the problem of malaria. From October 1878 to May 1879 Italy was drenched by the heaviest rains in living memory, creating ideal conditions for a major upsurge in malaria, which duly occurred in the summer of 1879. Francesco Ladelci, *Intorno alle febbri di periodo* (Rome, 1880), 4.

7. *Carta della malaria dell'Italia illustrata* (Florence, 1882); *Il curato di campagna e la malaria dell'Italia: Quindici dialoghi* (Rome, 1884).

8. *Atti della Giunta per l'Inchiesta Agraria sulle condizioni della classe agricola,* 15 vols. (Rome, 1881–1886).

9. *Atti della Giunta per l'Inchiesta Agraria,* vol. XI, tomo 1, *Provincie di Roma e Grosseto* (1883), 70. This work was explicitly singled out for praise by Angelo Celli, *Come vive il campagnolo nell'Agro Romano* (Rome, 1900), 14.

10. *Atti della Giunta per l'Inchiesta Agraria,* vol. XII, tomo 1 (1884), 295–296; and vol. XI, tomo 1 (1883), 28.

11. *Atti della Giunta per l'Inchiesta Agraria,* vol. XIV, tomo 1 (1885), 9.

12. *Intorno alle febbri di periodo,* 4.

13. Classic statements of the miasmatic position include Carlo Pavesi, *Le risaie ed il vasto disboscamento dei terreni* (Rome, 1874); Francesco Puccinotti, *Opere mediche,* 2 vols. (Milan, 1855–1856); Pietro Roberti, *Manuale di cognizioni utili concernenti la patologia, la profilassi e la terapia della malaria* (Lagonegro, 1906); Antonio Selmi, *Il miasma palustre: Lezioni di chimica igienica* (Padua, 1870); and Tommasi-Crudeli, *The Climate of Rome.* For a survey of scientific opinion regarding the etiology of malaria on the eve of the biological discoveries at the end of the century, see Guido Baccelli, "La malaria di Roma," in Ministero di Agricoltura, Industria e Commercio: Direzione Generale della Statistica, *Monografia della città di Roma,* vol. I (Rome, 1881), 149–195. The Ministry of Agriculture defined malaria as "a miasma . . . probably consisting of microscopic organic germs that are produced in stagnant waters, or . . . also in the soil and subsoil when they are soaked with stagnant water" (ibid., lvii).

14. *The Climate of Rome,* 53.

15. Edwin Klebs and Corrado Tommasi-Crudeli, "On the Nature of Malaria," trans. Edward Drummond, *New Sydenham Society* (1888), 1–56.

16. Angelo Celli, "L'epidemiologia e la profilassi della malaria," *L'arte medica,* I, nos. 45–47 (1890), 10–11; Errico De Renzi, "Relazione sulla campagna antimalarica condotta in Provincia di Caserta nell'anno 1907," ACS, MI, DGS (1882–1915), b. 95, fasc. "Studi sulla malaria in provincia di Caserta. Relazioni del Prof. De Renzi," 13.

17. Francesco Scalzi, *La meteorologia in rapporto alle febbri malariche e alle flogosi polmoniche studiate negli ospedali di Santo Spirito e del Laterano nell'anno 1878* (Rome, 1879), 12; Ettore Marchiafava and Amico Bignami, *La infezione malarica* (Milan, 1904), 167–168. For a discussion of Max von Pettenkofer, see Frank M. Snowden, *Naples in the Time of Cholera, 1884–1911* (Cambridge, England, 1995), esp. chapters 1 and 5.

18. "L'infezione malarica," *Giornale della malaria,* I (1907), 146–147.

19. Classic discussions of the pathology of malaria as explained in miasmatic terms are Ladelci, *Intorno alle febbri;* Giuseppe Pinto, *Cura delle complicazioni nelle febbri di periodo* (Rome, 1868); and Puccinotti, *Opere mediche.* For a brief survey of traditional factors that were considered "predisposing" or "occasional" causes of malaria, see Marchiafava and Bignami, *La infezione malarica,* 146–148.

20. Torelli's findings were confirmed by the parliamentary enquiry of 1885 conducted by Agostino Bertani. Its results are summarized in MI, DGS, *La malaria in Italia ed i risultati della lotta antimalarica* (Rome, 1924), 10–12.

21. The estimate of one hundred thousand is that of Giovanni Battista Grassi, *Difesa contro la malaria nelle zone risicole* (Milan, 1905), 5.

22. Angelo Celli et al., *La malaria* (Turin, 1934), 25–26.

23. "Senato del Regno," 5.

24. Eugenio Di Mattei, "La malaria in Italia nei lavoratori della terra e nei loro figli," *Malaria e malattie dei paesi caldi,* IV (1913), 243.

25. Mario Panizza, *Risultati dell'inchiesta istituita da Agostino Bertani sulle condizioni sanitarie dei lavoratori della terra in Italia: Riassunto e considerazioni* (Rome, 1890), 21.

26. The fairy tale analogy was also adopted by Jacini, who referred to Italy as "poor Cinderella." "Tornata del 27 aprile 1885," *Atti parlamentari della Camera dei senatori, Discussioni, Legislatura XV, sessione 1882–83–84,* 3549.

27. On the devastating epidemic of 1879, see Ladelci, *Intorno alle febbri,* 4.

28. See the WHO's information and advocacy Web site for the Roll Back Malaria program, http://www.rbm.who.int/newdesign2/poverty/poverty.

29. Ministero dell'Agricoltura: Ispettorato Generale del Bonificamento, della Colonizzazione e del Credito Agrario, *I consorzi antianofelici e il risanamento delle terre malariche* (Rome, 1918), 27.

30. Medico Provinciale, "Relazione sulla campagna antimalarica svoltasi nella Provincia di Girgenti nell'anno 1924," ACS, MI, DGS (1896–1934), b. 58, fasc. "Relazione sulla campagna antimalarica."

31. Medico Provinciale Albertazzi, "Relazione sull'applicazione della legge contro la malaria durante l'anno 1906," ACS, MI, DGS (1882–1915), b. 116, fasc. "Foggia"; "Roma," ACS, MI, DGS (1882–1915), b. 122, fasc. "Roma: Applicazione della legge sulla malaria," 10; "Provvedimenti pel servizio sanitario all'Agro Romano," *Atti del consiglio comunale di Roma dell'anno 1900,* I (1900), 488.

32. G. Pecori and G. Escalar, "Relazione sulla campagna antimalarica dell'anno 1930: Ufficio d'Igiene e Sanità del Governatorato di Roma," *Rivista di malariologia,* X (1931), 588.

33. The conservative leader Sidney Sonnino denounced the scandalous housing of day laborers in the Roman Campagna. See *Atti del parlamento italiano, Camera dei deputati, sessione del 1882–83, 1a della XV Legislatura, Discussioni,* IV, 2903–2904; and Celli, *Come vive il campagnolo nell'Agro Romano.*

34. *Inchiesta parlamentare sulle condizioni dei contadini nelle province meridionali e nella Sicilia,* 8 vols. (Rome, 1908–1911).

35. "Proposta del signor consigliere Pericoli di nominare una commissione d'inchiesta sulle condizioni dei lavoratori della campagna romana e sulle provvidenze opportune per migliorarle," *Atti del consiglio comunale di Roma dell'anno 1881* (Rome, 1882), 256–257.

36. "Campagna malarica del 1912," 8 May 1913, ACS, MI, DGS (1910–1920), b. 97 bis, fasc. "Caltanissetta."

37. *Il curato di campagna,* 44.

38. Bartolommeo Gosio, "Relazione sulla campagna antimalarica del 1906," ACS, MI, DGS (1882–1915), b. 95, fasc. "Studi sulla malaria nelle Calabrie e Basilicata. Relazione de. Prof. Gosio."

39. *Inchiesta sulle condizioni dei contadini in Basilicata e in Calabria (1910)* in *Scritti sulla questione meridionale,* vol. IV, 50–54 and 87–110.

40. Ministero per l'Agricoltura: Ispettorato Generale del Bonificamento, della Colonizzazione e del Credito Agrario, *I Consorzi antianofelici,* 16.

41. *La malaria e le risaie in Italia* (Milan, 1905), 6.

42. "Relazione dell'Ufficio Centrale composto dei senatori Pantaleoni, Moleschott, Verga e Torelli, relatore. Bonificamento delle regioni di malaria lungo le ferrovie d'Italia," *Atti parlamentari, Senato del Regno, sessione del 1880–81–92, documenti,* no. 19–A, 2. For other accounts asserting that malaria was one of the important factors promoting emigration, see Giacomo Rossi and Giuseppe Guarini, *La bonifica del Vallo di Diano nei suoi rapporti colla malaria* (Rome, 1906), 309; and F. Bertarelli, "Ancora i risultati della nostra legislazione antimalarica," *Critica sociale,* XVII (1907), 365–366.

43. On the effect of malaria on the army, see Generale Medico Chiaiso, "Note sulla malaria nell'esercito negli anni 1902–1903," *Atti della Società per gli Studi della Malaria,* V (1904), 723–744; and Torelli, *Il curato di campagna,* 50–55.

44. Emile Zola, *Rome* (Rome, 1907), 402.

45. On the effect of malaria on pregnant women, see Errico De Renzi, "Relazione sulla campagna antimalarica nella provincia di Caserta (agosto-dicembre 1911)," ACS, MI, DGS (1882–1915), b. 89, 11.

46. *Atti del consiglio comunale di Roma degli anni 1872–1873* (Rome, 1873), 781. For examples of racial anxiety in the press, see G. Cavasola, "Contro la malaria," *Corriere della sera,* 27–28 Mar. 1901; and "Il Chinino di Stato," *Corriere della sera,* 9–10 Jan. 1902.

47. Letter of Ernesto Ara and Riccardo Vella to Comm. Villetti, 26 Oct. 1922, ACC, Archivio Ripartizione VIII "Igiene," b. 159, fasc. 1 ("Anno 1922: Campagna antimalarica").

48. Antonio Sergi, "Sulla profilassi chininica scolastica," *Malariologia,* serie II, I (1915), 59.

49. Marchiafava and Bignami, *La infezione malarica,* 155–156.

50. Arcangelo Ilvento, "Sul servizio medico-scolastico rurale della Croce Rossa Giovanile," MI, DGS, *Organizzazioni antimalariche alla luce delle nuove dottrine* (Rome, 1925), part 2, chapter 2, 40.

51. This point was made by Giovanni Battista Grassi. See *Atti del Congresso Risicolo* (Vercelli, 1903), 233. A copy of the *Atti* is to be found in ACS, MI, DGS (1882–1915), b. 750.

52. *Atti della Giunta per l'Inchiesta Agraria,* vol. XII, fasc. 1, *Relazione del commissario Barone Giuseppe Andrea Angeloni, Deputato al Parlamento, sulla quarta circoscrizione (Provincie di Foggia, Bari, Lecce, Chieti, Teramo e Campobasso)* (1884), 294.

53. *Atti del Congresso Risicolo* (1903), 233.

54. On the differences between northern and southern malaria, see MI, DGS, *La malaria in Italia ed i risultati della lotta antimalarica,* 22–32. For the description of the "two Italies," see Antonio Tropeano, "La profilassi della malaria con l'uso quotidiano del chinino: Relazione all'Assemblea dell'Ordine dei Sanitari di Catanzaro e Provincia (dicembre 1906)," *Giornale della malaria,* II (1908), 276.

55. Oreste Bordiga, "La produzione ed il commercio del riso," *Atti del 20 Congresso Risicolo Internazionale: Mortara, 1–3 ottobre 1903* (Mortara-Vigevano, 1904), 50. A copy of the *Atti* is located in ACS, MI, DGS (1882–1915), b. 750. In rank order, the leading provinces for rice production in Italy at the turn of the century were Pavia, Novara, Milan, Verona, Mantua, Bologna, Rovigo, Reggio Emilia, and Ravenna. "La coltura del riso e le diverse operazioni agricole," ACS, MI, DGS (1882–1915), b. 748, fasc. "Legge sulla risicoltura," 14–15. On the history of rice production in Italy, see Luigi Faccini, "Lavoratori della risaia fra '700 e '800: Condizioni di vita, alimentazione, malattie," *Studi storici,* XIV, no. 3 (July 1974), 545–588.

56. The provisions of the Cantelli law and the subsequent legislation regulating rice cultivation are outlined in Giovanni Lorenzoni, *I lavoratori delle risaie* (Milan, 1904), 137–166. The texts of the provincial regulations completing the Cantelli law in the major

rice-producing provinces can be found in ACS, MI, DGS (1882–1915), b. 750, fasc. "Risicoltura: Affari generali (1895)." On the events leading to the ban at Parma, see Luigi Pagliani and C. Guerci, *Relazione intorno alla coltivazione delle risaie nell'Agro Parmense* (Rome, 1895).

Chapter 2. From Miasma to Mosquito

1. On the highly malarial island of Sicily, which was representative of conditions prevailing in the South as a whole, a similar problem arose for the theory of paludism. Out of a total surface area of 27,000 square kilometers, 10,000 square kilometers were classified as malarial areas. But the major permanent swamps in Sicily covered only 242 square kilometers. F. Salpietra, "La malaria," *Rivista sanitaria siciliana,* XIV, no. 21 (Nov. 1926), 1034, 1040.

2. L. W. Hackett, *Malaria in Europe: An Ecological Study* (Oxford, 1937), 11.

3. An important discussion of "wet" and "dry" malaria, and of the misleading association of the disease with swamps, is Eliseo Jandolo, "Gli indirizzi della legislazione attuale sulle bonifiche," *Rivista di malariologia,* XI (1932), 52–62.

4. For outlines of the annual cycle of malaria, see Giovanni Battista Grassi, *Relazione dell'esperimento di preservazione dalla malaria fatto sui ferrovieri nella piana di Capaccio* (Milan, 1901); and Saverio Santori, "La malaria nella provincia di Roma nel decennio 1888–1897," *Atti della Società per gli Studi della Malaria,* I (1899), 113–114.

5. "Relazione dell'Ufficio Centrale composto dai senatori Pantaleoni, Moleschott, Verga C. E Torelli, relatore. Bonificamento delle regioni di malaria lungo le ferrovie d'Italia," *Atti parlamentari: Senato del Regno, sessione del 1880–81–82, documenti,* no. 19–A, allegato 13. On the eve of the First World War, the physicians directing the antimalarial campaign in Sardinia confirmed Torelli's account of deforestation. Elderly inhabitants reported that deforestation had become intense after about 1850. Alessandro Lustig, Achille Sclavo, and Michele Alivia, *Relazione sommaria della campagna antimalarica condotta nella Provincia di Sassari nel 1910: Contributo alla conoscenza delle condizioni igieniche-sociali della Sardegna* (Florence, 1911), 19.

6. Cesare Lombroso, *Crime: Its Causes and Remedies,* trans. P. Horton (Boston, 1911), 248–249. A recent study of the deforestation of mountains in the Mediterranean is John Robert McNeill, *The Mountains of the Mediterranean World: An Environmental History* (Cambridge, England, 1992).

7. *Il curato di campagna e la malaria dell'Italia: Quindici dialoghi* (Rome, 1884), 47–48. Statistics on the development of railroads are provided by "Progetto di legge presentato dal senatore Torelli: Bonificamento delle regioni di malaria lungo le ferrovie d'Italia," *Atti parlamentari: Senato del Regno, sessione del 1880, documenti,* vol. I, no. 19, 1. On the role of the notorious excavation ditches (*cave di prestito*) in the etiology of malaria, see Angelo Celli, "L'epidemiologia e la profilassi della malaria," *L'arte medica,* I, nos. 45–47 (1890), 12. On "man-made malaria," a classic discussion is Paul F. Russell, Luther S. West, and Reginald D. Manwell, *Practical Malariology* (Philadelphia, 1946), chapter 26, 533–545.

8. "Relazione dell'Ufficio Centrale," allegato 26.

9. Ibid., allegato 15.

10. On popular means of self-protection against malaria, see Angelo Celli, "Sull'immunità dall'infezione malarica," *Atti della Società per gli Studi della Malaria,* I (1899), esp. 52–54.

11. For discussion of malaria's effects on the pattern of settlement in the South, see *Inchiesta parlamentare sulle condizioni dei contadini nelle provincie meridionali e nella Sicilia,* vol. II, *Abruzzo e Molise, Tomo I, Relazione del delegato tecnico dott. Cesare Jarach* (Rome, 1909), 181–182, 201, 275; and vol IV, *Campania, Tomo I, Relazione del delegato tecnico prof. Oreste Bordiga* (Rome, 1909), 37. See also Francesco Saverio Nitti, *Inchiesta sulle condizioni dei contadini in Basilicata e in Calabria (1910)* in *Scritti sulla questione meridionale,* vol. IV (Bari, 1968), 1, 20, 26, 43, 58, 87–110. The two most influential malariologists of the Giolittian era, Grassi and Celli, also stressed the widespread awareness of the protective value of altitude and its effect on the pattern of settlement. See Giovanni Battista Grassi, "Considerazioni epidemiologiche," USR, AG, b. 21, fasc. 5 ("Fiumicino 1918") n.d., 2–3; and Celli, "Sull'immunità dall'infezione malarica," 52–53.

12. *Inchiesta parlamentare,* vol. I, *Sicilia, Tomo I, Relazione del delegato tecnico prof. Giovanni Lorenzoni* (Rome, 1910), 17.

13. *The Climate of Rome and the Roman Malaria,* trans. Charles Cramond Dick (London, 1892), 131.

14. On the persistent belief in the protective value of wine and steak in the Roman Campagna, see Nicola Giusti, "La campagna antimalarica nell'Agro Romano: Stazione sanitaria di Decimo," *Atti della Società per gli Studi della Malaria,* V (1904), 618. On the "doctrine of signatures," see Redcliffe N. Salaman, *The History and Social Influence of the Potato* (Cambridge, England, 1949), 110–113; and Roy Porter, *The Greatest Benefit to Mankind* (London, 1997), 201–205, 282.

15. On this point, see Bernardino Fantini, "*Unum facere et alterum non omittere:* Antimalarial Strategies in Italy, 1880–1930," *Parassitologia,* XL (1998), esp. 92–95.

16. On the Baccarini Law, see Giuseppe Tassinari, *La bonifica integrale nel decennale della legge Mussolini* (Rome, 1939), 147–148; and Elisabetta Novello, *La bonifica in Italia: Legislazione, credito e lotta alla malaria dall'Unità al Fascismo* (Milan, 2003), 40–48. For a history of land reclamation in Italy since the eighteenth century, see Pietro Bevilacqua and Manlio Rossi Doria, eds., *Le bonifiche in Italia dal '700 a oggi* (Rome, 1984). With special reference to the Roman Campagna after unification, see Ministero di Agricoltura, Industria e Commercio: Direzione Generale dell'Agricoltura, *Il bonificamento dell'Agro Romano* (Rome, 1915).

17. Vincenzo Gioberti, *Del primato morale e civile degli italiani,* 3 vols. (Turin, 1920–1932; 1st ed. 1843); Giuseppe Tropeano, *La malaria nel Mezzogiorno d'Italia* (Napoli, 1908), 31.

18. On the troubling questions arising with regard to miasmatism, see Ettore Marchiafava and Amico Bignami, *La infezione malarica* (Milan, 1904), 122–126.

19. On the initial discovery of the plasmodium, see Alphonse Laveran, *Prophylaxie du paludisme* (Paris, n.d.), 1–14.

20. Among the works on the pathology of malaria that inform the discussion here are the following: Mark F. Boyd, *Malariology: A Comprehensive Survey of All Aspects of This Group of Diseases from a Global Standpoint* (Philadelphia, 1949); Robert Gold-

smith and Donald Heyneman, *Tropical Medicine and Parasitology* (Norwalk, Conn., 1989); Gordon Harrison, *Mosquitoes, Malaria and Man: A History of the Hostilities since 1880* (New York, 1978); Franklin A. Neva and Harold W. Brown, *Basic Clinical Parasitology,* 6th ed. (Norwalk, Conn., 1994); and Walter H. Wernsdorfer and Ian McGregor, *Malaria: Principles and Practice of Malariology* (Edinburgh, 1988). Contemporary accounts include Vittorio Ascoli, *La malaria* (Turin, 1915); Patrick Manson, *Tropical Diseases* (London, 1914); Ronald Ross, *The Prevention of Malaria* (London, 1910); and Giuseppe Sanarelli, *Lo stato attuale del problema malarico: Rilievi e proposte* (Rome, 1925). Although the pathology of malaria at the molecular level is still imperfectly understood, research suggests that one of the most serious causes of suffering and death is an autoimmune response of the body involving the release of proteins known as cytokines, the most important and best studied of which is "tumor necrosis factor" (TNF). The overabundant production of TNF as an immune response of the body has been identified as a principal factor in the pathophysiology of human malaria. On this issue, see I. A. Clark, "Cell-Mediated Immunity in Protection and Pathology of Malaria," *Parasitology Today,* III (1987), 300–305; I. A. Clark and G. Chaudhri, "Tumor Necrosis Factor May Contribute to the Anaemia of Malaria by Causing Dyserythropoiesis and Erythrophagocytosis," *British Journal of Haematology,* LXX (1988), 99–103; Ian A. Clark, William B. Cowden, and Geeta Chaudhri, "Possible Roles for Oxidants, through Tumor Necrosis Factor in Malarial Anemia," in John W. Eaton, Steven R. Meshnick, and George J. Brewer, eds., *Malaria and the Red Cell: Proceedings of the Second Workshop on Malaria and the Red Cell, Held in Ann Arbor, Michigan, October 24, 1988* (New York, 1989), 73–82; I. A. Clark and W. B. Cowden, "Roles of TNF in Malaria and Other Parasitic Infections," *Immunology,* series LVI (1992), 365–407; and I. M. Schlichtherle et al., "Molecular Aspects of Severe Malaria," *Parasitology Today,* XII (1996), 329–332.

21. On the work of Camillo Golgi, see his collected papers, *Gli studi di Camillo Golgi sulla malaria,* ed. Aldo Perroncito (Rome, 1929).

22. Since he lived and worked at Pavia rather than Rome, Golgi is best described as a member of the Italian School rather than of the Rome School.

23. "Italy in the History of Malaria," *Rivista di parassitologia,* XIII (1952), 93, 99.

24. In the tropical world there is a fourth species, *Plasmodium ovale,* but it is replaced in Europe by *Plasmodium malariae.*

25. Brief overviews of the society's activities are F. Jerace, "L'opera della Società per gli Studi della Malaria," *Rivista di malariologia,* XVII (1938), 206–207; and Margherita Bettini Prosperi and Gilberto Corbellini, "Una tradizione malariologica durata settant'anni (1898–1967)," in Giuliana Gemelli, Girolamo Ramunni, and Vito Gallotta, eds., *Isole senza arcipelago: Imprenditori scientifici, reti e istituzioni tra Otto e Novecento* (Bari, 2003), 55–82. Given the disputes that divided the Rome School and the absence of a collective institutional incarnation, there are scholars who debate whether the school actually existed. The most important revisionist assessment is that of Gilberto Corbellini, "I malariologi italiani: Storia scientifica e istituzionale di una comunità conflittuale," in Antonio Casella et al., *Una difficile modernità: Tradizioni di ricerca e comunità scientifiche in Italia, 1890–1940* (Pavia, 2000), 299–327.

26. Banco di Napoli, "Relazione sull'operato dell'istituto per combattere la malaria: Anno 1904," Mar. 1905, ACS, MI, DGS (1910–1920), b. 106, fasc. "Banco di Napoli: Azione per la lotta contro la malaria."

27. Grassi explains the financial resources that were made available to him as he carried out his experiments to prove the mosquito theory of transmission in *Studi di uno zoologo sulla malaria* (Rome, 1901), 6.

28. On the issue of anophelism without malaria, see Hackett, *Malaria in Europe*, 10–12; and Scuola Superiore di Malariologia, *Lezioni del Prof. A. Missiroli* (Rome, 1929), 3–6, 28–32.

29. Grassi's account of the development of the mosquito theory of transmission is *Studi di uno zoologo.*

30. For an account by Ross of his work, see *The Prevention of Malaria*, 10–29.

31. For Grassi's account of this experiment, see *Studi di uno zoologo*, 21–26. See also Laveran, *Prophylaxie du paludisme*, 27–30. Grassi defined his "doctrine" as consisting of the following points: (1) "Human malaria is transmitted exclusively by means of anophelines, and where they are lacking, it cannot take hold"; (2) "At their birth anophelines are not harmful; they become so only after biting an infected human"; (3) "To become infective, an anopheline requires a temperature that is not too low"; (4) "The parasites of human malaria can live only in anophelines, or in man." For Italian conditions specifically, there were two additional points: (1) "There is here an annual and almost total truce in the epidemic of malaria. It lasts approximately from the start of January to the end of the first week of June. We call this the interepidemic period"; (2) "All the anophelines from the previous year die in the early spring so that there is hardly one left by the middle of April." Giovanni Battista Grassi, "La lutte contre le paludisme à Fiumicino" (1924), USR, AG, b. 22, fasc. 3.

32. G. B. Grassi, A. Bignami, and G. Bastianelli, "Ciclo evolutivo delle semilune nell' 'Anopheles Claviger' ed altri studi sulla malaria dall'ottobre 1898 al maggio 1899," *Annali d'igiene sperimentale, nuova serie*, IX (1899), 258–270; Grassi, *Studi di uno zoologo*, 30. On *anofelismo senza malaria*, see Giovanni Battista Grassi, "A proposito del paludismo senza malaria," *Rendiconti della R. Accademia dei Lincei*, X (1901), 2 sem., serie 5, fasc. 6, 123–131.

33. *Relazione dell'esperimento di preservazione dalla malaria fatto sui ferrovieri nella piana di Capaccio* (Milan, 1901), 1.

34. Grassi's account of the experiment at Capaccio is *Relazione dell'esperimento.*

35. Giovanni Battista Grassi, *Difesa contro la malaria nelle zone risicole* (Milan, 1905), 5. For corroborating experiments in Sicily and the Pontine Marshes, see Eugenio Di Mattei, "La profilassi malarica colla protezione dell'uomo dalle zanzare," *Annali d'igiene sperimentale, nuova serie*, XI (1901), 107–114; and C. Fermi and U. Cano-Brusco, "Esperienze profilattiche contro la malaria istituite allo Stagno di Liccari," *Annali d'igiene sperimentale, nuova serie*, XI (1901), 121–124.

36. Medico Provinciale di Bari, "Relazione sull'applicazione delle leggi contro la malaria durante il 1916," ACS, MI, DGS (1910–1920), b. 111, fasc. "Bari." Grassi's discussion of the issues is in "Relazione dell'esperimento antimalarico di Fiumicino," 18 Dec. 1918, ACS, MI, DGS (1910–1920), b. 103, fasc. "Commissione per lo studio delle opere di piccola bonifica: Relazione del prof. Battista Grassi," 32–34.

37. On the experiment at Ostia, see Giovanni Battista Grassi, *Aggiunte all'opera 'Studi di uno zoologo sulla malaria': Relazione riassuntiva* (Rome, 1902). At Ostia Grassi made use of the commercial product known as Esanofele, which had quinine as its active ingredient, plus compounds of arsenic and iron as tonics.

38. A history of the medicinal uses of quinine is M. L. Duran-Reynals, *The Fever Bark Tree: The Pageant of Quinine* (Garden City, N.Y., 1946).

39. On the "divine medicine," see Dott. Fazio, "Relazione" (1915), ACS, MI, DGS (1896–1934), b. 57.

40. *Atti della Società per gli Studi della Malaria,* I (1899), vi.

41. *Aggiunte all'opera,* 10.

42. On this dispute, see Corbellini, "I malariologi italiani," 305, 307–308.

43. Daniel 2:24–45 (New English Bible).

44. "La lutte contre le paludisme à Fiumicino."

45. *Difesa contro la malaria nelle zone risicole,* 6.

46. For Grassi's estimate of the time and money required to free Italy from malaria, see *Difesa contro la malaria nelle zone risicole,* 5–6; Grassi, "La lutte contre le paludisme à Fiumicino."

47. "Malaria in Italy in 1903," *Lancet,* II (1904), 1371.

48. Ry, "Legislazione antimalarica," *Corriere della sera,* 30–31 Dec. 1900.

Chapter 3. A Nation Mobilizes

1. Giovanni Battista Grassi, *Difesa contro la malaria nelle zone risicole* (Milan, 1905), 5–7.

2. Ministero dell'Interno, Direzione Generale della Sanità Pubblica, *La malaria in Italia ed i risultati della lotta antimalarica* (Rome, 1924), 33. This point was also stressed by Antonio Labranca, inspector general of the Department of Health. In his words, "The fundamental characteristic [of the antimalarial legislation] is the recognition of malaria as an infectious and occupational disease, in that it is linked with work and with residence in unhealthy localities for reasons of work. Therefore, the expenses necessary for the measure contemplated for the cure and prevention of malaria—both among the rural population and among the workers employed in public works—are charged respectively to landlords and farmers on the one hand and to companies and public agencies on the other." "La legislazione e l'organizzazione sanitaria per la lotta contro la malaria in Italia," *Rivista di malariologia,* VII (1928), 719.

3. Ministero dell'Interno, *La malaria in Italia.* This work provides an overall survey of the antimalarial campaign in the Liberal period. One of the few modern articles devoted to this subject is Paola Corti, "Malaria e società contadina nel Mezzogiorno," in Franco Della Peruta, ed., *Storia d'Italia, Annali 7: Malattia e medicina* (Turin, 1984), 635–680.

4. Sardinia was an example of a region in which many localities did not appoint public health doctors. Medico Provinciale, "Relazione della campagna antimalarica dell'anno 1908," ACS, MI, DGS (1882–1915), b. 120, fasc. "Sassari."

5. "Roma," n.d., ACS, MI, DGS (1882–1915), b. 122 bis, fasc. "Roma: Applicazione della legge sulla malaria," 15.

6. Letter of Roberto Villetti to Gabinetto dell'on. Sindaco, 16 Feb. 1922, ACC, Archivio Ripartizione VIII "Igiene," b. 159, fasc. 1 ("Anno 1922: Campagna antimalarica"). On the leading role of Rome, see also Donato Vitullo, "Andamento dell'endemia malarica nell'Agro Romano in relazione ai metodi di lotta usati," *Rivista di malariologia,* XXXI (1952), 30–32.

7. An interesting article on the early phases of the campaign by a leading figure is Alessandro Lustig, "Questioni del giorno," *Minerva,* XXX (Dec. 1909–Dec. 1910), 87–90, 111–113.

8. Lodovico Violini Nogarola, *L'opera del Comitato Antimalarico Veronese dal 5 agosto 1912 al 31 dicembre 1913* (Verona, 1914), 5–13.

9. On the establishment and functions of rural health stations in the Roman Campagna, see "Proposta di assistenza sanitaria nell'Agro Romano," *Atti del consiglio comunale di Roma degli anni 1872–1873* (Rome, 1873), 710–714; "Istituzione di nuove stazioni sanitarie nell'Agro romano," *Atti del consiglio comunale di Roma dell'anno 1881,* I (Rome, 1881), 314–333; and "Progetto di riforma per i servizi di assistenza sanitaria nel suburbio ed Agro Romano," *Atti del consiglio comunale di Roma dell'anno 1907,* I (Rome, 1907), 800–859. On the use of the experience of the municipality of Rome as a model for the national campaign, see letter of Assessore per l'Igiene to Gabinetto dell'On.le Sindaco, 16 Feb. 1922, ACC, Archivio Ripartizione VIII "Igiene," b. 159, fasc. 1 ("Anno 1922: Campagna antimalarica"). The numbers of health stations are provided by Alberto Lutrario, "Epidemiologia e profilassi generale: La lotta antimalarica in Italia," *Bolletino Malariologico,* II (1923), 5.

10. Lustig, "Questioni del giorno," 90.

11. Grassi particularly stressed the need for dispensaries to provide a full medical service. Giovanni Battista Grassi, "La malaria nell'Agro Pontino e l'opera dell'Istituto Antimalarico Pontino," 21 Feb. 1925, ASL, CPA, b. 18 (1). For a description of the dispensary at Quadrato in the Pontine Marshes, see Istituto Nazionale pel Risanamento Antimalarico della Regione Pontina, "Relazione sanitaria del direttore dell'ambulatorio del Quadrato, dott. Vincenzo Giannelli, luglio 1923–giugno 1924," ASL, CPA, b. 18 (1), fasc. "Relazioni: Attività IAP, 1923–1926," 4. See also ASL, CPA, Comitato antimalarico: Relazione medici, b. 18 (1), fasc. "Relazioni: Attività IAP, 1923–1926"; Grassi, "La malaria nell'Agro Pontino e l'opera dell'Istituto Antimalarico Pontino"; and Dott. Pericle Pozzilli, "La Campagna antimalarica compiuta dal Municipio di Tivoli nell'Agro tiburtino nel 1906," ACS, MI, DGS (1882–1915), b. 122 bis, fasc. "Roma: Applicazione della legge sulla malaria."

12. On the role of health stations in the campaign against malaria, see Gaetano Rummo and Luigi Ferrannini, "La Campagna antimalarica nella provincia di Benevento durante il 1910: Relazione a S.E. Il Ministro dell'Interno," ACS, MI, DGS (1882–1915), b. 88, fasc. "On. Rummo," sottofasc. "Prov. Di Benevento"; and Alessandro Lustig, Achille Sclavo, and Michele Alivia, *Relazione sommaria della campagna antimalarica condotta nella Provincia di Sassari nel 1910: Contributo alla conoscenza delle condizioni igieniche-sociali della Sardegna* (Firenze, 1911), 6–10. See also letter of Bartolommeo Gosio to Ministero dell'Interno, Direzione General della Sanità, 11 Aug. 1904, ACS, MI, DGS (1882–1915), b. 91, fasc. "Prof. Gosio." Gosio wrote, "Above all I must report the excellent results already achieved by the dispensaries, especially those located in the countryside. This institution is greeted everywhere with real enthusiasm both by doctors and by patients. I am ever more convinced that this is the only system that can produce positive, lasting, and demonstrable results in malarial areas."

13. The official report on the involvement of the Red Cross is Paolo Postempski, *La Campagna antimalarica compiuta dalla Croce Rossa Italiana nell'Agro Romano nel 1900* (Rome, 1901).

14. A brief summary of the role of central government in the campaign is that of Lutrario, "Epidemiologia e profilassi generale," 3–5.

15. The list of *commissari* is in ACS, MI, DGS (1882–1915), b. 94, fasc. "Convocazioni," sottofasc. "Riunione di scienziati convocati dal Ministro Giolitti per la lotta contro la malaria." On the financial contributions of central government, see letter of Prefect of Venice to On. Ministero dell'Interno, Direzione Generale della Sanità, 5 Oct. 1909, ACS, MI, DGS (1882–1915), b. 127.

16. Domenico Migliori, *Sanatorii antimalarici nella provincia di Cosenza* (Cosenza, 1911); Giuseppe Zagari, "Relazione" (1909), ACS, MI, DGS (1882–1915), b. 93; Arnaldo Trambusti, *La lotta contro la malaria in Sicilia* (Palermo, 1910), 47; Lutrario, "Epidemiologia e profilassi generale"; B. Gosio, "Sanatorî per bambini malarici," *Rivista di malariologia,* XV (1936), 345–357; Umberto Gabbi, "I Sanatori montani per I bambini malarici," *Malaria e malattie dei paesi caldi,* II (1911), 93–98.

17. On the establishment of sanatoriums in Basilicata by the National League against Malaria, see Medico Provinciale di Potenza, "Relazione sulla lotta antimalarica nell'anno 1912," ACS, MI, DGS (1910–1920), b. 115, fasc. "Potenza: Relazione sulla lotta contro la malaria." On sanatoriums in general, see also Gosio, "Sanatorî per bambini malarici," 345–357. On the sanatoriums in Calabria, see Migliori, *Sanatorii antimalarici.* For the Roman Campagna, see letter of Mayor of Rome to S.E. Il Ministro dell'Interno, Sept. 1919, ACC, Archivio Ripartizione VIII "Igiene," b. 157, fasc. 4 ("Anno 1919: Campagna antimalarica").

18. Quoted in "Il Governo contro la malaria," *L'avvenire sanitario,* 10 Mar. 1910. On Giolitti's commitment to the campaign, see ACS, MI, DGS (1882–1915), b. 94, fasc. "Convocazioni," sottofasc. "Riunione di scienziati convocati dal Ministro Giolitti per la lotta contro la malaria"; Giolitti, "Dispaccio telegrafico ai prefetti," 4 Sept. 1903, ACS, MI, DGS (1882–1915), b. 124, fasc. "Chinino di Stato: Affari generali"; letter of Giolitti to Signori Prefetti del Regno, 20 Jan. 1904, ACS, MI, DGS (1882–1915), b. 125, fasc. "Acquisto di chinino a prezzo ordinario," no. 20500–3.

19. Ufficiale Sanitario di Marsala, "Relazione" (1910), ACS, MI, DGS (1882–1915), b. 93; letter of Ministro delle Finanze to On. Ministero dell'Interno, Dec. 1902, ACS, MI, DGS (1882–1915), b. 125, fasc. "Prezzo del chinino: Istruzioni circa la vendita al pubblico da parte di farmacisti, droghieri, ecc.," no. 16201.

20. On social medicine as an integral part of the antimalarial campaign, see "Medicina sociale e malaria in Italia," *Avanti!,* 29 July 1901; Tullio Rossi-Doria, "Nuovi tempi e medici nuovi," *Avanti!,* 6 Dec. 1900; and Giuseppe Badaloni, *La lotta contro la malaria: Relazione al Consiglio superiore di Sanità presentata nella seduta dell'11 agosto, 1909* (Rome, 1910), 80–82.

21. For an example of an educational speech delivered by a physician at Ostia in the Roman Campagna, see Augusto Maggi, *Scritti d'un medico dell'Agro Romano* (Rome, 1912), 81–197. Maggi employs the term *apostles* to describe physicians. Alessandro Marcucci, one of the leading figures in the rural school movement, describes Angelo Celli as a modern "Peter the Hermit" leading a "holy crusade" against the "bondage" (*schiavitù*) of the farm laborers. *La scuola di Giovanni Cena* (Pavia, 1956). Pietro Castellino, who directed the antimalarial campaign in Apulia, aspired to the "resurrection" of the malarial population. "La campagna antimalarica nelle Puglie durante l'anno 1906," ACS,

MI, DGS (1882–1915), b. 91, fasc. "Relazioni: On. Castellino." See also Medico Provinciale di Foggia Albertazzi, "Relazione sull'applicazione della legge contro la malaria durante l'anno 1908," b. 116, fasc. "Foggia." Albertazzi writes of the physicians as possessing the "faith of apostles" and of acting as "fervent apostles" of the new doctrine. See also Bartolommeo Gosio, "Considerazioni generali," in Direzione Generale della Sanità Pubblica, *Organizzazioni antimalariche alla luce delle nuove dottrine* (Rome, 1925), chapter 1, 5.

22. Letter of Prefect of Sassari to Ministero dell'Interno, Direzione Generale della Sanità, 22 Dec. 1910, ACS, MI, DGS (1882–1915), b. 93, fasc. "Lotta contro la malaria: Spese complessive." In Foggia province as well physicians purchased quinine from their own funds when the townships failed to supply adequate quantities. Medico Provinciale Albertazzi, "Relazione sull'applicazione della legge contro la malaria durante l'anno 1908," ACS, MI, DGS (1882–1915), b. 116, fasc. "Foggia."

23. For sample texts of speeches given by Tropeano to the rural poor in Apulia, see Giuseppe Tropeano, "L'educazione popolare e le conferenze antimalariche nel Mezzogiorno," *Giornale della malaria,* III (1909), 193–226, 241–273, 433–473, and 481–500.

24. For a history of the anarcho-syndicalist movement in Apulia, see my *Violence and Great Estates in the South of Italy: Apulia, 1900–1922* (Cambridge, England, 1984). On the political impetus behind the leagues, see Gilberto Corbellini, "I malariologi italiani: Storia scientifica e istituzionale di una comunità conflittuale," in Antonio Casella et al., *Una difficile modernità: Tradizioni di ricerca e comunità scientifiche in Italia, 1890–1940* (Pavia, 2000), 299–327.

25. Zagari, "Relazione," ACS, MI, DGS (1882–1915), b. 90.

26. Zagari, "Relazione sulla campagna antimalarica nella provincia di Sassari per l'anno 1909," ACS, MI, DGS (1882–1915), b. 93, fasc. "Relazioni," 11. For similar conclusions in the province of Catanzaro, see Dott. V. Ferenico, Incaricato per la sorveglianza della lotta antimalarica nella Prov. di Catanzaro, "Relazione della lotta antimalarica dell'anno 1908," 30 June 1909, ACS, MI, DGS (1882–1915), b. 114.

27. Zagari, "Relazione sulla campagna antimalarica nella provincia di Sassari per l'anno 1909," 20.

28. Lustig, Sclavo, and Alivia, *Relazione sommaria,* 82. F. Salpietra made a similar observation with regard to Sicily. In his view, "In order fully to understand the malaria problem as it affects Sicily and the whole of the Mezzogiorno, one cannot be content with examining the hydrological, telluric, and entomological sources of the disease. It is obvious that here malaria is less a disaster imposed by nature than the result of the state of total neglect or primitive utilization in which the land of Sicily has been left for centuries." "La Malaria," *Rivista sanitaria siciliana,* XIV, no. 21 (1 Nov. 1926), 1046. See also Dott. Alivia, Medico Provinciale, "Relazione sull'applicazione delle leggi contro la malaria nel 1906," ACS, MI, DGS (1882–1915), b. 120, fasc. "Sassari."

29. Conditions prevailing in the Sicilian sulfur mines in the 1880s are memorably described by the Jacini inquiry. See *Atti della Giunta per l'Inchiesta Agraria sulle condizioni della classe agricola,* vol. XIII, tomo 1, fasc. 3, *Relazione del Commissario Abele Damiani, Deputato al Parlamento, sulla prima circoscrizione (Provincie di Caltanissetta, Catania, Girgenti, Messina, Palermo, Siracusa e Trapani): Relazione generale* (Rome, 1885), 646–666.

30. "Riassunti di monografie sul lavoro: Italia. I carusi delle solfare di Sicilia," *Bollettino dell'Ufficio del Lavoro, nuova serie,* I (1913), 276–277.

31. On the conditions of Sicilian miners as discussed before the mosquito theory of disease, see *Atti della Giunta per l'Inchiesta Agraria,* vol. XIII, tomo 1, fasc. 3, *Relazione del Commissario Abele Damiani,* 646–666. For a consideration of malaria as an occupational disease based on the doctrine, see speech of Dott. Ignazio Di Giovanni, "La Malaria nelle Miniere di Zolfo," 3 Oct. 1926, ACS, MI, DGS (1896–1934), b. 58. Printed in *Rivista sanitaria siciliana,* XIV, no. 21 (1 Nov. 1926), 1072–1076.

32. For the history of the Sardinian mining industry, see Francesco Sanfelice and V. E. Malato Calvino, "Le miniere della Sardegna: Ricerche sperimentali sull'aria e statistiche sugli operai," *Annali d'igiene sperimentale, nuova serie,* XII (1902), 1–49; and Commissione parlamentare d'inchiesta sulla condizione degli operai delle miniere della Sardegna, *Atti della commissione,* 4 vols. (Rome, 1910–1911).

33. Commissione parlamentare d'inchiesta sulla condizione degli operai delle miniere della Sardegna, *Atti della commissione,* vol. I, *Relazione riassuntiva e allegati* (Rome, 1910), 67. On average a Sardinian miner lost 7.7 days a year through illness, as compared with 6.6 in Tuscany, 5.0 in Sicily, and 3.7 in Piedmont.

34. "Patologia e igiene del lavoro: La lotta antimalarica nelle miniere dell'Iglesiente," *Bollettino dell'Ufficio del Lavoro, nuova serie,* I (1913), 142.

35. On malaria as a probable cause of industrial accidents among sulfur miners, see I. Bertolio, "La campagna antimalarica nell'Iglesiente mineraria," n.d., ACS, MI, DGS (1882–1915), b. 90, fasc. "Sassari."

36. P. Marginesu, "Relazione sul funzionamento dell'ambulatorio di Gonnesa nell'estate 1919," 20 Dec. 1919, ACS, MI, DGS (1910–1920), b. 104, fasc. "Cagliari: Bonifiche antimalariche"; Sanfelice and Calvino, "Le miniere della Sardegna," 40; Commissione parlamentare d'inchiesta sulla condizione degli operai delle miniere della Sardegna, *Atti della commissione,* vol. II, *Studi, statistiche e documenti allegati alla relazione generale* (Rome, 1910), 464.

37. Commissione parlamentare d'inchiesta sulla condizione degli operai delle miniere della Sardegna, *Atti della commissione,* vol. I, *Relazione riassuntiva e allegati* (Rome, 1910), 35.

38. Gildo Frongia, *Lotta antimalarica nella provincia di Cagliari nel 1914 diretta dall'Ispettore Generale Medico Comm. Serafino Ravacini in collaborazione con il Cav. Lamberto Salaroli, medico provinciale, e il Dott. Gildo Frongia, medico provinciale aggiunto* (Cagliari, 1915), 14.

39. Bertolio, "La campagna antimalarica nell'Iglesiente mineraria."

40. Trambusti, *La lotta contro la malaria in Sicilia,* 41–44, 86ff.

41. Quoted in Giuseppe Tropeano, "Rivista critica della stampa," *Giornale della malaria,* I (1907), 93–94.

42. The account here of the opposition of peasants to state quinine is based above all on the following reports in the files of ACS, MI, DGS (1882–1915): letter of Giuseppe Zagari, Augusto Ott, Mario Colombo, Giacomo Cobelli, and G. Loria, "Relazione sulla campagna antimalarica condotta nel 1910: Sassari," b. 90, fasc. "Sassari (Prof. Zagari)"; Giuseppe Zagari, "Relazione sulla campagna antimalarica nella provincia di Sassari per l'anno 1909," b. 93, fasc. "Relazioni"; Medico Provinciale di Catanzaro, "Relazione

sulla lotta antimalarica del 1909," b. 114, fasc. "Catanzaro"; Prefect of Catanzaro Facciolati, "Relazione sulla campagna antimalarica del 1905," 22 Feb. 1906, b. 114, fasc. "Catanzaro"; Medico Provinciale Albertazzi, "Relazione sull'applicazione della legge contro la malaria durante l'anno 1908," b. 116, fasc. "Foggia"; Medico Provinciale, "Campagna antimalarica 1907," b. 119, fasc. 53 ("Applicazione della legge sulla malaria: Reggio Calabria"); Ispettore Generale Medico Ravicini, "Appunto per l'Illmo Signor Direttore Generale della Sanità Pubblica," 15 May 1909, b. 124, fasc. "Chinino di Stato: Affari generali." See also Medico Provinciale, "Relazione sanitaria letta al Consiglio Sanitario Provinciale nella Seduta del 13 febbraio 1925," ACS, MI, DGS (1896–1934), b. 58, fasc. "Girgenti." Classic works stressing the role of rumor in epidemics of plague are Alessandro Manzoni, *I promessi sposi* (Milan, 1903; 1st ed. 1840–1842); and *Storia della colonna infame* (Naples, 1928; 1st ed. 1842). For cholera, see Giovanni Verga, *Mastro-Don Gesualdo* (Milan, 1979).

43. Istituto Nazionale pel Risanamento Antimalarico della Regione Pontina, "Relazione sanitaria del direttorio dell'ambulatorio del Quadrato, dott. Vincenzo Giannelli, luglio 1923–giugno 1924," ASL, CPA, b. 18 (1), fasc. "Relazioni: Attività IAP, 1923–1926," 4–5. See also Giuseppe Zagari, Augusto Ott, Mario Colombo, Giacomo Cobelli, and G. Loria, "Relazione sulla campagna antimalarica condotta nel 1910: Sassari," ACS, MI, DGS (1882–1915), b. 90.

44. Ministero dell'Interno, Direzione Generale della Sanità Pubblica, *Consigli popolari per la difesa individuale contro la malaria* (Rome, 1907), 10.

45. Dott. Gustavo Foà, "Relazione sanitaria del direttore dell'ambulatorio Colonia Elena (agosto 1923–aprile 1924)," ASL, CPA, Comitato antimalarico: Relazioni medici, b. 18 (1), fasc. "Relazioni: Attività IAP, 1923–1926," 5. Quadrato is the location where Littoria (now Latina) later arose.

46. On popular misgivings with regard to quinine, see Medico Provinciale di Reggio Calabria, "Campagna antimalarica 1907," ACS, MI, DGS (1882–1915), b. 119, fasc. "Reggio Calabria"; Medico Provinciale di Milano, "Relazione sulla lotta contro malaria nel 1912," ACS, MI, DGS (1910–1920), b. 114, fasc. "Milano"; Lustig, Sclavo, and Alivia, *Relazione sommaria,* 20, 49, 55, 59–61, 75; Francesco Martirano, "La profilassi della malaria nel Mezzogiorno d'Italia durante il 1904," *Atti della Società per gli Studi della Malaria,* VI (1905), 445; and Medico Provinciale Fradelle, "Relazione sull'andamento della lotta antimalarica dell'anno 1910," ACS, MI, DGS (1910–1920), b. 117 bis, fasc. "Roma: Relazioni sulla lotta contro la malaria."

47. Ministero delle Finanze, Direzione Generale delle Privative, *Relazione e bilancio industriale dell'azienda del chinino di stato per l'esercizio dal 1 luglio 1905 al 30 giugno 1906* (Rome, 1907), 9–10; Prefect of Catanzaro Facciolati, "Relazione sulla campagna antimalarica del 1905," 22 Feb. 1906, ACS, MI, DGS (1882–1915), b. 114, fasc. "Catanzaro"; Lustig, Sclavo, and Alivia, *Relazione sommaria,* 49.

48. A consideration of remedies previously advocated is Giovanni Battista Grassi, *Relazione dell'esperimento di preservazione dalla malaria fatto sui ferrovieri nella piana di Capaccio* (Milan, 1901), 6. On the problem of intolerance of quinine and its side effects, see Errico De Renzi, "Relazione sulla campagna antimalarica condotta in Provincia di Caserta nell'anno 1907," ACS, MI, DGS (1882–1915), b. 95, fasc. "Studi sulla malaria in provincia di Caserta"; and Prefetto di Pavia, "Relazione sulla campagna anti-

malarica attuata col chinino di Stato nelle squadre fisse dei mondarisi dell'agro pavese," 30 Aug. 1904, ACS, MI, DGS (1882–1915), b. 188 bis, fasc. "Pavia: Applicazione della legge sulla malaria." See also Patrick Manson, *Tropical Diseases,* 5th ed. (London, 1914), 118–135. For the use of quinine as an abortifacient and spermicidal medication, see Maria Sophia Quine, *Population Politics in Twentieth-Century Europe* (London, 1996), 6.

49. Pietro Castellino, "La campagna antimalarica nelle Puglie durante l'anno 1906," ACS, MI, DGS (1882–1915), b. 91, fasc. "Relazioni (on. Castellino)," 183.

50. Ibid., 184. Banfield's famous work is *The Moral Basis of a Backward Society* (New York, 1958).

51. Ispettore Generale Medico Ravicini, "Appunto per l'Illmo Signor Direttore Generale della Sanità Pubblica," 15 May 1909, ACS, MI, DGS (1882–1915), b. 124, fasc. "Chinino di Stato: Affari generali."

52. On popular reactions to screening, see Grassi, *Difesa contro la malaria nelle zone risicole,* 8–10; and Maggi, *Scritti d'un medico dell'Agro romano,* 62.

53. An example of such a pamphlet is Società per gli Studi della Malaria, *Istruzioni popolari per difendersi dalla malaria* (Rome, 1904).

54. Medico Provinciale di Campobasso, "Relazione sulla applicazione della legge contro la malaria durante il 1907," ACS, MI, DGS (1882–1915), b. 114, fasc. "Campobasso."

55. Gaetano Rummo and Luigi Ferrannini, "La Campagna antimalarica nella provincia di Benevento durante il 1910: Relazione a S.E. il Ministro dell'Interno," ACS, MI, DGS (1882–1915), b. 88, fasc. "On. Rummo." See also letter of Prefect of Sassari to S.E. Il Ministro dell'Interno, 6 May 1907, ACS, MI, DGS (1882–1915), b. 120, fasc. "Sassari," no. 201836.

56. Letter of Augusto Maggi to Prof. Marchiafava, 12 Aug. 1918, ACC, Archivio Ripartizione VIII "Igiene," b. 158, fasc. 2 ("Anno 1920").

57. L. W. Hackett and F. W. Knipe, "Annual Report on the Work of the International Health Division of the Rockefeller Foundation in Italy and Albania and in Entomological Research in Germany, 1931," RAC, Record Group 1.1, Series 751 Italy, box 248, 48.

58. Ernesto Cacace, "L'insegnamento antimalarico e la profilassi antimalarica scolastica: Relazione al III Congresso Internazionale d'Igiene Scolastica in Parigi," *Rivista pedagogica,* V, no. 2 (1911), 179–187.

59. Angelo Celli, "Portiamo l'alfabeto ai contadini dell'Agro Romano," *I Diritti della scuola,* 5 Oct. 1906.

60. On the early history of the peasant schools, see Marcucci, *La scuola;* and Pacifico Passerini, *Le scuole rurali di Roma e il bonificamento dell'Agro Romano* (Rome, 1908). The early financing is discussed in Giovanni Cena, *Opere,* vol. 2, *Prose critiche,* ed. Giorgio De Rienzo (Rome, 1968), 306–307.

61. Marcucci, *La scuola,* 19.

62. Alberto Missiroli, "La scuola primaria e la sua nuova disciplina nella lotta antimalarica," in Direzione Generale della Sanità Pubblica, *Organizzazioni antimalariche alla luce delle nuove dottrine* (Rome, 1925), part 3, chapter 1, 19.

63. Marcucci, *La scuola,* 35–40.

64. Cacace, "L'insegnamento antimalarico," 179; and "Scuole rurali: Diario di didattica pratica," *Corriere delle maestre,* 4 Jan. 1914, 177–180.

65. Medico Provinciale di Sassari, "Relazione della campagna antimalarica dell'anno 1908," ACS, MI, DGS (1882–1915), b. 120, fasc. "Sassari."

66. "Scuole rurali: Diario di didattica pratica," *Corriere delle maestre,* 4 Oct. 1914, 1–5; Alessandro Marcucci, "La scuola rurale in Italia," in Associazione Nazionale Educatori Benemeriti, ed., *Scuola e maestri d'Italia* (Rome, 1957), 195.

67. "Attività femminile in Italia," *Unione femminile,* I, no. 10 (1901), 107; and Nogarola, *L'opera del Comitato Antimalarico Veronese,* 10–11.

68. Cacace, "L'insegnamento antimalarico," 181.

69. Alessandro Marcucci, "La scuola ambulante nell'Agro Romano," *La cultura popolare,* 1913, 253.

70. Istituto Nazionale pel Risanamento Antimalarico della Regione Pontina, "Relazione sanitaria del direttore dell'ambulatorio del Quadrato, dott. Vincenzo Giannelli, luglio 1923–giugno 1924," ASL, CPA, b. 181 (1), fasc. "Relazioni: Attività IAP, 1923–1926," 1.

71. Cena, *Opere,* vol. 2, *Prose critiche,* 306; Medico Provinciale, "Relazione della campagna antimalarica dell'anno 1908," ACS, MI, DGS (1882–1915), b. 120, fasc. "Sassari."

72. Alessandro Marcucci, *Il programma didattico* (Rome, n.d.), 5.

73. Marcucci, *La scuola,* 25; Werner Peiser, "Scuole rurali nella Campagna Romana," *Rivista pedagogica,* XXVI (1938), 113; Bonaventura Campari, "Il problema scolastico popolare," *Corriere delle maestre,* 1 Feb. 1914, 123.

74. N. Badaloni, "Per finire," n.d., ACS, MI, DGS (1882–1915), b. 94, fasc. "Nomina," 4–5.

75. "Relazione sulla campagna antimalarica del 1909," n.d., ACS, MI, DGS (1882–1915), b. 120, fasc. 55 ("Applicazione della legge sulla malaria: Rovigo"); and Alfredo Conti, "Relazione sulla malaria," 19 Nov. 1909, ACS, MI, DGS (1882–1915), b. 119, fasc. 52 ("Applicazione della legge sulla malaria: Ravenna"), 2–4. For a similar discussion of the effects of land reclamation in the province of Campobasso (Abruzzi), see Medico Provinciale di Campobasso, "Relazione sulla campagna antimalarica del 1909," ACS, MI, DGS (1882–1915), b. 114, fasc. "Campobasso."

76. Gaetano Rummo, "La campagna antimalarica del 1909 nelle provincie di Benevento e Napoli," 15 Dec. 1909, ACS, MI, DGS (1882–1915), b. 95, fasc. "Studi sulla malaria per le provionce di Napoli e Benevento," 20.

77. "Relazione al Consiglio Superiore di Sanità," 11 Aug. 1909, ACS, MI, DGS (1882–1915), b. 96. The report was written by N. Badaloni.

78. The literature on Italian emigration is voluminous. Important studies of the phenomenon on which I have relied for the discussion here include Francesco Paolo Cerase, *Sotto il dominio dei borghesi: Sottosviluppo ed emigrazione nell'Italia meridionale, 1860–1910* (Rome, 1975); Domenico Demarco, *Per una storia economica dell'emigrazione italiana* (Geneva, 1978); Foerster, *The Italian Emigration of Our Times;* Alan M. Kraut, *Silent Travelers: Germs, Genes, and the "Immigrant Menace"* (New York, 1994); Ercole Sori, *L'emigrazione italiana dall'Unità alla seconda guerra mondiale* (Bologna, 1979).

79. See Chapter 1.

80. *Inchiesta parlamentare sulle condizioni dei contadini nelle provincie meridionali e nella Sicilia,* vol. II, *Abruzzi e Molise: Relazione del delegato tecnico dott. Cesare Jarach,* 2 vols. (Rome, 1909).

81. Ibid., vol. II, 6.

82. On the improved conditions in the Abruzzi that resulted from mass emigration, see *Inchiesta parlamentare,* vol. II, *Abruzzi e Molise,* vol. I, esp. 18, 23, 50, 86, 95–96, 118–119, 157–158, 197, 205; and vol. II, 7–8, 14. The conditions described by the parliamentary investigation were confirmed and related to malaria by the medical officers of health. See, for example, Medico Provinciale, "Relazione sulla campagna antimalarica del 1909," ACS, MI, DGS (1882–1915), b. 114, fasc. "Campobasso"; and Errico De Renzi, "Relazione sulla campagna antimalarica nella provincia di Caserta (agosto–dicembre 1911)," ACS, MI, DGS (1882–1915), b. 87, fasc. "On. De Renzi: Provincia di Caserta," 10.

83. *Inchiesta parlamentare,* vol. VI, *Sicilia, Tomo 1 (Parte I e II), Relazione del delegato tecnico prof. Giovanni Lorenzoni* (Rome, 1910), 705–706.

84. *Inchiesta parlamentare,* vol. VI, *Sicilia, Tomo 1 (Parte III, IV e V), Relazione del delegato tecnico prof. Giovanni Lorenzoni,* 9.

85. Medico Provinciale, "Relazione sull'applicazione delle leggi contro la malaria durante il 1906," ACS, MI, DGS (1882–1915), b. 117, fasc. "Messina."

Chapter 4. From Quinine to Women's Rights

1. Giovanni Battista Grassi, "Risultati della lotta antimalarica in seguito alle nuove scoperte," 25 Mar. 1925, USR, AG, b. 17.

2. Ibid.

3. Consiglio Superiore di Sanità, "Seduta plenaria del 6 giugno 1929," ACS, MI, DGS (1896–1934), b. 60, fasc. "Smalarina."

4. A. Missiroli, "La prevenzione della malaria nel campo pratico," *Rivista di malariologia,* VII (1928), 447.

5. Naturally, the statistics for quinine "distributed" do not correspond to the amount of quinine effectively consumed. Frequently those who received quinine hoarded, sold, or otherwise disposed of it. The amount of quinine actually swallowed or injected is unknowable.

6. Ministero dell'Interno, Direzione Generale della Sanità Pubblica, *La malaria in Italia ed i risultati della lotta antimalarica* (Rome, 1924), 22.

7. Medico Provinciale Albertazzi, "Relazione sull'applicazione della legge contro la malaria durante l'anno 1908," ACS, MI, DGS (1882–1915), b. 116, fasc. "Foggia."

8. Giovanni Battista Grassi, "Risultati della lotta antimalarica in seguito alle nuove scoperte," 25 Mar. 1925, USR, AG, b. 17, fasc. 17, 6.

9. Domenico Migliori, Medico Provinciale di Cosenza, "Relazione sullo svolgimento della campagna antimalarica del 1912," ACS, MI, DGS (1910–1920), b. 113.

10. Errico De Renzi, "Relazione all'Ill.mo Sig. Direttore Generale della Sanità Pubblica sulla campagna antimalarica in Terra di Lavoro nell'anno 1910," ACS, MI, DGS (1882–1915), b. 93, fasc. "Caserta: Relazioni," 3–4.

11. Medico Provinciale, "Relazione sulla campagna antimalarica del 1909," ACS, MI, DGS (1882–1915), b. 120, fasc. 55 ("Applicazione della legge sulla malaria: Rovigo").

12. On the recession of malaria in certain provinces, see the following documents in ACS, MI, DGS (1910–1920): Ispettore Generale Medico, "La malaria in provincia di

Benevento," 25 July 1916, b. 97, fasc. "Benevento: lotta antimalarica"; Prefect of Cremona, "Relazione circa l'applicazione delle leggi durante l'anno 1912," 24 July 1913, b. 113, fasc. "Cremona: Relazioni sulla lotta contro la malaria," no. 20183.4; Medico Provinciale di Novara, "Relazione sull'applicazione della legge sulla malaria nell'anno 1912," b. 114 bis, fasc. "Novara"; Medico Provinciale, "Relazione sulla campagna antimalarica del 1912," b. 116 bis, fasc. "Sondrio."

13. Giovanni Battista Grassi, "Risultati della lotta antimalarica in seguito alle nuove scoperte," 25 Mar. 1925, USR, AG, b. 17, 6. As Grassi requested, his body is buried "modestly" at the cemetery of Fiumicino, so he was indeed there when the disease was eradicated after the Second World War.

14. Giovanni Battista Grassi, "Risultati della lotta antimalarica in seguito alle nuove scoperte," 25 Mar. 1925, USR, AG, b. 17, fasc. 46. Consiglio Superiore di Sanità, "Seduta plenaria del 6 giugno 1929," ACS, MI, DGS (1896–1934), b. 60, fasc. "Smalarina."

15. Giuseppe Sanarelli, *Lo stato attuale del problema malarico: Rilievi e proposte* (Rome, 1925), 15–16, 41. Sanarelli was the director of the Istituto Antimalarico Pontino, and Grassi had served as medical director of one of its subsidiary health stations. See Gustavo Foà, "Annotazioni sull'uso della Cinconina nella lotta antimalarica durante la stagione interepidemica nell'anno 1924–25," *Rivista di malariologia,* V (1926), 3.

16. Ronald Ross, *The Prevention of Malaria* (London, 1910), vii–viii.

17. Prefect of Girgenti, "Relazione sulla campagna antimalarica," ACS, MI, DGS (1882–1915), b. 115.

18. F. Soper, "Malaria South of the Sahara," 17 June 1966, NLM, Fred L. Soper Papers, 1919–1975, box 53.

19. Sanarelli, *Lo stato attuale.*

20. Gaetano Rummo, "La campagna antimalarica del 1909 nelle provincie di Benevento e Napoli," 15 Dec. 1909, ACS, MI, DGS (1882–1915), b. 95, 7–8.

21. Medico Provinciale di Siracusa, "Campagna antimalarica 1912," ACS, MI, DGS (1910–1920), b. 116 bis, fasc. "Siracusa: Relazioni sulla lotta contro la malaria."

22. "Estratto della Relazione del Prefetto di Cagliari sulle malattie infettive relative al III trimestre del 1905," ACS, MI, DGS (1882–1915), b. 113, fasc. "Cagliari."

23. Giovanni Battista Grassi, "Relazione dell'esperimento antimalarico di Fiumicino," 18 Dec. 1918, ACS, MI, DGS (1910–1920), b. 103, fasc. "Commissione per lo studio delle opere di piccola bonifica," sottofasc. "Relazione del prof. Battista Grassi." See also the following documents in ACS, MI, DGS (1882–1915): Medico Provinciale, "Relazione sull'applicazione delle leggi contro la malaria durante il 1907," b. 117, fasc. "Messina"; Medico Provinciale di Potenza, G. Pica, "Relazione sulle applicazioni delle leggi contro la malaria durante il 1906," b. 119, fasc. 51 ("Potenza: Applicazione della legge sulla malaria"); Medico Provinciale, "Relazione sulla lotta antimalarica del 1906," b. 119, fasc. 53 ("Reggio Calabria: Applicazione della legge sulla malaria").

24. Giuseppe Tropeano, "Per la lotta contro la malaria (La scheda C)," *Giornale della malaria,* I (1907), 40–42.

25. Ministero dell'Interno, Direzione Generale della Sanità, *La malaria in Italia,* 11–13. The malaria-free provinces at that date were Ancona, Arezzo, Belluno, Brescia, Cuneo, Florence, Forlì, Genoa, Lucca, Macerata, Massa-Carrara, Modena, Parma, Pesaro-Urbino, Piacenza, Porto Maurizio, and Turin.

26. Gaetano Rummo, "Relazione (1909)," ACS, MI, DGS (1882–1915), b. 93.

27. The standard recommendations for therapy were drawn up in Ministero dell'Interno, Direzione Generale della Sanità Pubblica, *Istruzioni tecniche per la cura della malaria* (Rome, 1926).

28. Giuseppe Badaloni, *La lotta contro la malaria: Relazione al Consiglio Superiore di Sanità presentata nella seduta dell'11 agosto 1909* (Rome, 1910), 26–29. On the same point with regard to the province of Rome see Ispettore Generale Medico Ravicini, "Appunto per l'Illmo Signor Direttore Generale della Sanità Pubblica," 15 May 1909, ACS, MI, DGS (1882–1915), b. 124, fasc. "Chinino di Stato: Affairi generali."

29. A representative and sober assessment of the limits of quinine prophylaxis is Gaetano Rummo and Luigi Ferrannini, "La campagna antimalarica nella provincia di Benevento durante il 1910: Relazione a S.E. il Ministro dell'Interno," ACS, MI, DGS (1882–1915), b. 88, fasc. "On. Rummo," sottofasc. "Provincia di Benevento."

30. Consiglio Superiore di Sanità, "Seduta plenaria del 6 giugno 1929," ACS, MI, DGS (1896–1934), b. 60, fasc. "Smalarina," 2–4.

31. Claudio Fermi, *Regioni malariche: Decadenza, risanamento e spesa: Sardegna,* vol. 1 (Rome, 1934), 245.

32. The standard daily dose was 40 centigrams for adults and 20 for children. The weekly dose was 1 gram for adults and 60 centigrams for children. Weekly administration was easier but enhanced the problem of side effects. Prefetto di Pavia, "Relazione sulla campagna antimalarica attuata col chinino di Stato nelle squadre fisse dei mondarisi dell'agro pavese," 30 Aug. 1904, ACS, MI, DGS (1882–1915), b. 118 bis, fasc. "Pavia: Applicazione della legge sulla malaria."

33. Letter of L. W. Hackett to F. F. Russell, 17 June 1927, RAC, Record Group 1.1, Series 751 Italy, box 7, folder 80, "Diary of L. W. Hackett—Italy, 1927–1928," no. 102; Badaloni, *La lotta contro la malaria.*

34. On the belief that quinine conferred immunity, see Gaetano Rummo, "La campagna antimalarica del 1909 nelle provincie di Benevento e Napoli," 15 Dec. 1909, ACS, MI, DGS (1882–1915), b. 95, fasc. "Studi sulla malaria per le province di Napoli e Benevento: Relazione del prof. Rummo"; and Bartolommeo Gosio, "Relazione sulla campagna antimalarica del 1906," ACS, MI, DGS (1882–1915), b. 95, fasc. "Studi sulla malaria nelle Calabrie e Basilicata."

35. In the province of Trapani, the medical officer of health reported that there were major inequalities. The amount of the quinine levy per hectare in the various townships (*comuni*) of the province varied as follows: Alcamo, 0.175 lire; Calatafimi, 0.102; Campobello di Mazzara, 0.133; Camporeale, 0.043; Castellammare del Golfo, 0.058; Castelvetrano, 0.010; Gibellina, 0.044; Marsala, 0.409; Mazzara del Vallo, 0.049; Monte S. Giuliano, 0.038; Paceco, 0.058; Partanna, 0.085; Poggioreale, 0.222; Salaparuta, 0.057; Salemi, 0.166; Santa Ninfa, 0.016; Trapani, 0.077. Medico Provinciale di Trapani Barone, "Relazione sulla campagna antimalarica del 1906," 22 June 1907, ACS, MI, DGS (1882–1915), b. 122, fasc. "Trapani."

36. Giovanni Battista Grassi, *Difesa contro la malaria nelle zone risicole* (Milan, 1905), 7.

37. Medico Provinciale di Reggio Calabria, "Relazione sulla campagna antimalarica del 1906," ACS, MI, DGS (1882–1915), b. 119, fasc. 53 ("Reggio Calabria").

38. On the persistent failure of local government to implement the quinine program, see the following documents in ACS, MI, DGS (1882–1915): Medico Provinciale di Caltanissetta, "Relazione sull'applicazione delle leggi contro la malaria durante il 1908," b. 113, fasc. "Caltanissetta"; Medico Provinciale di Catanzaro, "Relazione sulla lotta antimalarica del 1909," b. 114, fasc. "Catanzaro"; Medico Provinciale, "Relazione sulla campagna antimalarica del 1909," b. 114, fasc. "Campobasso"; Medico Provinciale Albertazzi, "Relazione sull'applicazione della legge contro la malaria durante l'anno 1908," b. 116, fasc. "Foggia"; Medico Provinciale, "Relazione sull'applicazione delle leggi contro la malaria durante il 1908," b. 116, fasc. "Girgenti"; Medico Provinciale, "Relazione sull'applicazione delle leggi contro la malaria durante il 1907," b. 117, fasc. "Messina"; Medico Provinciale, "Relazione della campagna antimalarica dell'anno 1906," b. 119, fasc. "Reggio Calabria"; and Medico Provinciale, "Relazione della campagna antimalarica dell'anno 1908" and "Relazione della campagna antimalarica dell'anno 1906," b. 120, fasc. "Sassari." See also Medico Provinciale Fradelle, "Relazione sull'andamento della lotta antimalarica dell'anno 1910," ACS, MI, DGS (1896–1934), b. 117 bis, fasc. "Roma: Relazioni sulla lotta contro la malaria."

39. Prefetto di Trapani, "Relazione sull'applicazione delle leggi contro la malaria durante il 1908," 11 June 1909, ACS, MI, DGS (1882–1915), b. 122, fasc. "Applicazione della legge sulla malaria, protocollo n. 20183.1/63 (Trapani)"; Medico Provinciale di Sassari, "Relazione della campagna antimalarica dell'anno 1908," ACS, MI, DGS (1882–1915), b. 120, fasc. "Sassari."

40. Pietro Castellino, "La campagna antimalarica nelle Puglie durante l'anno 1906," ACS, MI, DGS (1882–1915), b. 91, fasc. "Relazioni: On. Castellino," 69–70.

41. Direttore Generale della Sanità Pubblica, "Relazione all'Onorevole Consiglio Superiore di Sanità," 12 July 1917, ACS, MI, DGS (1896–1934), b. 57 bis, fasc. "Malaria: Affari generali e di massima," no. 20183–4.

42. Angelo Celli, "Ostacoli all'applicazione delle leggi contro la malaria e proposte per rimuoverli," n.d., USR, AC, b. 7, fasc. "Società per gli Studi della Malaria."

43. An ardent champion of nationalization was Giuseppe Tropeano. See his article "La campagna antimalarica nel Mezzogiorno (verso la nazionalizzazione)," *Giornale della malaria,* I (1907), 268–279.

44. Delegato Governativo Dott. Giuseppe Spagnolio, "Relazione sulla campagna antimalarica in provincia di Messina, anno 1910," ACS, MI, DGS (1882–1915), b. 93, fasc. "Relazioni," 10.

45. "Relazione sulla campagna antimalarica del 1912," ACS, MI, DGS (1910–1920), b. 116, fasc. "Sondrio."

46. Voltaire, *Candide ou l'optimisme* in *Candide et autres contes* (Paris, 1992).

47. "Il terremoto in Calabria e in Sicilia," *Avanti!,* 12 Sept. 1905.

48. On the 1908 earthquake, see John Dickie, "The Smell of Disaster: Scenes of Social Collapse in the Aftermath of the Messina-Reggio Calabria Earthquake, 1908," in John Dickie, John Foot, and Frank M. Snowden, eds., *Disastro! Disasters in Italy since 1860: Culture, Politics, Society* (New York, 2002), 237–255.

49. Medico Provinciale, "Relazione sull'applicazione delle leggi contro la malaria durante il 1906," ACS, MI, DGS (1882–1915), b. 115, fasc. "Cosenza." See also B. Gosio, *Un triennio di lotta antimalarica nelle Calabrie e Basilicata: Studi e proposte* (Rome,

1908), 30–31; Cesare Lombroso, "Il flagello dei temporali dopo il terremoto," *Avanti!*, 23 Sept. 1905; Oddino Morgari, "Insufficienza e lentezza dei soccorsi in Calabria," *Avanti!*, 25 Sept. 1905; and "Nei paesi del terremoto," *Corriere della sera*, 24 Sept. 1905.

50. For discussion of malaria following the earthquake of 1908, see the following documents in ACS, MI, DGS (1882–1915): Giuseppe Spagnolio, "Relazione sulla campagna antimalarica in provincia di Messina, anno 1910," b. 93, fasc. "Relazioni"; V. Ferenico, "Relazione della lotta antimalarica dell'anno 1908," June 1909, b. 114, fasc. "Catanzaro"; Medico Provinciale, "Relazione sulla lotta antimalarica dell'1909," b. 119, fasc. 53 ("Applicazione della legge sulla malaria: Reggio Calabria").

51. *Naples in the Time of Cholera, 1884–1911* (Cambridge, England, 1995).

52. Medico Provinciale di Siracusa, "Relazione sulla campagna antimalarica del 1911," ACS, MI, DGS (1910–1920), b. 116 bis, fasc. "Siracusa."

53. Ibid.

54. Medico Provinciale di Caltanissetta, "Campagna malaria del 1912," 8 May 1913, ACS, MI, DGS (1910–1920), b. 97 bis, fasc. "Caltanissetta: Lotta antimalarica."

55. Letter of Prefect of Avellino to Ministero dell'InternoDirezione Generale della Sanità, 10 Aug. 1912, ACS, MI, DGS (1910–1920), b. 97, fasc. "Avellino: Lotta antimalarica," n. 24550.

56. Medico Provinciale di Potenza, "Relazione sulla lotta antimalarica nell'anno 1912," ACS, MI, DGS (1910–1920), b. 115, fasc. "Potenza: Relazioni sulla lotta contro la malaria."

57. Medico Provinciale di Ferrara, "Relazione sulla campagna antimalarica nel 1911," ACS, MI, DGS (1910–1920), b. 113, fasc. "Ferrara: Relazioni sulla lotta contro la malaria."

58. Letter of Prof. Alfonso Di Vestea to Sig. Direttore Generale della Sanità Pubblica, 18 June 1912, ACS, MI, DGS (1882–1915), b. 92, fasc. "Prov. Di Pisa e Grosseto: Prof. Di Vestea," sottofasc. "Prov. Di Grosseto."

59. Prof. Pietro Castellino, "La campagna antimalarica nelle Puglie durante l'anno 1906," ACS, MI, DGS (1882–1915), b. 91, fasc. "Relazioni: On. Castellino," 76–81.

60. Ibid.

61. On the "framing" of disease and its importance as a political factor, see Charles F. Rosenberg, *Explaining Epidemics and Other Studies in the History of Medicine* (Cambridge, England, 1992), esp. chapter. 15, 305–318.

62. Associazione fra gli Agricoltori del Vercellese, *Sulle condizioni dell'agricoltura e degli agricoltori* (Vercelli, 1901), 10–11. On the hiring of women, see "La coltura del riso e le diverse operazioni agricole," ACS, MI, DGS (1882–1915), b. 748, fasc. "Legge sulla risicoltura," 14, 16; see also fasc. "Relazione della Commissione per le risaie nominata con Decreto 28 Agosto 1906," sottofasc. "Commissione per le reisaie: Verbali delle sedute."

63. Prefetto di Pavia, "Relazione sulla campagna antimalarica attuata col chinino di stato nelle squadre fisse dei mondarisi dell'agro pavese," 30 Aug. 1904,.ACS, MI, DGS (1882–1915), b. 120, fasc. "Pavia: Applicazione della legge sulla malaria," 15–16.

64. Ibid., 18.

65. For the 1905 report commissioned by the Ministry of the Interior, see "La coltura del riso e le diverse operazioni agricole," ACS, MI, DGS (1882–1915), b. 748, fasc.

"Legge sulla risicoltura." The deliberations of the Consiglio Superiore della Sanità can be found in ACS, MI, DGS (1882–1915), b. 747 bis, fasc. "Progetto di legge sulla coltivazione delle risaie." For the final report of its committee of inquiry, see Camillo Golgi, Alfonso Di Vestea, and Arnaldo Maggiora, "Relazione della Commissione nominata dal Consiglio Superiore di Sanità per stabilire d'accordo col Consiglio del Lavoro la durata della giornata di lavoro nella mondatura del riso," 28 Jan. 1904, ACS, MI, DGS (1882–1915), b. 750. Conditions in the rice fields of Pavia province are well described by the prefect in a 1904 report: Prefetto di Pavia, "Relazione sulla campagna antimalarica attuata col chinino di Stato nelle squadre fisse dei mondarisi dell'agro pavese," 30 Aug. 1904, ACS, MI, DGS (1882–1915), b. 120, fasc. "Pavia: Applicazione della legge sulla malaria." The conditions prevailing in the rice fields were also the subject of a series of reports for *Critica sociale.* See Giulio Casalini, "Leggi sociali in gestazione: La legge sul lavoro risicolo," *Critica sociale,* XIV (1904), 55–58, 77–80, 127–128, 140–141.

66. S. P. James, "The Disappearance of Malaria from England," *Proceedings of the Royal Society of Medicine,* XXXIII, part 1 (1929–1930), esp. 77–85. James wrote with regard to *Anopheles maculipennis,* the group to which *Anopheles labranchiae* was believed to belong. Nicholas H. Swellengrebel and A. De Buck, *Malaria in the Netherlands* (Amsterdam, 1938), 142–144, 172–177. On the critical importance of housing in the transmission of malaria, see B. Gosio, "Malaria di Grosseto nell'anno 1899," *Policlinico, Sezione Medica,* VII (1900), 180, 186.

67. On the effects of malaria on pregnancy, see Errico De Renzi, "Relazione sulla campagna antimalarica nella provincia di Caserta (agosto–dicembre 1911)," ACS, MI, DGS (1882–1915), b. 87, fasc. "On. De Renzi: Prov. di Caserta," 10–11.

68. On the effects of malaria on pregnancy, see the WHO's Web site for the Roll Back Malaria program, where there is a link devoted to "Preventing Malaria during Pregnancy," http://www.rbm.who.int/newdesign2/pregnancy/pregnancy.

69. ACS, MI, DGS (1882–1915), b. 747, fasc. "Relazione della commissione per le risaie nominata con Decreto 28 agosto 1906," sottofasc. "Commissione per le risaie: Verbali delle sedute," no. 1, 39.

70. Letter of Ministro delle Finanze to On. Ministero dell'Interno, Dec. 1902, ACS, MI, DGS (1882–1915), b. 125, fasc. "Prezzo del chinino: Istruzioni circa la vendita al pubblico," no. 16201.

71. "Dopo il congresso medico di Milano," *Avanti!,* 12 Oct. 1909; "La riunione del Consiglio Generale della Federaz. lavoratori della terra," *Avanti!,* 2 Nov. 1909.

72. *I lavoratori delle risaie* (Milan, 1904), 131–133. For an earlier author who worried in 1814 about the "dark and shameful deeds" committed by rice workers both by day and by night, see Luigi Angeli, "Delle risaie e dei loro pessimi effetti," in Luigi Faccini, ed., *Uomini e lavoro in risaia: Il dibattito sulla risicoltura nel '700 e nell '800* (Milan, 1976), esp. 107–109.

73. For the text of the law of 1907, the bill originally presented by Giolitti to parliament in 1905, and the papers in its support, see ACS, MI, DGS (1882–1915), b. 747, fasc. "Risicoltura: Atti parlamentari"; and b. 747 bis, fasc. "Progetto di legge sulla coltivazione delle risaie." For the supplementary general and special regulations, see b. 749, fasc. "Regolamenti per l'esecuzione della legge sulla risicoltura." An important example of the provincial regulations that completed the protective structures created in 1907 is that of

the province of Novara, "Testo del regolamento per la coltivazione del riso nella Provincia di Padova," 16 July 1909, ACS, MI, DGS (1882–1915), b. 749 bis.

74. *Il Monopolio dell'uomo* (Palermo, 1979). On Anna Kuliscioff's part in the campaign to pass protective legislation on behalf of rice workers, see Maria Casalini, "Femminismo e socialismo in Anna Kuliscioff, 1890–1907," *Italia contemporanea*, Apr.–June 1981, esp. 40–43. Two useful biographies of Kuliscioff are Maria Casalini, *La signora del socialismo italiano: Vita di Anna Kuliscioff* (Rome, 1987); and Marina Addis Saba, *Anna Kuliscioff: Vita privata e passione politica* (Milan, 1993).

75. "Questioni di ordine pubblico: Cenni storici sulle agitazioni agrarie dal 1898 a 1905 e sulle cause di esse," ACS, MI, DGS (1882–1915), b. 748, fasc. "Legge sulla risicoltura," 1.

76. "Il Congresso dei contadini," *Avanti!*, 25 Nov. 1901. Similarly, the socialist deputy Angelo Cabrini stressed the role of women and their unionization as crucial to the establishment of the provincial federation of Federterra in the rice-growing province of Mantua. Angelo Cabrini, "I Lavoratori della terra," *Avanti!*, 24 Feb. 1901.

77. "Molinella," *Avanti!*, 10 May 1901.

78. Medico Provinciale Albertazzi, "Relazione sull'applicazione della legge contro la malaria durante l'anno 1908," ACS, MI, DGS (1882–1915), b. 116, fasc. "Foggia."

Chapter 5. The First World War and Epidemic Disease

1. Goffredo Bellonci, "L'urto di classe nel Parmense-Stato d'assedio," *Il giornale d'Italia*, 4 May 1908; and "Un'intervista col presidente dell'Agraria," *Il resto del carlino*, 12 May 1908.

2. Goffredo Bellonci, "Il fiero contrasto delle due solidarietà nel Parmense," *Il giornale d'Italia*, 8 May 1908.

3. Medico Provinciale di Caltanissetta, "Relazione sull'applicazione delle leggi contro la malaria durante il 1917," ACS, MI, DGS (1910–1920), b. 112 bis, fasc. "Caltanissetta."

4. Claudio Fermi, "Alcuni schiarimenti alle critiche mosse dal Prof. Canalis ai risultati da me ottenuti nelle campagne antianofelo-malariche a Terranova nel 1916 e 1917," ACS, MI, DGS (1910–1920), b. 104 bis, fasc. "Sassari: Bonifiche Terranova e Siniscola (Prof. Fermi)," 10.

5. Ministero dell'Interno, Direzione Generale della Sanità Pubblica, *La malaria in Italia ed i risultati della lotta antimalarica* (Rome, 1924), 23.

6. Giorgio Mortara, *La salute pubblica in Italia durante e dopo la guerra* (Bari, 1925), 250.

7. All of the following materials are in ACS, MI, DGS (1910–1920): Report of Prefect of Caltanissetta to On. Min. Dir. Gen. Sanità Pubblica, 25 Mar. 1918, b. 97 bis, fasc. "Caltanissetta: Lotta antimalarica," no. 2655; letter of Prefect of Caltanissetta to On. Min. Dir. Gen. Sanità Pubblica, 25 June 1918, b. 97 bis, fasc. "Caltanissetta: Lotta antimalarica," no. 6342; letter of Prefect of Cosenza to Min. Int. Dir. Gen. Sanità, 24 Jan. 1919, b. 98, fasc. "Cosenza: Lotta antimalarica," no. 726; Reports of Prefect of Foggia of 19 Mar. 1918 and 9 Apr. 1918, b. 98, fasc. "Foggia: Lotta antimalarica"; Medico Provinciale di Bari, "Relazione sull'applicazione delle leggi contro la malaria durante il 1917,"

b. 111, fasc. "Bari"; "Relazione sull'applicazione delle leggi contro la malaria durante in 1915," b. 112, fasc. "Cagliari: Relazioni sulla malaria"; Medico Provinciale di Caltanissetta, "Relazione sull'applicazione delle leggi contro la malaria durante il 1917," b. 112 bis, fasc. "Caltanissetta."

8. League of Nations Health Organisation: Malaria Commission, *Report on Its Tour of Investigation in Certain European Countries in 1924* (Geneva, 1925), 17, 19.

9. Claudio Fermi, "Alcuni schiarimenti alle critiche mosse dal Prof. Canalis ai risultati da me ottenuti nelle campagne antianofelo-malariche a Terranova nel 1916 e 1917," ACS, MI, DGS (1910–1920), b. 104 bis, fasc. "Sassari: Bonifiche Terranova e Siniscola," 10.

10. It was reported from Sassari in 1918 that "in general it is a question of multiple infections, so that, in the majority of cases, the fever is quotidian." Medico Provinciale di Sassari, "Lotta antimalarica 1918," ACS, MI, DGS (1910–1920), b. 116, fasc. "Sassari: Relazione sulla lotta contro la malaria."

11. Giovanni Battista Grassi, "La lotta antimalarica a Fiumicino," *Symposia genetica,* IV (1956), 370.

12. John R. Schindler, *Isonzo: The Forgotten Sacrifice of the Great War* (Westport, Conn., 2001), xii.

13. Letter of Segretariato Generale per gli Affari Civili, R. Esercito Italiano, Comando Supremo, 6 Oct. 1917, ACS, MI, DGS (1910–1920), b. 94, fasc. "Norme di profilassi antimalarica della Direzione di Sanità della 3a Armata," no. 104691.

14. "Profilassi antimalarica nell'Esercito Italiano durante la guerra," *Annali d'igiene,* XXIX (1919), 536.

15. Ibid.

16. Letter of Augusto Maggi, 1918, ACC, Archivio Ripartizione VIII "Igiene," b. 158, fasc. 2.

17. Letter of Prefect of Venice to On. Min. Int., Direzione Generale della Sanità, 20 May 1918, ACS, MI, DGS (1910–1920), fasc. "Malaria e bonifica," no. 1481 Sanità; Prefect of Udine, "Lotta antimalarica: Relazione sulla campagna del 1916," 2 June 1917, ACS, MI, DGS (1910–1920), b. 117, fasc. "Udine: Relazioni sulla lotta contro la malaria," no. 1577.

18. On the defeat of Caporetto, there is a large scholarly literature. See, for example, Giovanna Procacci, "The Disaster of Caporetto," John Dickie, John Foot, and Frank M. Snowden, eds., *Disastro! Disasters in Italy since 1860: Culture, Politics, Society* (New York, 2002), 141–161. The defeat and its aftermath are also the subject of Ernest Hemingway, *A Farewell to Arms* (New York, 1929).

19. "Relazione sulla campagna antimalarica nella provincia di Udine nell'anno 1920," ACS, MI, DGS (1910–1920), b. 117, fasc. "Udine," 1.

20. Mortara, *La salute pubblica,* 81.

21. Ibid., 249. Here I have grouped together the mainland South and the islands.

22. Report of Prefect of Caltanissetta to Ministero dell'Interno, Direzione Generale della Sanità, 25 Mar. 1918, ACS, MI, DGS (1910–1920), b. 97 bis, fasc. "Caltanissetta: Lotta antimalarica," no. 2655. The medical officer of health for the province provided a strongly concurring analysis. See Report of Medico Provinciale di Caltanissetta, "Relazione sull'applicazione delle leggi contro la malaria durante il 1917," ACS, MI, DGS (1910–1920), b. 112 bis, fasc. "Caltanissetta: Relazioni sulla lotta contro la malaria."

23. Letter of Direttore Generale della Sanità to Com. Serafino Ravicini, 7 Aug. 1917, ACS, MI, DGS (1910–1920), b. 94, fasc. "Norme di profilassi antimalarica alla direzione di sanità della 3a Armata," no. 20183; letter of Segretario Generale, Comando Supremo, R. Esercito italiano: Segretariato Generale per gli affari civili to Min. Int. Dir. Gen Sanità, 6 Oct. 1917, ACS, MI, DGS (1910–1920), b. 94, fasc. "Norme di profilassi antimalarica alla direzione di sanità della 3a armata," no. 104691.

24. Colonello medico Giambattista Mariotti Bianchi, "La malaria e l'esercito," in Scuola Superiore di Malariologia, *Conferenze* (Rome, 1927), 3. Spring infections were vivax malaria, and estivo-autumnal infections were falciparum. See also ACS, MI, DGS (1910–1920), b. 114, fasc. "Milano."

25. Medico Provinciale di Potenza, "Relazione sull'applicazione delle leggi contro la malaria durante il 1917," 26 Apr. 1918, ACS, MI, DGS (1910–1920), b. 115, fasc. "Potenza: Relazioni sulla lotta contro la malaria."

26. *Malaria in Europe: An Ecological Study* (Oxford, 1937), 2.

27. Ibid.

28. Ibid.

29. Scuola Superiore di Malariologia, *Conferenze,* 3.

30. All of the following materials are in ACS, MI, DGS (1910–1920): Report of the Prefect of Caltanissetta, b. 97 bis; Report of the Medico Provinciale, 1917, b. 112 bis, fasc. "Caltanissetta"; Report of the Medico Provinciale, 1917, b. 114, fasc. "Girgenti"; Report of the Prefect of Caserta, 1919, b. 97 bis, fasc. "Caserta."

31. Report of Prefect of Foggia, 9 Apr. 1918, ACS, MI, DGS (1910–1920), b. 98, fasc. "Foggia: Lotta antimalarica." The prefect of Foggia reported all of these factors as important in the epidemic that engulfed the province during the war years.

32. Letter of Prefect of Foggia to MI, DGS, 19 Mar. 1918, ACS, MI, DGS (1910–1920), b. 98, fasc. "Foggia: Lotta antimalarica," Mar. no. 2979.

33. Arrigo Serpieri, *La guerra e le classi rurali italiane* (Bari, 1930), 219.

34. Ministero dell'Interno, Direzione Generale della Sanità Pubblica, and Ministero dell'Economia Nazionale, Direzione Generale dell'Agricoltura, *La risicoltura e la malaria nelle zone risicole d'Italia* (Rome, 1925), vi.

35. Letter of the Prefect of Cagliari, 20 Apr. 1916, ACS, MI, DGS (1910–1920), b. 97 bis, fasc. "Cagliari."

36. "Relazione sull'applicazione delle leggi contro la malaria durante il 1916," ACS, MI, DGS (1910–1920), b. 117 bis, fasc. "Verona."

37. "Relazione sull'applicazione delle leggi contro la malaria durante il 1917," ACS, MI, DGS (1910–1920), b. 112, fasc. "Cagliari: Relazioni sulla malaria."

38. Medico Provinciale di Siracusa, "Relazione della campagna antimalarica del 1916," ACS, MI, DGS (1910–1920), b. 116 bis, fasc. "Siracusa."

39. B. Gosio, "Considerazioni generali," in Direzione Generale della Sanità Pubblica, *Organizzazioni antimalariche alla luce delle nuove dottrine* (Rome, 1925), 9–10.

40. Letter of Prefect of Caserta to Ministero dell'Interno, Direzione Generale della Sanità, 24 Jan. 1919, ACS, MI, DGS (1910–1920), b. 97, fasc. "Caserta: Applicazione leggi contro la malaria," no. 852. In a similar spirit, the city of Rome informed the prefect that "the exceptional conditions of the times have caused serious difficulties to the city authorities, especially with regard to the need to replace the many public health doctors

of the Agro Romano. When they were called to military service, they had to be replaced with doctors on short-term contracts who lacked the necessary knowledge of the locale. They also lacked zeal and took little interest in the performance of the tasks linked to their temporary posts." Quoted in letter of Prefect of Rome to Ministero dell'Interno, Direzione Generale della Sanità, 9 Aug. 1916, ACS, MI, DGS (1910–1920), b. 102 bis, fasc. "Roma: Lotta antimalarica," no. 43332.

41. Letter of Roberto Villetti, 16 Feb. 1922, ACC, Archivio Ripartizione VIII "Igiene," b. 159, fasc. 1 ("Anno 1922: Campagna antimalarica"). On the reestablishment of the society, see "Resoconti: Società per gli Studi della Malaria," *Rivista di malariologia,* V (1926), 740–745.

42. Letter of Roberto Villetti, 27 June 1922, ACC, Archivio Ripartizione VIII "Igiene," b. 159, fasc. 1 ("Anno 1922: Campagna antimalarica"); Prof. Adriano Valenti, "China-alcaloidi della china e malaria," n.d., ACS, MI, DGS (1896–1934), b. 57, fasc. "Coltivazione dell'albero della china."

43. "Relazione circa studi e ricerche per una piantagione di Chincone (Chine) per conto del Governo Italiano," n.d., ACS, MI, DGS (1886–1934), b. 57, fasc. "Coltivazione dell'albero della china."

44. Letter of Prefect of Caltanissetta to Ministero dell'Interno, Direzione Generale della Sanità, 24 June 1918, ACS, MI, DGS (1910–1920), b. 97 bis, fasc. "Caltanissetta: Lotta antimalarica," no. 6342.

45. Giuseppe Sanarelli, *Lo stato attuale del problema malarico: Rilievi e proposte* (Rome, 1925), 20, 36–37.

46. Letter of Roberto Villetti, 6 June 1922, ACC, Archivio Ripartizione VIII "Igiene," b. 159, fasc. 1 ("Anno 1922: Campagna antimalarica").

47. Ettore Marchiafava, "Esperimento di distruzione di zanzare e larve malariche," *Atti del consiglio comunale di Roma dell'anno 1917,* II (Rome, 1917), 230.

48. Appunto pei Gabinetti delle SS.EE. Ministro e Sottosegretario di Stato, "Diffusione e distribuzione geografica," n.d., ACS, MI, DGS (1910–1920), b. 180, fasc. "Epidemia influenzale." Useful discussions of the international pandemic are Alfred W. Crosby, Jr., *Epidemic and Peace* (Westport, Conn., 1976); Richard Collier, *The Plague of the Spanish Lady: The Influenza Pandemic of 1918–1919* (New York, 1974); K. David Patterson, *Pandemic Influenza, 1700–1900: A Study in Historical Epidemiology* (Totowa, N.J., 1986); and W. I. B. Beveridge, *Influenza: The Last Great Plague* (New York, 1977).

49. For a survey of the course of the epidemic in 1918, see Appunti pei Gabinetti delle SS.EE. Ministro e Sottosegretario di Stato, "Seguito dell'appunto sull'influenza in data 29 settembre 1918" and "Diffusione e distribuzione geografica," n.d., ACS, MI, DGS (1910–1920), b. 180, fasc. "Epidemia influenzale."

50. Letter of Prefect of Caserta to Ministero dell'Interno, Direzione Generale della Sanità, 24 Jan. 1919, ACS, MI, DGS (1910–1920), b. 97, fasc. "Caserta: Applicazione leggi contro la malaria," no. 852.

51. Letter of Prefect of Cosenza to MI, DGS, 24 Jan. 1919, ACS, MI, DGS (1910–1920), b. 98, fasc. "Cosenza: Lotta antimalarica," no. 726.

52. Report of Prefect of Caserta, 1919, ACS, MI, DGS (1910–1920), b. 97 bis, fasc. "Caserta."

53. Letter of Prefect of Cosenza to Ministero dell'Interno, Direzione Generale della

Sanità, 24 Jan. 1919, ACS, MI, DGS (1910–1920), b. 98, fasc. "Cosenza: Lotta antimalarica," no. 726.

54. Report of the Prefect of Cosenza, 1919, ACS, MI, DGS (1910–1920), b. 98, fasc. "Cosenza"; Appunto pei Gabinetti delle SS.EE. Ministro e Sottosegretario di Stato, "Diffusione e distribuzione geografica," n.d., ACS, MI, DGS (1910–1920), b. 180, fasc. "Epidemia influenzale." On the attempt to place restrictions on the use of quinine, see letter of Direttore Generale della Sanità Pubblica to S.E. Il Prof. Alberto De Stefani, 20 Aug. 1923, ACS, MI, DGS (1886–1934), b. 57, fasc. "Coltivazione dell'albero della china."

55. Alberto Missiroli, "Malaria in Italy during the War and Proposed Control Measures for the Year 1945," RAC, Record Group 1.2, Series 700 Europe, box 12, folder 102, 7.

56. Comitato Romano per l'Assistenza Antimalarica, *L'opera del Comitato Romano per l'Assistenza Antimalarica dal 1921 al 1935* (Rome, 1938), 6–7; League of Nations Health Organisation: Malaria Commission, *Report on Its Tour of Investigation in Certain European Countries in 1924* (Geneva, 1925), 27.

57. Mortara, *La salute pubblica,* 49.

58. Ibid., 51–56.

59. S. P. James, "Advances in Knowledge of Malaria since the War," *Transactions of the Royal Society of Tropical Medicine and Hygiene,* XXXI (1937), 263–264.

60. Sanarelli, *Lo stato attuale,* 20.

61. Ibid., 31–44.

62. ACS, MI, DGS (1896–1934), b. 60, fasc. "Smalarina." On X-ray therapy, see b. 57 bis, fasc. "Radioterapia della malaria."

63. For the reports on Fermi's experiments with piccola bonifica, see the following documents in ACS, MI, DGS (1910–1920), b. 103, fasc. "Commissione per lo studio delle opere di piccola bonifica": "Relazione a S.E. Il Ministro dell'Interno," 2 Jan. 1919; Lazzaro Trincas, "Esperimenti di profilassi antimalarica nei comuni di Portotorres e Sorso," 25 Dec. 1918; Donato Ottolenghi, "Io Rapporto Sommario sugli esperimenti di lotta antimalarica in provincia di Cagliari," 22 June 1918; P. Canalis, S. Ravicini, and D. Ottolenghi, "Risultati della lotta contro le zanzare anofeline e delle opere di piccola bonifica in Terranova Pausania (Sassari) negli anni 1916 e 1917," 17 Jan. 1918; and Ulisse Zaniboni, Capitano Medico, "Campagna antianofelo-malarica del 1917," 11 Aug. 1917. Fermi's own reply to criticisms is "Alcuni schiarimenti alle critiche mosse dal Prof. Canalis ai risultati da me ottenuti nelle campagne antianofelo-malariche a Terranova nel 1916 e 1917," ACS, MI, DGS (1910–1920), b. 104 bis, fasc. "Sassari (Provincia): Bonifiche Terranova e Siniscola (Prof. Fermi)." Fermi also gives an extensive account of piccola bonifica in *Regioni malariche: Decadenza, risanamento e spesa: Sardegna,* vol. 1 (Rome, 1934), 488–492, 535–658.

64. Alessandro Marcucci, "La scuola ambulante nell'Agro Romano," *La cultura popolare,* 1913, 252.

65. "Colonie di bonifica per i bambini malarici," in Direzione Generale della Sanità Pubblica, *Organizzazioni antimalariche alla luce delle nuove dottrine* (Rome, 1925), 58.

66. This discussion of the metaphors employed by the antimalarial campaign is influenced by Susan Sontag, *Illness as Metaphor* (New York, 1978).

67. Ministero per l'Agricoltura: Ispettorato Generale del Bonificamento, della Colo-

nizzazione e del Credito Agrario, *I Consorzi antianofelici e il risanamento delle terre malariche* (Rome, 1918), 82.

68. Alessandro Marcucci, *La scuola di Giovanni Cena* (Pavia, 1958), 18.

69. Ibid., 107.

Chapter 6. Fascism, Racism, and Littoria

1. The classic study of the gradual consolidation of power by the Fascist movement throughout the 1920s remains Adrian Lyttelton, *The Seizure of Power: Fascism in Italy, 1919–1929* (London, 1973). Ironically in 1924 Mussolini was congratulated by feminists for giving women the vote. He did in fact institute equality by abolishing elections for everyone.

2. On therapeutic strategies with regard to cholera, see my *Naples in the Time of Cholera, 1884–1911* (Cambridge, England, 1995), 121–138.

3. ACS, MI, DGS (1896–1934), b. 60, fasc. "Smalarina: Trattamento curativo ed immunizante."

4. The report by Peroni himself is *Malaria: Profilassi e cura in quattro anni di continuate esperienze antimalariche in bonifiche dell'Opera Nazionale per i Combattenti* (Milan, 1933). A favorable interim report by the veterans' association is ONC, "Relazione sulla campagna antimalarica 1927 nelle bonifiche della Stornara (Taranto), di S. Cataldo (Lecce) e di Sanluri (Cagliari)," 1928, ACS, MI, DGS (1896–1934), b. 59, fasc. "Smalarina: Relazioni." Another positive assessment is H. E. Driessen, *Malaria: La valeur de la quinine et du mercure dans son traitement et dans la lutte contre le paludisme* (Rome, 1929).

5. Letter of Missiroli to Presidente della Commissione per gli Studi sulla Smalarina, 5 Dec. 1930, ACS, MI, DGS (1896–1934), b. 60, fasc. "Smalarina," sottofasc. "Rapporto e documenti dello esperimento attuato dalla Stazione Sperimentale per la Lotta Antimalarica in Posada."

6. "Adunanza del 6 Dicembre 1930 della Commissione nominata dal Consiglio Superiore di Sanità per l'esame dei risultati dello esperimento di lotta antimalarica eseguito dall'On. Opera Nazionale Combattenti: Verbali," ACS, MI, DGS (1896–1934), b. 60, fasc. "Smalarina."

7. ACS, MI, DGS (1896–1934), b. 60, fasc. "Smalarina," sottofasc. "Commisione per lo studio dei risultati di lotta antimalarica alla 'Stornara.' "

8. Giulio Alessandrini, Report to S.E. il Presidente Generale della CRI, 9 Jan. 1934, ASCRI, b. 578, Corrispondenza Agro Pontino, fasc. "Inchiesta Rotelli Guido"; Nallo Mazzocchi Alemanni, "La trasformazione agraria" in ONC, *L'Agro Pontino: Anno XVIII* (Rome, 1940), 45–46, 102; Arnaldo Cortesi, "The Former Pontine Marshes Turned into Smiling Fields," *New York Times*, 30 Oct. 1932.

9. Alemanni, "La trasformazione agraria," 102. A discussion of the Pontine Marshes between 1900 and 1934 is Annibale Folchi, *L'Agro Pontino, 1900–1934* (Rome, 1994). For a discussion of the reclamation effort of Pius VI, see Piero Bevilacqua and Manlio Rossi Doria, "Lineamenti per una storia delle bonifiche in Italia dal XVIII al XX secolo," in Piero Bevilacqua and Manlio Rossi Doria, eds., *Le bonifiche in Italia dal '700 a oggi* (Rome, 1984), 28–36.

10. Cortesi, "The Former Pontine Marshes."

11. *Atti parlamentari, Camera dei Deputati, Legislatura XXVII, 1a Sessione, Discussioni, Tornata del 6 dicembre 1928,* 9629; *Tornata del 8 dicembre 1928,* 9766–9769. A recent example of a brief positive mention of the Fascist project in the Pontine Marshes as a successful policy of public health is Leonard Jan Bruce-Chwatt and Julian de Zuluetta, *The Rise and Fall of Malaria in Europe: A Historico-Epidemiological Study* (Oxford, 1980), 3–4.

12. Natale Prampolini, "La Bonifica idraulica delle Paludi Pontine," *Roma,* XIII (1935), 157; Giuseppe Tassinari, *La bonifica integrale nel decennale della legge Mussolini* (Rome, 1939), 18–19. In contexts not primarily concerned with public health, the idea that bonifica needed to become a far more expansive enterprise than land drainage alone had emerged within the community of economists, agronomists, and engineers, and was explicitly articulated as early as the Regional Congress for Venetian Bonifications held at San Donà di Piave in March 1922. Elisabetta Novello, *La bonifica in Italia: Legislazione, credito e lotta alla malaria dall'Unità al fascismo* (Milan, 2003), 198–211.

13. For the use of the expression *bonfica integrale* by the ONC, see "Consiglio di Stato," Adunanza di 10 febbraio 1922, ACS, ONC, Servizio Ingegneria: Progetti, b. 1. On the development of the idea by Alessandro Messea as early as 1922, see letter of Consigliere Delegato dell'Istituto Nazionale pel Risanamento Antimalarico della Regione Pontina to Dott. Alessandro Messea, 25 Mar. 1927, ACS, MI, DGS (1886–1934), b. 58 bis, fasc. "Istituto Nazionale pel Risanamento Antimalarico della regione pontina." The term was also used in 1924 by Giovanni Battista Grassi. Grassi, "La lutte contro le paludisme à Rome," unpublished ms., 1924, USR, AG, b. 22, fasc. 3.

14. Giacomo Rossi, "Tre anni di lotta antimalarica a Maccarese durante l'effettuazione della 'Bonifica integrale,'" *Rivista di malariologia,* VIII (1929), 1–27.

15. Istituto Nazionale pel Risanamento Antimalarico della Regione Pontina, "Organizzazione della lotta alla malaria e dei servizi igienici e demografici nell'Agro Pontino: Progetto di Massima," ACS, MI, DGS (1896–1934), b. 58 bis, fasc. "Istituto Nazionale pel Risanamento Antimalarico della Regione Pontina."

16. Eliseo Jandolo, "Gli indirizzi della legislazione attuale sulle bonifiche," *Rivista di malariologia,* XI (1932), 56. On the long legacy from the Liberal period that lay behind the adoption of bonifica integrale by the Fascist regime, see Novello, *La bonifica in Italia,* 11–15.

17. Prampolini, "La Bonifica idraulica delle Paludi Pontine," 158.

18. Tassinari, *La bonifica integrale,* 16.

19. The leading proponent of zooprophylaxis as a solution to Italy's malarial problem was Domenico Falleroni, Chief Medical Inspector at the Department of Health. A clear statement of his views is "Per la soluzione del problema malarico italiano," *Rivista di malariologia,* VI (1927), 344–409. On the use of the strategy of animal deviation in the Roman Campagna, see G. Pecori and G. Escalar, "Relazione sulla campagna antimalarica nell'Agro Romano durante l'anno 1932," *Rivista di malariologia,* XII (1933), 902–903. See also L. W. Hackett, *Malaria in Europe: An Ecological Study* (Oxford, 1937), 63–65.

20. On the plan to introduce fish as an antilarval measure, see Istituto Nazionale pel Risanamento Antimalarico della Regione Pontina, "Organizzazione della lotta alla malaria e dei servizi igienici e demografici nell'Agro Pontino," ACS, MI, DGS (1896–1934),

b. 58 bis. On the use of gambusie in Littoria province, see "Verbale dell'adunanza del 21 febbraio 1938," ASL, CPA, b. 3/1, fasc. 2/1 ("Anno 1938: Adunanze del comitato"). Fourteen thousand fish were released into the canals of the province in the summer of 1937. A clear explanation of the background and first introduction of the fish to Italy is Gianfranco Donelli and Enrica Serinaldi, *Dalla lotta alla malaria alla nascita dell'Istituto di Sanità Pubblica: Il ruolo della Rockefeller Foundation in Italia, 1922–1934* (Rome, 2003), 76–77.

21. There are authorities who prefer the term *bonifica sociale* ("social bonification"). An example is Francesco D'Erme, an engineer with extensive knowledge of the hydraulic reclamation of the Pontine Marshes. Interview, 15 July 2003.

22. Alessandro Messea, "Malaria: I provvedimenti del Governo Nazionale per la stirpe," *Gerarchia,* VIII (1928), 213.

23. Antonio Labranca, "La legislazione e l'organizzazione sanitaria per la lotta contro la malaria in Italia," *Rivista di malariologia,* VII (1928), 721–722.

24. A. Missiroli, E. Mosna, and M. Alessandrini, "La lotta antianofelica nell'Agro Pontino: Rapporto per gli anni 1945–1947," *Rendiconti dell'Istituto Superiore di Sanità,* XI (1948), part 3, 759–790.

25. Alemanni, "La trasformazione agraria," 107.

26. Adunanza del 3/11/1939: ordine del giorno, n. 1 comunicazione dela presidenza, ASL, CPA, b. 3/1, fasc. 2/1 1939 ("Adunanza del Comitato. Comitato Prov. Antimalarico di Littoria").

27. Patrizia Dogliani, *L'Italia fascista, 1922–1940* (Milan, 1999), 202.

28. Carlo Vallauro, "I lavoratori agricoli nel Lazio tra le due guerre: Il costo umano della modernizzazione," in Carlo Vellauro, ed., *Fascio e aratro* (Rome, 1985), 15. For a discussion of bonifica integrale and its place among the initiatives of the Fascist regime, see also Renzo De Felice, *Mussolini il duce,* vol. 1, *Gli anni del consenso, 1929–1936* (Turin, 1974), 134–158.

29. Ugo Todaro, "Relazione," 1 Dec. 1932, ACS, ONC, Servizio Ingegneria: Progetti, b. 10, fasc. "Bonifica Integrale dell'Agro Pontino: Progetto esecutivo del centro comunale di Littoria," sottofasc. "Relazioni," 7.

30. For a brief overview of the construction of homesteads, see ONC, *L'Agro Pontino,* 46–47.

31. Enzo Fede, "Alloggiamenti operai in Agro Pontino: Relazione," 30 Sept. 1933, ACS, ONC, Servizio Ingegneria: Progetti, b. 4, fasc. "Fabbricati Colonici: progetto secondo lotto," sottofasc. "Relazioni," 1–2.

32. Ibid., 9.

33. Croce Rossa Italiana, Comitato Centrale, "Relazione sui servizi sanitari dell'Agro Pontino, quadrimestre gennaio-aprile 1934 a cura della Direzione dei Servizi Sanitari," ASCRI, b. 578: Corrispondenza Agro Pontino, 2–3.

34. On the condition of workers on the project of bonifica integrale, see Oscar Gaspari, *L'emigrazione veneta nell'Agro Pontino durante il periodo fascista* (Brescia, 1985), 13–70.

35. Letter of Consoli to Davanti, 25 July 1934, ASCRI, b. 578: Corrispondenza Agro Pontino, fasc. "Misc.," 2.

36. Letter of Giulio Alessandrini to Signori Direttori delle stazioni sanitarie della Croce

Rossa Italiana nell'Agro Pontino, 26 Dec. 1933, ASCRI, b. 578: Corrispondenza Agro Pontino, fasc. "Misc.," 2.

37. CPA, "Verbale dell'adunanza del 16 marzo 1935," ASL, CPA, b. 3/1, fasc. 2/1 ("Anno 1935: Adunanze comitato").

38. Interview, 15 July 2003.

39. Edmondo Rossoni, *Direttive fasciste all'agricoltura* (Rome, 1939), 21–22.

40. Unsigned letter to On. Luigi Razza, 22 Dec. 1933, ASCRI, b. 578: "Corrispondenza Agro Pontino," fasc. "Inchiesta Rotelli Guido."

41. "La malaria nell'Agro Pontino e l'opera dell'Istituto Antimalarico Pontino," 21 Feb. 1925, ASL, Consorzio della Bonifica di Littoria, Comitato Antimalarico: Relazioni mediche, b. 18 (1), fasc. "Relazioni attività IAP, 1923–1926."

42. On recruitment and settlement of peasants from the Veneto, see Gaspari, *L'emigrazione veneta.*

43. L. W. Hackett, "Annual Report for 1930: Paris Office, International Health Division," 16 Mar. 1931, RAC, Record Group 5, Series 3, subseries 751.1, box 248, no. 248.

44. For an overview of the project and statistics on the work undertaken, see ONC, *L'Agro Pontino.*

45. Ugo Todaro, "L'edilizia urbana e rurale," in ONC, *L'Agro Pontino,* 68. Two helpful studies of the "new towns" built by the regime are Diane Ghirardo, *Building New Communities: New Deal America and Fascist Italy* (Princeton, 1989); and Renato Besana et al., eds., *Metafisica costruita: Le città di fondazione degli anni trenta dall'Italia all'Oltremare* (Milan, 2002).

46. On borgate, see Todaro, "L'edilizia urbana e rurale," 76–78.

47. Ibid., 68.

48. An official discussion of the achievements of the regime in the Pontine Marshes is Tassinari, *La bonifica integrale,* 77–147.

49. Ing. Ugo Todaro, "Progetto di trasformazione fondiaria dell'Agro Pontino: II lotto. Relazione," 1 Jan. 1933, ACS, ONC, Servizio Ingeneria: Progetti, b. 4, fasc. "Fabbricati Colonici, progetto secondo lotto," sottofasc. "Relazioni," 9.

50. *Christ Stopped at Eboli,* trans. Frances Frenaye (New York, 1947).

51. For the celebrations of the Decennale and the attention given to the Pontine Marshes, see the special edition of the Fascist newspaper *Popolo d'Italia* for 28 Oct. 1932. On the exhibition of 1938 in the Circus Maximus, see "La Mostra della bonifica si inaugurerà prossimamente," *Tribuna,* 8 Dec. 1938; and "La Mostra delle Bonifiche inaugurata ieri dal Duce," *Tribuna,* 24 Dec. 1938.

52. Giovanni Biadene, "La Prima Mostra Nazionale delle Bonifiche," *Illustrazione Italiana,* LIX (1932), 862–863.

53. On the exhibits of bonifica integrale, see ASL, CPA, b. 18, fasc. "Esposizioni e Mostre." An example of the literature produced to accompany the exhibits is Comitato Provinciale Antimalarico di Littoria, *Realizzazioni sanitarie del regime fascista in Agro Pontino: la vittoria sulla malaria* (Milan, 1938), which was the official pamphlet of the Mostra delle Bonifiche for 1938.

54. See, for example, Arrigo Serpieri, *La legge sulla bonifica integrale nel quinto anno di applicazione* (Rome, 1935); and Tassinari, *La bonifica integrale.* An article by Serpieri to celebrate the tenth anniversary of Fascism is "La bonifica integrale," *Popolo d'Italia,* 28 Oct. 1932.

55. Comitato Romano per l'Assistenza Antimalarica, *L'opera del Comitato Romano per l'Assistenza Antimalarica dal 1921 al 1935* (Rome, 1938), 3.

56. Quoted in "Notizie: La redenzione dell'Agro Pontino," *Rivista di malariologia,* XIV (1935), sezione II, 252–253.

57. Elaine Mancini, *Struggles of the Italian Film Industry during Fascism, 1930–1935* (Ann Arbor, 1985), 136.

58. For a review of "Camicia Nera," see Corrado d'Errico, "Camicia Nera: Film della guerra e della Rivoluzione. Dal 1914 al 1933: dalle febbri della palude al sole di Littoria," *Tribuna,* 21 Mar. 1933.

59. Il Duce's words are prominently inscribed in marble above the balcony of the Latina (formerly Littoria) city hall.

60. Ruth Ben-Ghiat, *Fascist Modernities: Italy, 1922–1945* (Berkeley, 2001), 80–81. On Blasetti, see Mancini, *Struggles,* 99–120.

61. Paolo Orano, *Il Fascismo* (Rome, 1940), vol. 2, 60–61.

62. Gioacchino Escalar, *L'organizzazione antimalarica: Corso per visitatrici fasciste* (Rome, n.d.), 1–2.

63. Tassinari, *La bonifica integrale.*

64. On these uses of the concept of *bonifica* by Mussolini's regime, see Ben-Ghiat, *Fascist Modernities,* 124–127.

65. There is an extensive literature on the postwar crisis in the countryside. See, for example, my *Violence and Great Estates in the South of Italy: Apulia, 1900–1922* (Cambridge, England, 1984); and *The Fascist Revolution in Tuscany, 1919–1922* (Cambridge, England, 1989), chapters 1 and 2. See also Anthony L. Cardoza, *Agrarian Elites and Italian Fascism: The Province of Bologna, 1901–1926* (Princeton, 1982); Luciano Casali, ed., *Movimento operaio e fascismo nell'Emilia romagna, 1919–1923* (Rome, 1973); Paul Corner, *Fascism in Ferrara, 1915–1925* (Oxford, 1975); Luigi Preti, *Le lotte agrarie nella valle padana* (Turin, 1955); and Renato Zangheri, *Lotte agrarie in Italia: La Federazione dei Lavoratori della Terra, 1901–1926* (Milan, 1960).

On the early history of the ONC, see Novello, *La bonifica in Italia,* 190–194; and G. Barone, "Statalismo e riformismo: L'Opera Nazionale Combattenti (1917–1923)," *Studi storici,* XXV (1984), 203–244.

66. Oscar Gaspari, "Bonifiche, migrazioni interne, colonizzazioni (1920–1940)," in Pietro Bevilacqua, Andreina De Clementi, and Emilio Franzina, *Storia dell'emigrazione italiana* (Rome, 2001), vol. 1, 325.

67. G. Pecori and G. Escalar, "Relazione sulla campagna antimalarica del 1926 dell'Ufficio d'Igiene del Governatorato di Roma," *Rivista di malariologia,* VI (1927), 245.

68. The expenses (in lire) for the antimalarial campaign of 1936 in Littoria province were as follows: health stations, 1,648,000; antimosquito services, 885,000; hospitalization in infirmaries, 800,000; summer camp for children, 240,000; and general expenses, 1,350,000. "Verbale della riunione per la lotta antimalarica nell'Agro Pontino," 12 Feb. 1935, ASL, CPA, b. 3/1, fasc. 2/1 ("Anno 1935: Adunanze comitato").

69. This era also witnessed the gradual introduction of the first synthetic antimalarials to replace quinine—atebrin, chinoplasmin, and plasmochin. On the early development of synthetic antimalarials, see Werner Schulemann, "Retrospections and Perspectives of Chemotherapy of Malaria," n.d., NLM, Fred L. Soper Papers, 1919–1975, box 57.

70. Pecori and Escalar, "Relazione sulla campagna antimalarica del 1926 dell'Ufficio d'Igiene del Governatorato di Roma," 245.

71. F. Carton, "La Scuola dell'Agro Romano," *Capitolium,* I (1925–1926), 733–742.

72. Alessandro Marcucci, "La scuola rurale in Italia," in Associazione Nazionale Educatori Benemeriti, ed., *Scuola e maestri d'Italia* (Rome, 1957), 192.

73. Alessandro Marcucci, *La scuola di Giovanni Cena* (Pavia, 1958), 15.

74. G. Escalar, "Nella scuola dell'Agro Romano," *Capitolium,* IV (1928), 441.

75. G. Escalar, "I balilla rurali del Governatorato nella difesa della malaria," *Capitolium,* VI (1930), 632.

76. Le Scuole per i Contadini dell'Agro Romano e delle Paludi Pontine, *Relazione (1929–1931)* (Rome, 1931).

77. Nicola Pende, "La Scuola fascista nella sua fase corporativa, imperiale e biologica," *Rivista pedagogica,* XXX (1937), 249–250.

78. Ibid., 253.

79. Marcucci, *La scuola,* 126–132.

80. On antimalarial instruction in the rural schools, see Escalar, "Nella scuola dell'Agro Romano," 439–444.

81. On the Asilo Marchiafava and its operations, see G. Escalar, "Il Sanatorio Antimalarico Governatoriale 'Ettore Marchiafava,'" *Capitolium,* IV (1928), 126–132.

82. "Verbale della riunione per la lotta antimalarica nell'Agro Pontino," 12 Feb. 1935, ASL, CPA, b. 3/1, fasc. 2/1 ("Anno 1935: Adunanze comitato").

83. CPA, "Adunanza del 28 febbraio 1939–XVII, ordine del giorno n. 6," ASL, CPA, b. 3/1, fasc. 2/1 ("1939: Adunanze del Comitato").

84. CPA, "Note illustrative al piano finanziario 1940," ASL, CPA, b. 3/1, fasc. 2/1 ("1939: Adunanze del Comitato"), 2.

85. The many agencies responsible for antimalarial activities in the Pontine Marshes are considered in CPA, "Verbale dell'aduanza del 16 marzo 1935," ASL, CPA, b. 3/1, fasc. 2/1 ("Anno 1935: Adunanze comitato"). Vincenzo Rossetti, the municipal officer of health for Littoria, pointed to the confusion confronting the CPA as it attempted to coordinate the campaign. CPA, "Ordine del giorno delle sedute del 26 ottobre 1936," ASL, CPA, b. 3/1, fasc. 2/1 ("Anno 1936: Adunanze del Comitato"), 5–7.

86. David Schoenbaum, *Hitler's Social Revolution: Class and Status in Nazi Germany, 1933–1939* (Garden City, N.Y., 1966).

87. CPA, "Ordine del giorno della seduta del 26 ottobre 1936–XIV," ASL, CPA, b. 3/1, fasc. 2/1 ("Anno 1936: Adunanze del Comitato"), 5. For an idea of the various agencies responsible for public health in the province, see "Verbale della riunione per la lotta antimalarica nell'Agro Pontino," 12 Feb. 1935, ASL, CPA, b. 3.1, fasc. 2/1 ("Anno 1935").

88. "Mattinata con i coloni di Littoria," *Tribuna,* 16 Dec. 1932.

89. *Atti del consiglio comunale di Roma degli anni 1872–73* (Rome, 1873), 781.

90. F. Salpietra, "La Malaria," *Rivista sanitaria siciliana,* XIV, no. 21 (1 Nov. 1926), 1033.

91. Franco Genovese, *La Malaria in provincia di Reggio Calabria* (Florence, 1924), v–vii.

92. Giuseppe Graziani, *La bonifica integrale e sua importanza antimalarica* (Padova, 1939).

93. On the racial anxieties Fascism exploited, see Ben-Ghiat, *Fascist Modernities,* 2–3, 148–157.

94. Nicola Pende, *Bonifica umana, nazione e biologia politica* (Bologna, 1933), 240.

95. "Mattinata con i coloni di Littoria," *Tribuna,* 16 Dec. 1932; and "Tutti i ragazzi di Littoria sono in camicia nera," *Tribuna,* 16 Feb. 1933. The newspaper slid easily from describing bonifica integrale as a means to defend health to describing it as a means to defend "the health of the race." "L'opera svolta dal Governo Fascista contro la malaria documentata alla Mostra delle Bonifiche," *Tribuna,* 12 Oct. 1932.

96. For classic statements of the dominant racial theory in Fascist Italy, see Giuseppe Sergi, *Da Alba Longa a Roma: Inizio dell'incivilimento in Italia* (Turin, 1934); Pende, *Bonifica umana* and *La politica fascista della razza* (Rome, 1940); and Enzo Rottini, *La purità della razza quale fattore di sviluppo demografico* (Città di Castello, 1940).

97. Mirko Ardemagni, "La rivoluzione fascista salverà la razza bianca," *Gerarchia,* XV (1935), 673–677.

98. A classic attempt to define the various racial currents that occupied the Italian peninsula was Sergi, *Da Alba Longa a Roma.* An interesting recent survey of Italian racial ideologies is Aaron Gillette, *Racial Theories in Fascist Italy* (London, 2002).

99. Pende, *Bonifica umana,* 241.

100. Gaspari, *L'emigrazione veneta,* 72.

101. Nicola Pende, "La terra, la donna e la razza," *Gerarchia,* XVIII (1938), 663.

102. Pende, *Bonifica umana,* 240; Nicola Pende, *Medicina e sacerdozio alleate per la bonifica morale della società* (Ancona, 1940), 12.

103. Pende, "La terra, la donna e la razza," 663–669.

104. Giulio Alessandrini, Report to S.E. Il Presidente Generale della CRI., 9 Jan. 1934, ASCRI, b. 578, Corrispondenza Agro Pontino.

105. See, for instance, U. Mellana, *Bonifica integrale: principii generali e realizzazioni pratiche* (Cuneo, 1930).

106. Benito Mussolini, *Agricoltura e bonifiche* (Rome, 1937), 113; Tassinari, *La bonifica integrale,* 9, 29–30, 37, 334. Il Duce made this declaration in a speech on bonifica integrale in 1929.

107. Mellana, *Bonifica integrale,* 20.

108. Ibid.

109. Nicola Pende, *La politica fascista della razza* (Rome, 1940), 4.

110. "Relazione della Giunta Generale del Bilancio (relatore Bolzon), Disegno di legge, Conversione in legge del Regio decreto-legge 4 ottobre 1934, n. 1682, concernente l'istituzione della provincia di Littoria," *Atti parlamentari, Legislatura XXIX, Sessione 1934, Documenti,* vol. 4, *Camera dei deputati,* no. 254–A, 1.

111. Giulio Alessandrini, *La lotta contra la malaria nell'Agro Pontino* (Bologna, 1935), 20.

112. Giuseppe Sanarelli, *Lo stato attuale del problema malarico: Rilievi e proposte* (Rome, 1925).

113. Ibid., 43–45.

114. Azeglio Filippini, "La stazione sperimentale per la lotta antimalarica," *Rivista di malariologia,* XIV (1935), sezione II, 1–2.

115. Mussolini was described as a "great doctor" to the official delegation of malar-

iologists from the League of Nations who visited Sicily in 1926. ACS, MI, DGS (1896–1934), b. 58.

116. Scuola Superiore di Malariologia, *Lezioni del Professor A. Missiroli* (Rome, 1929), 118.

117. On the foundation of the experimental research stations in Calabria and Sardinia, see Filippini, "La stazione sperimentale," 1–4.

118. "Gli scopi della sanità pubblica," 1929, RAC, Record Group 1.1 Projects, Series 751 Italy, box 1, folder 5, 2–3.

119. On the involvement of William Hackett and the Rockefeller Foundation in Italy, see Gianfranco Donelli and Enrica Serinaldi, *Dalla lotta alla malaria alla nascita dell'Istituto di Sanità Pubblica: Il ruolo della Rockefeller Foundation in Italia, 1922–1934* (Rome, 2003).

120. Letter of Dr. Hackett to Dr. Strode, 13 Apr. 1932, RAC, Record Group 1.1, Series 751 Italy, box 6, folder 75, 1.

121. "Diary of L. W. Hackett—Italy, 1927–1928," RAC, Record Group 1.1, Series 751 Italy, box 7, folder 80, 4. The entry in question is for 13 October 1927.

122. Filippini, "La stazione sperimentale," 1–2. Initially the institute was named the Scuola Superiore di Malariologia.

123. RAC, Record Group 1.1 Projects, Series 751 Italy, box 1, folder 4.

124. R. A. Lambert, "Impressions of Italian Medicine," 8 Feb. 1933, RAC, Record Group 1.1 Projects, Series 751 Italy, box 1, folder 25, 1.

125. John B. Grant, "Italian Health Survey," 22 Sept. 1948, RAC, Record Group 1.1 Projects, Series 751 Italy, box 1, folder 9.

126. G. Izar, "La malaria secondo le moderne concezioni," *Rivista di malariologia,* XXVI (1947), 83.

Chapter 7. Creating Disaster

1. A. Treves, *L'emigrazione interna nell'Italia fascista* (Turin, 1976), 301–302.

2. Felice Jerace, "Prospettive della lotta antimalarica in Italia, *Rivista di malariologia,* XVII (1948), 96.

3. For brief discussions of the conditions that led to the upsurge in malaria as a result of the war, see Lorenza Merzagora, Gilberto Corbellini, and Mario Coluzzi, *L'altra battaglia di Cassino: Contro la malaria a cinquant'anni dall'epidemia della Valle del Liri* (Gaeta, 1996), esp. 57–75; and Bartolo Alosi, "La malaria in Sicilia dopo cinque campagne antimalariche," *Rivista di malariologia,* XXV (1946), 19–30. With regard to the Veneto, see Istituto Interprovinciale per la lotta Antimalarica nelle Venezie, "Relazione tecnica sulla campagna antimalarica, 1 novembre 1943–30 settembre 1944 nelle Provincie Venete," n.d., ACS, II (1927–1973), b. 1.

4. United Nations Relief and Rehabilitation Administration: Italian Mission, *Survey of Italy's Economy* (Rome, 1947), 167.

5. Alberto Missiroli, "Malaria in Italy during the War and Proposed Control Measures for the Year 1945," RAC, Record Group 1.2, Series 700 Europe, box 12, folder 102 (Rockefeller Foundation Health Commission—Typhus, Malaria, 1944 [November–December]), 1.

6. Useful studies of the Italian reversal of alliances are F. W. Deakin, *The Brutal*

Friendship: Mussolini, Hitler, and the Fall of Italian Fascism (London, 1962); Richard Lamb, *War in Italy, 1943–1945: A Brutal Story* (London, 1993); and Friedrich-Karl von Plehwe, *The End of an Alliance: Rome's Defection from the Axis in 1943* (London, 1971).

7. Lamb, *War in Italy,* 24.

8. Karl Wolff, the supreme commander for the SS and police in occupied Italy, explained the German disregard for complaints from Mussolini about the mistreatment of Italian civilians. Giving clear expression to the contempt in which the German leadership held Italians, Wolff said under interrogation at Nuremberg in 1945 that "Il Duce was just an Italian like any other Italian and all his statements or complaints were full of the typical Latin exaggerations. Undoubtedly you have had the same experience with the Italians. . . . Reports by Il Duce can be generally dismissed. He would take the word of any maid, of any person that came running to tell him some grotesquely inflated story and accept it as truth and pass it on in the form of a report or complaint." "Testimony of Karl Wolff," 26 Oct. 1945, PRO, WO 208/4671.

9. Kesselring's order of 17 June 1944 stated that, "The fight against the partisans must be carried on with all means at our disposal and with the utmost severity. I will protect any commander who exceeds our usual restraint in the choice and severity of the methods he adopts against the partisans. In this connection, the old principle holds good that a mistake in choice of method in executing one's orders is better than failure or neglect to act. Only the most prompt and severe handling is good enough as punitive and deterrent measures to nip in the bud outrages on a greater scale." "Testimony of Karl Wolff," 26 Oct. 1945, PRO, WO 208/4671, 8.

10. On the German "war against civilians," see Michele Battini, *Peccati di memoria: La mancata Norimberga italiana* (Rome, 2003); Michele Battini and Paolo Pezzino, *Guerra ai civili: Occupazione tedesca e politica del massacro, Toscana 1944* (Venice, 1997); Giovanni Contini, *La memoria divisa* (Milan, 1997); Philip Cooke, "Recent Work on Nazi Massacres in Italy," *Modern Italy,* V, no. 2 (2000), 211–218; Leonardo Paggi, ed., *Le memorie della repubblica* (Scandicci, 1999); Lamb, *War in Italy;* and Paolo Pezzino, *Anatomia di un massacro: Controversia sopra una strage tedesca* (Bologna, 1997). See also Luca Baldissara and Paolo Pezzino, eds., *Crimini e memorie di guerra: Violenze contro le popolazioni e politiche del ricordo* (Naples, 2004); Enzo Collotti and Lutz Klinkhammer, *Il fascismo e l'Italia in guerra* (Rome, 1996), 127–145; Lutz Klinkhammer, *L'occupazione tedesca, 1943–1945* (Turin, 1996); and Gerhard Schreiber, *La vendetta tedesca, 1943–1945: Le rappresaglie naziste in Italia,* trans. Marina Buttarelli (Milan, 2000). On the British investigation of German war crimes and their intention of prosecuting, see "United Nations War Crimes Commission: Progress Report, 19 September 1944," PRO, WO 204/2190; and "German Generals Case," PRO, WO 310/123. The interrogation of Karl Wolff, the supreme commander of the SS and police in Italy, is especially revealing. See "Testimony of Karl Wolff," 26 Oct. 1945, PRO, WO 208/4671.

11. "Relazione sulle cause della recrudescenza malarica nella stagione epidemica 1942," 16 Aug. 1942, ASL, CPA, Categoria IV (Servizi), b. 12/4, no. 1516.

12. Giuseppe Giustolisi, "Relazione del medico provinciale nella riunione del CPA del 26/10/1942," ASL, CPA, b. 3/1, fasc. "Anno 1942: Adunanze del Comitato," 2.

13. Paul F. Russell, "Italy in the History of Malaria," *Rivista di parassitologia,* XIII (1952), 98.

14. On the twisted career of Erich Martini, see Rainer Hering, "Nazi Persecution and the Pursuit of Science: Correspondence between Erich Martini and Otto Hecht, 1946–47," *Jewish Culture and History,* III, no. 1 (Summer 2000), 95–124. There is a brief mention of the biological warfare unleashed by the Wehrmacht in Gilberto Corbellini, "I malariologi italiani: Storia scientifica e istituzionale di una comunità conflittuale," in Antonio Casella et al., *Una difficile modernità: Tradizioni di ricerca e comunità scientifiche in Italia, 1890–1940* (Pavia, 2000), 320.

15. Missiroli, "Malaria in Italy during the War and Proposed Control Measures for the Year 1945," 12. See also Alberto Missiroli, Report of 19 Jan. 1945, ACS, MS, ISS, Laboratorio di Parassitologia, b. 6, fasc. 19, sottofasc. "Maccarese."

16. Missiroli, "Malaria in Italy during the War and Proposed Control Measures for the Year 1945," 12–13.

17. Missiroli, Report of 19 Jan. 1945, 3.

18. Missiroli, "Malaria in Italy during the War and Proposed Control Measures for the Year 1945," 13.

19. Ibid., 5.

20. Letter of E. Mosna to Direttore Generale dell'Istituto, 29 Nov. 1943, ACS, MS, ISS, Laboratorio di Parassitologia, b. 6, fasc. 19, sottofasc. "Maccarese: Difesa antimalarica." There is an English version of this letter in RAC, Record Group 1.2, Series 700 Europe, folder 102 (Rockefeller Foundation Health Commission—Typhus, Malaria, 1944 [November–December]). Here I have used my translation.

21. Article 22; for the text of the Hague Convention, see James Brown Scott, *The Hague Peace Conferences of 1899 and 1907* (Baltimore, 1909), vol. 2. For the "Regulations Respecting the Laws and Customs of War on Land" adopted in 1907, see 377–401.

22. Ibid., Article 23, 387–389.

23. The text of the Geneva Protocol, signed on 17 June 1925 and entered into force on 8 February 1928, is available at the Web site of the Harvard Sussex Program on Chemical and Biological Warfare Armament and Arms Limitation, http://www.fas.harvard.edu/~hsp/1925.html.

24. Kesselring's trial is well treated in Battini, *Peccati di memoria,* esp. 73–88. For the charges against Kesselring, see "United Nations Charges against German War Criminals: Albert Kesselring, 23 December 1946, 244A," PRO, WO 32/14566. In addition to the Ardeatine Caves atrocity, Kesselring was convicted on the charge that he "incited the German Armed Forces and German Police Forces in Italy under his command to kill Italian civilians as reprisals" between June and August 1944.

25. Paul F. Russell, "Memorandum on Malaria and Its Control in Liberated Italy, 1 January–30 September 1944," 11 Oct. 1944, RAC, Record Group 1.2, Series 700 Europe, box 12, folder 101 (Rockefeller Foundation Health Commission—Typhus, Malaria, 1944 [February–October]), 2–3.

26. Henry W. Kumm, "Malaria Control West of Rome during the Summer of 1944," 26 Jan. 1945, RAC, Record Group 1.2, Series 700 Europe, box 12, folder 102, 2. Similarly, Fred Soper noted of the Tiber delta that, "The drainage works for this area had been deliberately sabotaged by the German military authorities before retreat." "The Use of DDT against Malaria Evaluated on a Rich-Benefit Basis," 3 Dec. 1970, NLM, Fred L. Soper Papers, 1919–1975, box 52, 2.

27. Kumm, "Malaria Control West of Rome during the Summer of 1944," 1.

28. Immediately after the events, the reporter Anne O'Hare McCormick wrote, "The Italian campaign has been fought against three enemies—the Germans, the terrain and the mosquito. Yesterday this correspondent went down to the mouth of the Tiber with Col. Paul Russell, chief of the malaria control branch of the Allied Control Commission, to see one of the battle fields where the Germans enlisted the mosquito as an ally in their bitter fight against the Allied armies and the Italian people. That they were out to punish both is evident in the furious demoliton along the beaches of Ostia and the scientific way wherein they smashed drainage pumps and blocked canals to flood the Agro Romano, the fertile plain between Rome and the sea that until fifty years ago was malarial swamp as deadly as the Pontine Marshes further southward." "Abroad: Undoing the German Campaign of the Mosquito," *New York Times,* 13 Sept. 1944.

29. Interview, 15 July 2003.

30. Diary of Alberto Coluzzi, 18–24, Private Archive of Mario Coluzzi. In Italy, the Todt organization was the agency responsible for providing Italian manpower to work in Germany.

31. Ibid.

32. Ibid.

33. Ibid.

34. Alberto Missiroli, "La malaria nella zona di Maccarese," 24 Jan. 1947, ACS, MS, ISS, Laboratorio di Parassitologia, b. 6, fasc. 19, sottofasc. "Maccarese: Difesa antimalarica."

35. On the successful protection of Allied troops from malaria, see Lieutenant-Colonel A.W. S. Thompson, "Malaria Control in Mobile Warfare. Italian Campaign 1943–1945," PRO, WO 222/159.

36. ACS, ONC, Servizio Ingegneria: Progetti, b. 77, fasc. "Stato di consistenza dei danni bellici subiti dalle opere fondiarie di pertinenza dell'O.N.C. nel Lazio," 15 July 1944, sottofasc. "Relazione," 2, 8.

37. On the damage to the environment in Littoria, see Alberto Missiroli, Report to Prefettura di Latina, 4 June 1946, ASL, CPA, Categoria IV (Servizi), b. 1/1, fasc. "Zone malariche," no. 500/1/1.

38. Leone Leppieri, "Piano tecnico per la campagna antimalarica 1945," 20 Nov. 1944, ASL, CPA, Categoria IV (Servizi), b. 12/4., fasc. "Relazioni mensili del malariologo per il 1944." See also Alberto Missiroli, Report of 14 Sept. 1945.

39. CPA, "Riunione del CPA del 19 ottobre 1946: Mario Alessandrini, 'Relazione,'" ASL, CPA, b.3/1, fasc. 2/1 ("Anno 1945: Adunanze del Comitato"), 3–6.

40. Ibid., 6–7.

41. Ibid., 3–4.

42. Russell, "Memorandum on Malaria and Its Control in Liberated Italy, 1 January–30 September 1944," 3.

Chapter 8. Fighting Disaster

1. CPA, "Riunione del Comitato Provinciale Antimalarico del 19 ottobre 1946," ASL, CPA, b. 2/1 ("Anno 1946: Adunanze del Comitato"), 6.

2. On the early history of the chemical, see G. Raffaele, "Il D.D.T.," *Rivista di malariologia,* XXIII (1944), 94–96.

3. Fred L. Soper, "The Use of DDT against Malaria Evaluated on a Rich-Benefit Basis," 3 Dec. 1970, NLM, Fred L. Soper Papers, 1919–1975, box 52.

4. Fischer's presentation speech at the award of the Nobel Prize in Physiology or Medicine in 1948 is available at the Nobel Prize Web site, http://nobelprize.org/medicine/laureates/1948/press.html.

5. Thomas H. G. Aitken, "A Study of Winter DDT House-Spraying and Its Concomitant Effect on Anophelines and Malaria in an Endemic Area," 5 Oct. 1945, NLM, Fred L. Soper Papers, 1919–1975, box 54.

6. "Fighting Malaria in Europe and Africa," Trustees' Confidential Bulletin of November 1944, RAC, Record Group 1.2, Series 700 Europe, box 12, folder 101 (Rockefeller Foundation Health Commission—Typhus, Malaria, 1944 [February–October]), 6.

7. Henry W. Kumm, "Malaria Control West of Rome during the Summer of 1944," 26 Jan. 1944, RAC, Record Group 1.2, Series 700 Europe, box 12, folder 102, 4.

8. On the place of Italy in the origins of the Cold War, see David W. Ellwood, *Italy, 1943–1945* (New York, 1985); Gabriel Kolko, *The Politics of War: The World and United States Foreign Policy, 1943–1945* (New York, 1968); and Paul Ginsborg, *A History of Contemporary Italy: Society and Politics, 1943–1988* (London, 1990).

9. L. W. Hackett, *Malaria in Europe: An Ecological Study* (Oxford, 1937), 108.

10. Commissario straordinario, "Campagna antimalarica 1955," ASL, CPA, Categoria IV (Servizi), b. 19/4.

11. CPA, "Riunione del CPA del 19 ottobre 1946: Mario Alessandrini, 'Relazione,'" ASL, CPA, b. 3/1, fasc. 2/1 ("Anno 1946: Adunanze del Comitato"), 4–6.

12. Letter of Leone Leppieri to Dirigenti i servizi sanitari dello Stato della Città del Vaticano, 11 Oct. 1944, ASL, CPA, Categoria IV (Servizi), b. 19/4, no. 219.

13. Istituto Interprovinciale per la Lotta Antimalarica nelle Venezie, Circolare, 6 Aug. 1943, ACS, II (1927–1973), b. 8, fasc. "Circolari," no. 389.

14. The text of the plan is in Istituto Interprovinciale, "Programma tecnico-finanziario relativo alla campagna antimalarica nelle province venete per l'anno 1945," ACS, II (1927–1973), b. 8, fasc. "Circolari." A description of the plan for 1946 by its technical director is Pietro Sepulcri, "La campagna antimalarica con il D.D.T. nel 1946 nelle provincie venete," *Rivista di malariologia,* XXVI (1947), 163–182.

15. On the importance attributed by the contemporary Venetian malariologists to the establishment of adequate nutrition through refectories for children, see Ugo De Negri, "Rapporti fra iponutrizione e malaria nel Delta del Po," *Rivista di malariologia,* XX (1941), sezione 1, 30–50.

16. "Resoconto seduta del Consiglio Direttivo," 31 Jan. 1946, ACS, II (1927–1973), b. 1, fasc. "Seduta del 31/1/1946."

17. Ibid., 7–8.

18. "Concetti direttivi del programma, 1945–46," ACS, II (1917–1973), b. 1, sottofasc. "Materiale per la seduta del Consiglio Direttivo del 31/1/46."

19. On the welfare initiatives undertaken under by the Allies, see United Nations Relief and Rehabilitation Administration: Italian Mission, *Survey of Italy's Economy* (Rome,

1947), 1–6, 167–200; and George Woodbridge, *UNRRA: The History of the United Nations Relief and Rehabilitation Administration,* 3 vols. (New York, 1950), esp. vol. 2, 257–294. UNRRA was founded in 1943, and continued its mission in Europe until June 1947. It was an agency of the "United Nations" — the term then used to designate the coalition of nations allied to fight the Axis powers.

20. Comitato Provinciale Antimalarico-Venezia, "Relazione sulla campagna antimalarica, 1 novembre 1944–31 ottobre 1945," ACS, II (1927–1973), b. 1, sottofasc. "Materiale per la seduta del Consiglio Direttivo del 31/1/46," 5.

21. On the Sardinia Project, an account by one of its directors is John A. Logan, *The Sardinia Project: An Experiment in the Eradication of an Indigenous Malarious Vector* (Baltimore, 1953). See also P. J. Brown, "Failure-as-Success: Multiple Meanings of Eradication in the Rockefeller Foundation Sardinia Project, 1946–1951," *Parassitologia,* XXXX (1998), 117–130; and J. A. Farley, "Mosquitoes or Malaria? Rockefeller Campaigns in the American South and Sardinia," *Parassitologia,* XXXVI (1994), 165–173. See also E. Tognotti, *Americani, comunisti e zanzare: Il piano di eradicazione della malaria in Sardegna tra scienza e politica negli anni della guerra fredda, 1946–1950* (Sassari, 1995); and *La malaria in Sardegna: Per una storia del paludismo nel Mezzogiorno, 1880–1950* (Milan, 1996).

22. Letter of Paul Russell to Alberto Missiroli, 3 Nov. 1949, RAC, Record Group 1.2, Series 700 Europe, box 14, folder 116. See also G. K. Strode, John B. Grant, John A. Logan, and Paul F. Russell, "Sardinian *Anopheles* Eradication Project: Statement to Clarify Objective," 17 Dec. 1948. For Fred Soper's account of the eradication, under his direction, of a nonindigenous vector in Brazil, see F. L. Soper and D. B. Wilson, *Anopheles Gambiae in Brazil, 1930–1949* (New York, 1943). The Sardinian project was, in part, an extension of the Brazilian experiment — an effort to eradicate an indigenous vector rather than a newly invading one.

23. "Mosquito Eradication and Malaria Control," Trustees Confidential Report, 1 Jan. 1954, RAC, Record Group 1.2, Series 700 Europe, box 12, folder 101 (Rockefeller Foundation Health Commission — Typhus, Malaria, 1944 [February–October]), 17.

24. The commitment of the Rockefeller Foundation to a high-tech, engineering approach to disease is discussed by Brown, "Failure-as-Success"; and J. A. Najera, *Malaria Control: Achievements, Problems and Strategies* (Geneva, 2000), 19–34.

25. C. Garrett-Jones, "Anopheles Eradication in Sardinia," 23 Mar. 1949, RAC, Record Group 1.2, Series 700 Europe, box 13, folder 113.

26. Letter of Paul Russell to Alberto Missiroli, 3 Nov. 1949, RAC, Record Group 1.2, Series 700 Europe, box 14, folder 116.

27. UNRRA, *Survey of Italy's Economy,* 178–184.

28. Garrett-Jones, "Anopheles Eradication in Sardinia," 10.

29. Garrett-Jones, "Anopheles Eradication in Sardinia," 4.

30. Letter of Marston Bates to G. K. Strode, 23 May 1949, RAC, Record Group 1.2, Series 700 Europe, box 13, folder 114.

31. UNRRA, *Survey of Italy's Economy,* 159.

32. An interesting early survey of the history of the campaign in the Roman Campagna stressing the multifaceted nature of the effort from beginning to end is Donato Vitullo, "Andamento dell'endemia malarica nell'Agro Romano in relazione ai metodi di lotta

usati," *Rivista di malariologia,* XXXI (1952), 27–39. A 2001 study of the eradication of malaria in the United States also stresses that the disappearance of the disease from the nation was not due primarily to the DDT spraying campaign of the 1940s but rather to long-term socioeconomic factors. See Margaret Humphreys, *Malaria: Poverty, Race, and Public Health in the United States* (Baltimore, 2001).

33. Alberto Missiroli, "Preventivo e previsioni per la profilassi antimalarica nel 1947," 8 Aug. 1946, ACS, Ministero della Sanità, Istituto Superiore di Sanità, Laboratorio di Parassitologia, b. 6, fasc. 19, sottofasc. "Preventivo Profilassi Antimalarica: Zona Roma-Caserta," 2.

34. WHO, Regional Office for Europe, *Prevention of the Reintroduction of Malaria in the Countries of the Western Mediterranean: Report on a WHO Meeting, Erice (Italy), 23–27 October 1979* (Geneva, 1979), 5; letter of Mariotti to Vincenzo Mele, 1 Apr. 1965, ASL, CPA, Categoria IV (Servizi), b. 1/1, fasc. "Zone malariche."

35. Missiroli, "Preventivo e previsioni per la profilassi antimalarica nel 1947," 2, 4.

36. Paul F. Russell, *Man's Mastery of Malaria* (New York, 1955), 40.

37. Najera, *Malaria Control,* 2.

38. Emilio Pampana, *A Textbook of Malaria Eradication* (London, 1969; 1st ed. 1963).

39. *Dynamics of Tropical Disease,* ed. L. J. Bruce-Chwatt and V. J. Glanville (London, 1973), esp. chapters 16–19, which are reprints of papers originally published in the 1960s that had a major influence in fostering confidence in the strategy chosen by the WHO.

40. *Malaria Control.*

41. For a critique of the WHO eradication program and an analysis of its difficulties, see Najera, *Malaria Control.* In Africa the failure of eradication was officially recognized as early as 1962 at the WHO Third Africa Malaria Conference. Botha de Meillon, "Conference on Anopheline Biology and Malaria Eradication (May 21–23, 1969)," *Mosquito Systematics Newsletter,* I, no. 3 (August 1969), 2.

42. Najera, *Malaria Control,* 83.

Conclusion

1. For statistics on the world burden of malaria, see World Health Organization (WHO), *Africa Malaria Report 2003,* chapter 1. The report is available at the WHO Web site for the Roll Back Malaria program, http://www.rbm.who.int/amd2003/amr2003/amr_toc.htm.

2. Kevin Marsh, "Malaria Disaster in Africa," *Lancet,* CCCLII (1998), 924.

3. For an assessment of the malarial problem of sub-Saharan Africa, see WHO, *Africa Malaria Report.*

4. On the establishment and goals of the WHO program, see the WHO Roll Back Malaria Web site, http://rbm.who.int/newdesign2.

5. *The Tomorrow of Malaria* (Karori, New Zealand, 1996).

6. David Alnwick, "Roll Back Malaria? The Scarcity of International Aid for Malarial Control: A Comment from WHO and the Roll Back Malaria Partnership Secretariat," 9 May 2003, http://www.malariajournal.com/content/2/1/8/comments.

7. Vasant Narashimhan and Amir Attaran, "Roll Back Malaria? The Scarcity of International Aid for Malaria Control," *Malaria Journal* II, no. 2 (2003), 8, available at http://www.malariajournal.com/content/2/1/8.

8. On the possibility of the reestablishment of transmission in Italy, see Roberto Romi, Guido Sabatinelli, and Giancarlo Majori, "Could Malaria Reappear in Italy?" *Emerging Infectious Diseases,* VII, no. 6 (Nov.–Dec. 2001), available at http://www.cdc.gov/ncidod/eid/citation.htm; and R. Romi, G. Pierdominici, C. Severini, A. Tamburro, M. Cocchi, D. Menichetti et al., "Status of Malaria Vectors in Italy," *Journal of Medical Entomology,* XXXIV, no. 3 (1997), 263–271. The fear of the reintroduction of malaria into Italy is also raised by Leonard Jan Bruce-Chwatt and Julian de Zulueta, *The Rise and Fall of Malaria in Europe: A Historico-Epidemiological Study* (Oxford, 1980), 101. Of the other two major vectors of malaria in the past, *An. superpictus* continues to flourish in densities that cause concern, while *An. sacharovi* is no longer present in relevant densities since the intervention with DDT.

9. On the role of agencies and associations in the antimalarial campaign, see Margherita Bettini Prosperi and Gilberto Corbellini, "Una tradizione malariologica durata settant'anni (1898–1967)," in Giuliana Gemelli, Girolamo Ramunni, and Vito Gallotta, *Isole senza arcipelago: Imprenditori scientifici, reti e istitutzioni tra Otto e Novecento* (Bari, 2003), 55–82.

10. Frederick Mugish and Jacqueline Arinaitwe, "Sleeping Arrangements and Mosquito Net Use among Under-Fives: Results from the Uganda Demographic and Health Survey," *Malaria Journal* II, no. 2 (2003), 40, available at http://www.malariajournal.com/content/2/1/40.

11. The classic environmentalist critique of DDT is Rachel Carson, *Silent Spring* (Boston, 1962).

12. *Malaria Control: Achievements, Problems and Strategies* (Geneva, 2000), 106.

13. K. Marsh and R. W. Snow, "30 Years of Science and Technology: The Example of Malaria," *Lancet,* CCCIL (1997), suppl. III, 2. For an overview of the directions of research in the field of malariology, the collection of papers presented at the Malaria Centenary Conference held at Rome in November 1998 is a good point of departure. See the special edition of the journal *Parassitologia,* XLI (Sept. 1999), nos. 1–3.

14. Bernardino Fantini, "*Unum facere et alterum non omittere:* Antimalarial Strategies in Italy, 1880–1930," *Parassitologia,* XL (1998), esp. 100.

15. Litsios, *The Tomorrow of Malaria,* 161.

16. *Italy: A Modern History* (Ann Arbor, 1959), 494.

17. On this point, see World Health Organization, *The World Health Report 2000: Health Systems: Improving Performance* (Paris, 2001). According to WHO calculations, Italy was third among all 191 member states in terms of the level of health of its citizens and second in terms of the performance of its health system. See annex table 1, 152–155.

Glossary

bonifica land drainage and reclamation
bonifica agraria agricultural reclamation
bonifica idraulica land drainage
bonifica igienica hygienic reclamation
bonifica integrale comprehensive reclamation including *bonifica idraulica, bonifica agraria,* and *bonifica igienica*
bonifica umana human reclamation, meaning either (1) complete or "radical" cure from malaria (as used by Grassi); or (2) eugenic improvement of the race (as used by the Fascists)
Il Duce Fascist leader (specifically, Benito Mussolini, comparable to *Führer* for Hitler)
latifondo great wheat-growing estate
paludismo swamp fever
piccola bonifica microenvironmental sanitation
risaia rice field

Select Bibliography

Archival Sources

Archivio Capitolino, Rome (ACC)
  Archivio Ripartizione VIII "Igiene"
Archivio Centrale dello Stato, Rome (ACS)
  Istituto Interprovinciale per la Lotta Antimalarica nelle Venezie (II)
  Ministero dell'Interno (MI)
    Direzione Generale della Sanità (DGS), 1882–1915
    Direzione Generale della Sanità (DGS), 1896–1934
    Direzione Generale della Sanità (DGS), 1910–1920
  Ministero Agricoltura e Foreste
  Ministero della Sanità (MS)
    Istituto Superiore della Sanità (ISS)
  Opera Nazionale Combattenti (ONC)
  Presidenza Zanardelli, Basilicata
Archivio di Stato di Latina, Latina (ASL)
  Fondo CBLT, Comitato Provinciale Antimalarico (CPA)
Archivio Storico della Croce Rossa Italiana, Rome (ASCRI)
Beinecke Rare Book and Manuscript Library, Yale University
  Papers of F. T. Marinetti
National Library of Medicine, Bethesda, Maryland (NLM)
  Fred L. Soper Papers
Private Archive of Mario Coluzzi, Rome

Alberto Coluzzi, Diary
Public Record Office, London (PRO)
War Office (WO)
Rockefeller Archive Center, North Tarrytown, New York (RAC)
Università degli Studi di Roma "La Sapienza," Rome (USR)
Dipartimento di Biologia Animale e dell'Uomo, Archivio Grassi (AG)
Dipartimento di Storia della Medicina, Archivio Celli (AC)

Books and Articles

Ackerknecht, Erwin H., *Malaria in the Upper Mississippi Valley, 1760–1900* (Baltimore, 1945).

Addis Saba, Marina, *Anna Kuliscioff: Vita privata e passione politica* (Milan, 1993).

Alatri, Giovanna, "Duilio Gambellotti: Un contributo artistico al processo educativo," *I problemi della pedagogia,* XXXVII, nos. 4–5 (July–Oct. 1991), 353–392.

Albertazzi, Alessandro, "La Campagna antimalarica in Capitanata," *Giornale della malaria,* I (1907), 49–54.

Alessandrini, Angelo, *Roma ed il Lazio dal punto di vista agrario ed igienico* (Rome, 1881).

Alessandrini, Giulio, *La lotta contro la malaria nell'Agro Pontino* (Bologna, 1935).

Alvaro, Corrado, *Terra nuova: Prima cronaca dell'Agro Pontino* (Rome, 1936).

Ambrogetti, Pietro, "La campagna antimalarica a Corcolle e Lunghezza nel 20 semestre 1902," *Atti della Società per gli Studi della Malaria,* IV (1903), 332–355.

Aquarone, Alberto, *L'Italia giolittiana* (Bologna, 1988).

Archivio Centrale dello Stato, *Fonti per la storia della malaria in Italia* (Rome, 2003).

Ardemagni, Mirko, "La rivoluzione fascista salverà la razza bianca," *Gerarchia,* XV (1935), 673–677.

Ascoli, Vittorio, *La malaria* (Turin, 1915).

——, "La malaria cronica," *Rivista di malariologia,* V (1926), 164–181.

——, "Le manifestazioni nervose da malaria," *Giornale della malaria,* II (1908), 443–449.

——, "Neuro-psicosi da malaria," *Giornale della malaria,* III (1909), 8–14.

Associazione fra gli Agricoltori del Vercellese, *Sulle condizioni dell'agricoltura e degli agricoltori* (Vercelli, 1901).

Associazione Nazionale Educatori Benemeriti, ed., *Scuola e maestri d'Italia* (Rome, 1957).

Atti del consiglio comunale di Roma.

Atti della Giunta per l'Inchiesta Agraria sulle condizioni della classe agricola, 15 vols. (Rome, 1881–1886).

Atti del parlamento italiano.

Atti del 20 Congresso Risicolo Internazionale: Mortara, 1–3 ottobre 1903 (Mortara-Vigevano, 1904).

Baccelli, Guido, "A proposito dei provvedimenti legislativi contro la malaria," *Giornale della malaria,* II (1908), 193–200.

Badaloni, Giuseppe, *La lotta contro la malaria: Relazione al Consiglio Superiore di Sanità presentata nella seduta dell'11 agosto 1909* (Rome, 1910).

Baldissara, Luca, and Pezzino, Paolo, eds., *Crimini e memorie di guerra: Violenze contro le popolazioni e politiche del ricordo* (Naples, 2004).

Balestra, Pietro, *L'hygiène dans la ville de Rome et dans la Campagne Romaine* (Rome, 1876).

Banfield, Edward, *The Moral Basis of a Backward Society* (New York, 1958).

Barone, G., "Statalismo e riformismo: L'Opera Nazionale Combattenti (1917–1923)," *Studi storici*, XXV (1984), 203–244.

Bastianelli, G., "Malaria," *Rivista di malariologia*, XXI (1942), 1–28.

Bastianelli, G., and Bignami, A., "Sulla struttura dei parassiti malarici e in specie dei gameti dei parassiti estivo-autunnali," *Annali d'igiene sperimentale, nuova serie*, IX (1899), 245–257.

Battini, Michele, *Peccati di memoria: La mancata Norimberga italiana* (Rome, 2003).

Battini, Michele, and Pezzino, Paolo, *Guerra ai civili: Occuapazione tedesca e politica del massacro, Toscana 1944* (Venice, 1997).

Ben-Ghiat, Ruth, *Fascist Modernities: Italy, 1922–1945* (Berkeley, 2001).

Besana, Renato, Carli, Carlo Fabrizio, Devoti, Leonardo, and Prisco, Luigi, eds., *Metafisica costruita: Le città di fondazione degli anni trenta dall'Italia all'Oltremare* (Milan, 2002).

Bettini Prosperi, Margherita, and Corbellini, Gilberto, "Una tradizione malariologica durata settant'anni (1898–1967)," in Giuliana Gemelli, Girolamo Ramunni, and Vito Gallotta, *Isole senza arcipelago: Imprenditori scientifici, reti e istitutzioni tra Otto e Novecento* (Bari, 2003), 55–82.

Beveridge, W. I. B., *Influenza: The Last Great Plague* (New York, 1977).

Bevilacqua, Pietro, De Clementi, Andreina, and Franzina, Emilio, eds., *Storia dell'emigrazione italiana*, 2 vols. (Rome, 2001).

Bevilacqua, Pietro, and Rossi Doria, Manlio, eds., *Le bonifiche in Italia dal '700 a oggi* (Rome, 1984).

Bianchini, Arturo, *La malaria e la sua incidenza nella storia e nell'economia della regione pontina* (Latina, 1964).

Biozzi, Silvio, *Malaria in Sardegna* (Sassari, 1937).

Bonelli, F., "La malaria nella storia demografica ed economica d'Italia: Primi lineamenti d'una ricerca," *Studi storici*, VII (1966), 659–687.

Borea, Luigi, "Campagna antimalarica nel Basso Ferrarese durante l'anno 1936," *Rivista di malariologia*, XVII (1938), sezione 1, 142–153.

Bortolotti, Franca Pieroni, *Sul movimento politico delle donne: Scritti inediti*, ed. Annarita Buttafuoco (Rome, 1987).

Boyd, Mark F., *Malariology: A Comprehensive Survey of All Aspects of This Group of Diseases from a Global Standpoint* (Philadelphia, 1949).

Brignone, Emiliano, "La malaria in Terranova Monferrato durante il quadriennio 1912–1915 con speciale menzione alla propaganda e profilassi antimalarica scolastica dell'anno 1915," *Malariologia*, Serie II, II (1916), 145–163.

——, "La propaganda e profilassi antimalarica nelle scuole comunali di Terranova Monferrato durante l'anno 1914," *Malariologia*, Serie II, I (1915), 63–72.

Brombilla, Giusseppe, *La malaria sotto l'aspetto economico-sociale* (Milan, n.d.).

Brown, P. J., "Failure-as-Success: Multiple Meanings of Eradication in the Rockefeller Foundation Sardinia Project, 1946–1951," *Parassitologia*, XL (1998), 117–130.

Bruce-Chwatt, Leonard Jan, and De Zulueta, Julian, *The Rise and Fall of Malaria in Europe: A Historico-Epidemiological Study* (Oxford, 1980).

Cacace, Ernesto, "L'insegnamento antimalarico e la profilassi antimalarica scolastica: Relazione al III Congresso Internazionale d'Igiene Scolastica in Parigi," *Rivista pedagogica,* V, no. 1 (1911), 179–187.

——, "Per la diffusione dell'insegnamento antimalarico e della profilassi antimalarica scolastica nei paesi malarici," *Malariologia,* Serie II, I (1915), 51–59.

Canevari, Alfredo, *Le agitazioni agrarie nel Lazio* (Rome, 1906).

Capanna, Ernesto, "Battista Grassi: Uno zoologo per la malaria," *Parassitologia,* XXXVIII, suppl. 1 (Dec. 1996), 3–47.

Caracciolo, Alberto, *Il movimento contadino nel Lazio (1870–1922)* (Rome, 1952).

Caraffa, Vincenzo, "L'infezione malarica," *Giornale della malaria,* I (1907), 145–157, 241–252.

Cardoza, Anthony L., *Agrarian Elites and Italian Fascism: The Province of Bologna, 1901–1926* (Princeton, 1982).

Casalini, Maria, *La signora del socialismo italiano: Vita di Anna Kuliscioff* (Rome, 1987).

Castellino, Pietro, "La malaria di fronte al bilancio del Ministero di A. I. E. C.," *Giornale della Malaria,* I (1907), 97–109.

——, "La profilassi chininica nella scienza e nella pratica," *Giornale della malaria,* III (1909), 49–54.

——, "Malaria e quesstione sociale: Riassunto della conferenza del Professor Pietro Castellino al Congresso Antimalarico di Foggia," *Giornale della malaria,* I (1907), 6–20.

Celli, Angelo, "Ancora sulla profilassi chininica: Risposte del Prof. A. Celli ai Professori P. Castellino e U. Gabbi," *Giornale della malaria,* II (1908), 216–220.

——, *Antagonismi igienico-economici: Lezioni di proemio al corso d'igiene e polizia sanitaria* (Rome, 1907).

——, *Come vive il campagnolo nell'Agro Romano* (Rome, 1900).

——, *Il tannato di chinina in cioccolattini per la profilassi e cura della malaria* (Naples, 1909).

——, "La malaria in Italia durante il 1902: Richerche epidemiologiche e profilattiche," *Atti della Società per gli Studi della Malaria,* IV (1903), 543–579.

——, "L'epidemiologia della malaria secondo le recenti vedute biologiche," *Atti della Società per gli Studi della Malaria,* II (1901), 76–129.

——, *Per la lotta contro la malaria* (Rome, 1902).

——, "Sull'immunità dall'infezione malarica," *Atti della Società per gli Studi della Malaria,* I (1899), 50–72.

Celli, Angelo, Celli-Fraentzel, Anna, Casagrandi, O., Escalar, G., Di Tucci, F., and Sepulcri, P., *La malaria* (Turin, 1934).

Celli-Fraentzel, Anna, "I riferimenti alla febbre palustre nella poesia," *Rivista di malariologia,* XIII (1934), 380–394.

—— [M. L. Heid, pseud.], *Uomini che non scompaiono* (Florence, 1944).

Cerase, Francesco Paolo, *Sotto il dominio dei borghesi: Sottosviluppo ed emigrazione nell'Italia meridionale, 1860–1910* (Rome, 1975).

Clark, Ian, "Cell-Mediated Immunity in Protection and Pathology of Malaria," *Parasitology Today,* III (1987), 300–305.

Clark, Ian, and Chaudhri, G., "Tumor Necrosis Factor May Contribute to the Anaemia of Malaria by Causing Dyserythropoiesis and Erythrophagocytosis," *British Journal of Haematology,* LXX (1988), 99–103.

Clark, Ian, and Cowden, W. B., "Roles of TNF in Malaria and Other Parasitic Infections," *Immunology,* series LVI (1992), 365–407.

Clark, Ian, Cowden, William B., and Chaudhri, Geeta, "Possible Roles for Oxidants, through Tumor Necrosis Factor in Malarial Anemia," in John W. Eaton, Steven R. Meshnick, and George J. Brewer, eds., *Malaria and the Red Cell: Proceedings of the Second Workshop on Malaria and the Red Cell, Held in Ann Arbor, Michigan, October 24, 1988* (New York, 1989).

Clark, Martin, *Modern Italy, 1871–1995* (London, 1998; 1st ed. 1984).

Collier, Richard, *The Plague of the Spanish Lady: The Influenza Pandemic of 1918–1919* (New York, 1974).

Collotti, Enzo, and Klinkhammer, Lutz, *Il fascismo e l'Italia in guerra* (Rome, 1996).

Colucci, V., "Osservazioni sul territorio del comune di Cerignola e sulle campagne antimalariche dal 1904 al 1906," *Giornale della malaria,* I (1907), 64–71.

Comitato Provinciale Antimalarico di Littoria, *Realizzazioni sanitarie del regime fascista in Agro Pontino: La vittoria sulla malaria* (Milan, 1938).

Comitato Romano per l'Assistenza Antimalarica, *L'opera del Comitato Romano per l'Assistenza Antimalarica dal 1921 al 1935* (Rome, 1938).

Commissariato Generale dell'Emigrazione, *L'emigrazione italiana dal 1910 al 1923,* 2 vols. (Rome, 1926).

Commissione parlamentare d'inchiesta sulla condizione degli operai delle miniere della Sardegna, *Atti della commissione,* 4 vols. (Rome, 1910–1911).

Comune di Roma, Ufficio d'Igiene, *Istruzioni ai medici per la profilassi e la cura dei malarici nell'Agro Romano* (Rome, 1900).

Consoli, Nicolò, "La lotta contro la malaria in Sicilia durante l'anno 1932 e l'azione svolta dal Provveditorato alle opere," *Rivista di malariologia,* XIII (1934), 487–530.

Cooke, Philip, "Recent Work on Nazi Massacres in Italy during the Second World War," *Modern Italy,* V, no. 2 (2000), 211–218.

Corbellini, Gilberto, and Merzagora, Lorenza, *La malaria tra passato e presente* (Rome, 1998).

———, "I malariologi italiani: Storia scientifica e istituzionale di una comunità conflittuale," in Antonio Casella, Alessandra Ferraresi, Giuseppe Giuliani, and Elisa Signori, *Una difficile modernità: Tradizioni di ricerca e comunità scientifiche in Italia, 1890–1940* (Pavia, 2000), 299–327.

Corner, Paul, *Fascism in Ferrara, 1915–1925* (Oxford, 1975).

Crollalanza, Araldo di, *L'epilogo vittorioso della bonifica pontina: Relazione al Duce* (Rome, 1941).

Crosby, Alfred W., Jr., *Epidemic and Peace* (Westport, Conn., 1976).

Deakin, F. W., *The Brutal Friendship: Mussolini, Hitler, and the Fall of Italian Fascism* (London, 1962).

De Faveri, Luigi, *L'infezione tubercolare nella zona malarica della provincia di Udine* (Udine, 1937).

De Felice, Renzo, *Mussolini il duce,* vol. 1, *Gli anni del consenso, 1929–1936* (Turin, 1974).

Della Paruta, Franco, ed., *Storia d'Italia, Annali 7: Malattia e medicina* (Turin, 1984).

Demarco, Domenico, *Per una storia economica dell'emigrazione italiana* (Geneva, 1978).

De Negri, Ugo, "La malaria nel delta del Po," *Rivista di malariologia,* XV (1936), 289–301.

Department of the Army, Historical Division, *Anzio Beachhead (22 January–25 May 1944)* (Washington, D.C., 1947).

D'Erme, Francesco, *Latina secondo Cencelli,* 3 vols. (Latina, n.d.).

Desowitz, Robert S., *The Malaria Capers* (New York, 1991).

Dickie, John, Foot, John, and Snowden, Frank M., *Disastro! Disasters in Italy since 1860: Culture, Politics, Society* (New York, 2002).

Di Mattei, Eugenio, "La malaria in Italia nei lavoratori della terra e nei loro figli," *Malaria e malattie dei paesi caldi,* IV (1913).

——, "La profilassi malarica colla protezione dell'uomo dalle zanzare," *Annali d'igiene sperimentale, nuova serie,* X (1900), 107–114.

Dionisi, Antonio, *Anatomia patologica della malaria* (Rome, 1927).

——, "La malaria di Maccarese dal marzo 1899 al febbraio 1900," *Atti della Società per gli Studi della Malaria,* III (1902), 1–67.

Direzione Generale della Sanità Pubblica, *Organizzazioni antimalariche alla luce delle nuove dottrine* (Rome, 1925).

Dogliani, Patrizia, *L'Italia fascista, 1922–1940* (Milan, 1999).

Donelli, Gianfranco, and Serinaldi, Enrica, *Dalla lotta alla malaria alla nascita dell'Istituto di Sanità Pubblica: Il ruolo della Rockefeller Foundation in Italia, 1922–1934* (Rome, 2003).

Driessen, H. E., *Malaria: La valeur de la quinine et du mercure dans son traîtement et dans la lutte contre le paludisme* (Rome, 1929).

Duran-Reynals, Marie Louise de Ayala, *The Fever Bark Tree: The Pageant of Quinine* (Garden City, N.Y., 1946).

Ellwood, David W., *Italy, 1943–1945* (New York, 1985).

Escalar, Gioacchino, *L'organizzazione antimalarica: Corso per visitatrici fasciste* (Rome, n.d.).

——, "Il Sanatorio Antimalarico Governatoriale 'Ettore Marchiafava,' " *Capitolium,* V (1929), 126–132.

——, "Nelle scuole dell'Agro Romano," *Capitolium,* IV (1928), 439–444.

——, "Piccola bonifica e lotta anti-anofelica," *Capitolium,* I (1925–1926), 510–514.

Evoli, Tiberio, "Campagna antimalarica del 1906," *Atti della Società per gli Studi della Malaria,* VIII (1907), 560–569.

Faccini, Luigi, "Lavoratori della risaia fra '700 e '800: Condizioni di vita, alimentazione, malattie," *Studi storici,* XIV, no. 3 (July 1974), 545–588.

Falcioni, D., "La campagna antimalarica nella bassa valle dell'Aniene durante il 1906," *Atti della Società per gli Studi della Malaria,* VIII (1907), 479–494.

Falleroni, Domenico, "Per la soluzione del problema malarico in Italia," *Rivista di malariologia,* VI (1927), 344–409.

Fantini, Bernardino, "Biologie, médecine et politique de santé publique: L'exemple historique du paludisme en Italie," thèse de doctorat en sciences historiques et philologiques, Ecole Pratique des Hautes Etudes, Sorbonne, Paris, 1992.

——, "*Unum facere et alterum non omittere:* Antimalarial Strategies in Italy, 1880–1930," *Parassitologia,* XL (1998), 91–101.

Farid, M. A., "The Malaria Program: From Euphoria to Anarchy," *World Health Forum,* I (1980), 8–22.

Farley, J., "Mosquitoes or Malaria? Rockefeller Campaigns in the American South and Sardinia," *Parassitologia,* XXXVI (1994), 165–173.

Federghini, A., *La malaria e cautele per evitarne le febbri: Suggerimenti agli impiegati delle ferrovie meridionali* (Ancona, 1875).

Fermi, Claudio, *Regioni malariche: Decadenza, risanamento e spesa: Sardegna,* 2 vols. (Rome, 1934).

Fermi, C., and Cano-Brusco, U., "Esperienze profilattiche contro la malaria istituiti allo Stagno di Liccari," *Annali d'igiene sperimentale, nuova serie,* XI (1901), 121–124.

Fichera, Filadelfo, *Il risanamento delle campagne italiane rispetto alla malaria, all'agricoltura, alla colonizzazione* (Milan, 1897).

Filippini, Azeglio, "La stazione sperimentale per la lotta antimalarica," *Rivista di malariologia,* XIV (1935), sezione II, 1–7.

Foà, Gustavo, "Annotazioni sull'uso della Cinconina nella lotta antimalarica durante la stagione interepidemica nell'anno 1924–1925," *Rivista di malariologia,* V (1926), 3–24.

Foerster, Robert F., *The Italian Emigration of Our Times* (New York, 1969; 1st ed. 1924).

Folchi, Annibale, *L'Agro Pontino, 1900–1934* (Rome, 1994).

Folchi, Giacomo, *Sull'origine delle intermittenti di Roma e sua campagna* (Rome, 1828).

Fortunato, Giustino, *Il Mezzogiorno e lo stato italiano,* 2 vols. (Florence, 1973).

——, *Pagine e ricordi parlamentari,* 2 vols. (Florence, n.d.).

Frongia, Gildo, *Lotta antimalarica nella provincia di Cagliari nel 1914 diretta dall'Ispettore Generale Medico Comm. Serafino Ravacini in collaborazione con il Cav. Lamberto Salaroli, medico provinciale, e il Dott. Gildo Frongia, medico provinciale aggiunto* (Cagliari, 1915).

Garofali, Filiberto, "Dieci mesi di lotta antimalarica in Amaseno (Lazio)," *Rivista di malariologia,* V (1926), 157–163.

Gaspari, Oscar, *L'emigrazione veneta nell'Agro Pontino durante il periodo fascista* (Brescia, 1985).

Genovese, Franco, *La malaria in provincia di Reggio Calabria* (Florence, 1924).

Gentile, Emilio, *The Sacralization of Politics in Fascist Italy,* trans. Keith Botsford (Cambridge, Mass., 1996).

Ghirardo, Diane, *Building New Communities: New Deal America and Fascist Italy* (Princeton, 1989).

Gillette, Aaron, *Racial Theories in Fascist Italy* (London, 2002).

Ginsborg, Paul, *A History of Contemporary Italy: Society and Politics, 1943–1988* (London, 1990).

Gioberti, Vincenzo, *Del primato morale e civile degli italiani,* 3 vols. (Turin, 1920–1932; 1st ed. 1843).

Goldsmith, Robert, and Heyneman, Donald, *Tropical Medicine and Parasitology* (Norwalk, Conn., 1989).

Golgi, Camillo, *Discorso di apertura del congresso per la fondazione di una Lega Nazionale contro la Malaria: 7 ottobre 1909* (Como, 1909).

——, *Gli studi di Camillo Golgi sulla malaria,* ed. Aldo Perroncito (Rome, 1929).

Gosio, B., *Guida alla lotta contro la malaria: Cinque lezioni per il personale ausiliario nella lotta contro la malaria* (Rome, 1920).

——, "Malaria di Grosseto nell'anno 1899," *Il Policlinico, Sezione medica,* VII (1900), 177–206, 253–272.

——, "I portatori di malaria: Appunti demoprofilatici," *Giornale della malaria,* II (1908), 337–347.

——, "Sanatorî per bambini malarici," *Rivista di malariologia,* XV (1936), 345–357.

——, *Un triennio di lotta antimalarica nelle Calabrie e Basilicata: Studi e proposte* (Rome, 1908).

Governatorato di Roma, Ufficio d'Igiene, *La piccola bonifica nell'Agro Romano* (Rome, 1930).

——, *Propaganda per la lotta contro la malaria: Il catechismo della malaria* (Rome, 1928).

——, *Propaganda per la lotta contro la malaria: Dialogo fra due sorelline* (Rome, 1928).

Grassi, Giovanni Battista, *Aggiunte all'opera "Studi di uno zoologo sulla malaria": Relazione riassuntiva* (Rome, 1902).

——, "Animali domestici e malaria," *Annali d'igiene,* XXXII (1922), fasc. 6, 1–95.

——, "A proposito del paludismo senza malaria," *Rendiconti della R. Accademia dei Lincei,* X (1901), 2 sem., serie 5, fasc. 6, 123–131.

——, *Bonifiche, laghi artificiali e malaria* (Rome, 1925).

——, *Cenni storici sulle recenti scoperte intorno alla trasmissione della malaria* (Rome, 1900).

——, *Difesa contro la malaria nelle zone risicole* (Milan, 1905).

——, "Osservazioni sulla biologia degli Anofeli," *Annali d'igiene,* XXXI (1921), fasc. 6, 3–23.

——, *Per la storia delle recenti scoperte sulla malaria* (Rome, 1900).

——, *Relazione dell'esperimento di preservazione dalla malaria fatto sui ferrovieri nella piana di Capaccio* (Milan, 1901).

——, *Relazione dell'esperimento di profilassi chimica contro l'infezione malarica fatta ad Ostia nel 1901* (Milan, 1902).

——, *Studi di uno zoologo sulla malaria* (Rome, 1901).

——, "The Transmission of Human Malaria," *Nature,* 1 March 1924, 1–10.

Grassi, G., Bignami, A., and Bastianelli, G., "Ciclo evolutivo delle semilune nell' 'Anopheles Claviger' ed altri studi sulla malaria dall'ottobre 1898 al maggio 1899," *Annali d'igiene sperimentale, nuova serie,* IX (1899), 258–270.

Graziani, Giuseppe, *La bonifica integrale e sua importanza antimalarica* (Padova, 1925).

Hackett, L. W., *Malaria in Europe: An Ecological Study* (Oxford, 1937).

Harrison, Gordon, *Mosquitoes, Malaria and Man: A History of the Hostilities since 1880* (New York, 1978).

Hemingway, Ernest, *A Farewell to Arms* (New York, 1929).
Humphreys, Margaret, *Malaria: Poverty, Race, and Public Health in the United States* (Baltimore, 2001).
Imparato, Luigi, "La campagna antimalarica dell'anno 1908 in Terra di Lavoro," *Giornale della malaria,* III (1908), 227–234.
Istituto di Studi Romani, *La bonifica delle paludi pontine* (Rome, 1935).
James, Henry, *Daisy Miller* (New York, 1900).
James, S. P., "Advances in Knowledge of Malaria since the War," *Transactions of the Royal Society of Tropical Medicine and Hygiene,* XXXI (1937), 263–278.
——, *Malaria at Home and Abroad* (London, 1920).
——, "The Disappearance of Malaria from England," *Proceedings of the Royal Society of Medicine,* XXXIII, part 1 (1929–1930), 71–87.
Jandolo, Eliseo, "Gli indirizzi della bonifica integrale nei rapporti con la malaria in Italia," *Rivista di malariologia,* XVII (1938), sezione 1, 462–474.
——, "Gli indirizzi della legislazione attuale sulle bonifiche," *Rivista di malariologia,* XI (1932), 52–62.
Jerace, Felice, "Il compito delle scuole rurali per la lotta antimalarica e per la propaganda dell'igiene," *Rivista di malariologia,* XVII (1938), sezione 1, 294–299.
——, "Il Papato Romano e la malaria," *Rivista di malariologia,* XIX (1940), sezione 1, 162–182.
Klebs, Edwin, and Tommasi-Crudeli, Corrado, "On the Nature of Malaria," trans. Edward Drummond, *New Sydenham Society* (1888), 1–56.
Klinkhammer, Lutz, *L'occupazione tedesca in Italia, 1943–1945* (Turin, 1996, 1st ed. 1993).
Kolko, Gabriel, *The Politics of War: The World and United States Foreign Policy, 1943–1945* (New York, 1968).
Kraut, Alan M., *Silent Travelers: Germs, Genes, and the "Immigrant Menace"* (New York, 1994).
Kuliscioff, Anna, *Il monopolio dell'uomo* (Palermo, 1979).
Labranca, Antonio, "La legislazione e l'organizzazione sanitaria per la lotta contro la malaria in Italia," *Rivista di malariologia,* VII (1928), 713–739.
Ladelci, Francesco, *Intorno alle febbri di periodo* (Rome, 1880).
Lamb, Richard, *War in Italy, 1943–1945: A Brutal Story* (London, 1993).
Laveran, Alphonse, *Prophylaxie du paludisme* (Paris, n.d.).
League of Nations Health Organisation, Malaria Commission, *Report on Its Tour of Investigation in Certain European Countries in 1924* (Geneva, 1925).
Levi, Carlo, *Christ Stopped at Eboli,* trans. Frances Frenaye (New York, 1947).
Litsios, Socrates, *The Tomorrow of Malaria* (Karori, New Zealand, 1996).
Logan, John A., *The Sardinia Project: An Experiment in the Eradication of an Indigenous Malarious Vector* (Baltimore, 1953).
Lombardi, G., "Importanza della campagna antimalarica in Capitanata," *Giornale della Malaria,* I (1907), 78–82.
Lombroso, Cesare, *Crime: Its Causes and Remedies,* trans. P. Horton (Boston, 1911).
Lorenzoni, Giovanni, *I lavoratori delle risaie* (Milan, 1904).
Lustig, Alessandro, "Questioni del giorno," *Minerva,* XXX (Dec. 1909–Dec. 1910), 87–90, 111–113.

Lustig, Alessandro, Sclavo, Achille, and Alivia, Michele, *Relazione sommaria della campagna antimalarica condotta nella Provincia di Sassari nel 1910: Contributo alla conoscenza delle condizioni igieniche-sociali della Sardegna* (Florence, 1911).

Lyttelton, Adrian, *The Seizure of Power: Fascism in Italy, 1919–1929* (London, 1973).

Macdonald, George, *Dynamics of Tropical Disease,* ed. L. J. Bruce-Chwatt and V. J. Glanville (London, 1973).

Mack Smith, Denis, *Italy: A Modern History* (Ann Arbor, 1959).

Maggi, Augusto, "La campagna antimalarica in Ostia nel secondo semestre 1902," *Atti della Società per gli Studi della Malaria,* IV (1903), 311–331.

——, "La campagna antimalarica nell'Agro romano durante il 1903. Stazione sanitaria di Ostia," *Atti della Società per gli Studi della Malaria,* V (1904), 629–645.

——, *Scritti d'un medico dell'Agro Romano* (Rome, 1912).

Mancini, Elaine, *Struggles of the Italian Film Industry during Fascism, 1930–1935* (Ann Arbor, 1985).

Manson, Patrick, *Tropical Diseases* (London, 1914).

Manzoni, Alessandro, *I promessi sposi* (Milan, 1903; 1st ed. 1840–1842).

——, *Storia della colonna infame* (Naples, 1928; 1st ed. 1842).

Marchiafava, Ettore, "Le gare d'igiene e la propaganda igienica nelle scuole del comune di Roma," *Capitolium,* I (1925–1926), 359–362.

——, "Le gare d'igiene nelle scuole del Governatorato di Roma," *Capitolium,* VII (1931), 365–371.

Marchiafava, Ettore, and Bignami, Amico, *La infezione malarica* (Milan, 1904).

Marcucci, Alessandro, *Il programma didattico* (Rome, n.d.).

——, *La scuola di Giovanni Cena* (Pavia, 1956).

——, *Per il contadino del Lazio: La nostra patria* (Rome, 1916).

Marinelli, Ferdinando, "La campagna antimalarica a Torremaggiore nel 1907," *Giornale della malaria,* II (1908), 112–120.

Marinetti, F. T., *Futurismo e fascismo* (Foligno, 1924).

Mario, Jessie White, *The Birth of Modern Italy: Posthumous Papers of Jessie White Mario,* ed. Duke Litta-Visconti-Arese (London, 1909).

Martirano, Francesco, "La malaria nel Mezzogiorno d'Italia," *Atti della Società per gli Studi della Malaria,* II (1901), 249–282; IV (1903), 440–468.

——, "La profilassi della malaria nel Mezzogiorno d'Italia durante il 1904," *Atti della Società per gli Studi della Malaria,* VI (1905), 335–348.

McNeill, John Robert, *The Mountains of the Mediterranean World: An Environmental History* (Cambridge, England, 1992).

Mellana, U., *Bonifica integrale: Principii generali e realizzazioni pratiche* (Cuneo, 1930).

Mennuni, Gioacchino, "La campagna antimalarica in Barletta durante l'anno 1908," *Giornale della malaria,* III (1909), 235–238.

——, "Su di alcune speciali e gravi cause di malaria nel comune di Barletta," *Giornale della malaria,* I (1907), 54–60.

Merzagora, Lorenza, Corbellini, Gilberto, and Coluzzi, Mario, *L'altra battaglia di Cassino: Contro la malaria a cinquant'anni dall'epidemia della Valle del Liri* (Gaeta, 1996).

Messore, Luigi, "Relazione della campagna antimalarica nel territorio di Marcianise nell'anno 1913," *Malariologia,* Serie II, I (1915), 119–130.

Migliori, Domenico, *Sanatorii antimalarici nella provincia di Cosenza* (Cosenza, 1911).

Ministero dell'Agricoltura, Ispettorato Generale del Bonificamento, della Colonizzazione e del Credito Agrario, *I consorzi antianofelici e il risanamento delle terre malariche* (Rome, 1918).

Ministero delle Finanze, Direzione Generale delle Privative, *Relazione e bilancio industriale dell'azienda del chinino di stato per l'esercizio dal 1 luglio 1905 al 30 giugno 1906* (Rome, 1907).

Ministero dell'Interno, Direzione Generale della Sanità Pubblica, *Consigli popolari per la difesa individuale contro la malaria* (Rome, 1907).

——, *Elenco delle zone malariche delimitate a tutto il 31 dicembre 1912* (Rome, 1913).

——, *Elenco delle zone malariche delimitate a tutto l'8 febbraio 1906 distribuite per provincie e comuni* (Rome, 1906).

——, *La campagna antimalarica dell'anno 1902 nella Maremma Toscana* (Rome, 1903).

——, *La malaria in Italia ed I risultati della lotta antimalarica* (Rome, 1924).

Ministero dell'Interno: Direzione Generale della Sanità Pubblica, and Ministero dell'Economia Nazionale: Direzione Generale dell'Agricoltura, *La risicoltura e la malaria nelle zone risicole d'Italia* (Rome, 1925).

Missiroli, Alberto, *La diagnosi differenziale dei parassiti malarigeni nei preparati colorati* (Rome, 1921).

——, "La prevenzione della malaria nel campo pratico," *Rivista di malariologia,* VII (1928), 413–455.

——, *Lezioni sulla epidemiologia e profilassi della malaria* (Rome, 1934).

Missiroli, A., Mosna, E., and Alessandrini, M., "La lotta antianofelica nell'Agro Pontino: Rapporto per gli anni 1945–1947," *Rendiconti dell'Istituto Superiore di Sanità,* XI, part 3 (1948), 759–790.

Monti, Antonio, *La bonifica dell'Agro Romano e la lotta contro la malaria nel pensiero e nell'azione del conte Luigi Torelli* (Milan, 1941).

Mortara, Giorgio, *La salute pubblica in Italia durante e dopo la guerra* (Bari, 1925).

Mussolini, Benito, *Agricoltura e bonifiche* (Rome, 1939).

Najera, Jose A., Liese, Bernhard H., and Hammer, Jeffrey, *Malaria: New Patterns and Perspectives* (Washington, D.C., 1992).

Negri, Adelchi, *Sul valore della bonifica umana come mezzo di lotta contro la malaria* (Pavia, 1909).

——, *Ulteriori osservazioni sul valore della "bonifica umana" come mezzo di lotta contro la malaria* (Pavia, 1910).

Neva, Franklin A., and Brown, Harold W., *Basic Clinical Parasitology,* 6th ed. (Norwalk, Conn., 1994).

Nitti, Francesco Saverio, *Scritti sulla questione meridionale,* 4 vols. (Bari, 1968).

Nogarola, Lodovico Violini, *L'opera del Comitato Antimalarico Veronese dal 5 agosto 1912 al 31 dicembre 1913* (Verona, 1914).

Novello, Elisabetta, *La bonifica in Italia: Legislazione, credito e lotta alla malaria dall'Unità al Fascismo* (Milan, 2003).

Opera Nazionale per i Combattenti, *L'Agro Pontino: Anno XVIII* (Rome, 1940).

Orano, Paolo, *Il fascismo* (Rome, 1940).

Orsi, Giovanni, "Contributo allo studio della malaria in provincia di Caserta," *Atti della Società per gli Studi della Malaria,* IX (1908), 295–303.

Ottolenghi, Donato, *Problemi igienici della bonifica integrale* (Florence, 1936).

Paggi, Leonardo, ed., *Le memorie della repubblica* (Scandicci, 1999).

Pagliani, Luigi, and Guerci, C., *Relazione intorno alla coltivazione delle risaie nell'Agro Parmense* (Rome, 1895).

Panizza, Mario, *Risultati dell'inchiesta istituita da Agostino Bertani sulle condizioni sanitarie dei lavoratori della terra in Italia: Riassunto e considerazioni* (Rome, 1890).

Pareto, Raffaele, *Relazione sulle condizioni agrarie ed igieniche della Campagna di Roma* (Florence, Genoa, 1872).

Passerini, Pacifico, *Le scuole rurali di Roma e il bonificamento dell'Agro Romano* (Rome, 1908).

Patterson, K. David, *Pandemic Influenza, 1700–1900: A Study in Historical Epidemiology* (Totowa, N.J., 1986).

Pavesi, Carlo, *Le risaie ed il vasto disboscamento dei terreni* (Rome, 1874).

Pecori, G., "La malaria dell'Urbe nei tempi passati e la sua salubrità attuale," *Capitolium,* I (1925–1926), 505–509.

Pecori, G., and Escalar, G., "Relazione sulla campagna antimalarica del 1926 dell'Ufficio d'Igiene del Governatorato di Roma," *Rivista di malariologia,* VI (1927), 244–267.

——, "Relazione sulla campagna antimalaria dell'anno 1927: Ufficio d'Igiene del Governatorato di Roma," *Rivista di malariologia,* VII (1928), 217–266.

——, "Relazione sulla campagna antimalarica dell'anno 1928: Ufficio d'Igiene del Governatorato di Roma," *Rivista di malariologia,* VIII (1929), 481–533.

——, "Relazione sulla campagna antimalarica dell'anno 1930: Ufficio d'Igiene e Sanità del Governatorato di Roma," *Rivista di malariologia,* X (1931), 545–610.

——, "Relazione sulla campagna antimalarica nell'Agro Romano durante l'anno 1931," *Rivista di malariologia,* XI (1932), 615–675.

——, "Relazione sulla campagna antimalarica nell'Agro Romano durante l'anno 1932," *Rivista di malariologia,* XII (1933), 910–952.

——, "Relazione sulla campagna antimalarica nell'Agro Romano durante l'anno 1933," *Rivista di malariologia,* XIII (1934), 622–668.

——, "Relazione della campagna antimalarica nell'Agro Romano durante l'anno 1934," *Rivista di malariologia,* XIV (1935), sezione 1, 469–519.

Pende, Nicola, *Bonifica umana, nazione e biologia politica* (Bologna, 1933).

——, *La mentalità mediterranea nella nuova medicina dell'Italia imperiale* (Rome, 1936).

——, *La politica fascista della razza* (Rome, 1940).

——, *La scuola fascista nella sua fase corporativa, imperiale e biologica* (Milan, 1937).

——, *Medicina e sacerdozio alleate per la bonifica morale della società* (Ancona, 1940).

Peroni, Giacomo, *Malaria: Profilassi e cura in quattro anni di continuate esperienze antimalariche in bonifiche dell'Opera Nazionale per I Combattenti* (n.p., 1933).

Pezzato, Ferdinando, *Tubercolosi e malaria* (Treviso, 1934).

Pezzino, Paolo, *Anatomia di un massacro: Controversia sopra una strage tedesca* (Bologna, 1997).

Pinto, Giuseppe, *Cura delle complicazioni nelle febbri di periodo* (Rome, 1868).

Pio Istituto di S. Spirito ed Ospedali Riuniti di Roma, *Rendiconto statistico-sanitario: Anno 1935—XIII* (Rome, 1936).
——, *Rendiconto statistico-sanitario: Anno 1936—XIV* (Rome, 1937).
——, *Rendiconto statistico-sanitario: Anno 1937—XV* (Rome, 1938).
Plehwe, Friedrich-Karl von, *The End of an Alliance: Rome's Defection from the Axis in 1943* (London, 1971).
Porter, Katherine Ann, *Pale Horse, Pale Rider: Three Short Novels* (New York, 1964; 1st ed. 1936).
Postempski, Paolo, *La Campagna antimalarica compiuta dalla Croce Rossa Italiana nell'Agro Romano nel 1900* (Rome, 1901).
Prampolini, Natale, "La bonifica integrale," *Rivista di malariologia,* XI (1932), 63–70.
Presidenza del Consiglio dei Ministri: Commissariato per le Migrazioni e la Colonizzazione Interna, *Le migrazioni interne in Italia nell'anno 1931* (Rome, 1932).
Preti, Luigi, *Le lotte agrarie nella valle padana* (Turin, 1955).
Puccinotti, Francesco, *Opere mediche,* 2 vols. (Milan, 1855–1856).
Quine, Maria Sophia, *Population Politics in Twentieth-Century Europe* (London, 1996).
Raffaele, Giulio, "Il D.D.T.," *Rivista di malariologia,* XXIII (1944), 94–96.
——, "La fase primaria dell'evoluzione monogonica dei parassiti malarici," *Rivista di malariologia,* XVII (1938), sezione 1, 331–343.
——, "Potere infettante del sangue durante l'incubazione della malaria aviaria," *Rivista di malariologia,* XV (1936), 77–87.
——, "Sul comportamento nel sangue dei parassiti della malaria aviaria," *Rivista di malariologia,* X (1931), 280–310.
——, "Sullo sviluppo iniziale dei parassiti malarici nell'ospite vertebrato," *Rivista di malariologia,* XVI (1937), sezione 1, 185–198.
Ravicini, S., "La campagna antimalarica in provincia di Roma durante il 1904," *Atti della Società per gli Studi della Malaria,* VI (1905), 335–348.
Regio Commissariato degli Ospedali Riuniti di Roma, *Statistica sanitaria degli Ospedali per gli anni 1892, 1893, 1894, 1895* (Rome, 1896).
——, *Statistica sanitaria dell'anno 1896* (Rome, 1897).
Ricchi, Teobaldo, *Nuova profilassi della malaria* (Bologna, 1900).
Ricciardi, Angelo, *La malaria nelle Puglie* (Noci, 1911).
Rizzi, Michele, "Cause dell'andamento dell'epidemia malarica nel 1907," *Giornale della malaria,* II (1908), 145–152.
Roberti, Pietro, *Manuale di cognizioni utili concernenti la patologia, la profilassi e la terapia della malaria* (Lagonegro, 1906).
Rosenberg, Charles F., *Explaining Epidemics and Other Studies in the History of Medicine* (Cambridge, England, 1992).
Ross, Ronald, *The Prevention of Malaria* (London, 1910).
Rossi, Giacomo, "Dell'influenza di alcune bonifiche sulla malaria in provincia di Napoli e Terra del Lavoro," *Atti della Società per gli Studi della Malaria,* IV (1903), 377–398.
——, "Tre anni di lotta antimalarica a Maccarese durante l'effettuazione della 'Bonifica integrale,'" *Rivista di malariologia,* VIII (1929), 1–27.
Rossi, Giacomo, and Guarini, Giuseppe, *La bonifica del Vallo di Diano nei suopi rapporti colla malaria* (Rome, 1906).

Rossoni, Edmondo, *Direttive fasciste all'agricoltura* (Rome, 1939).
Rottini, Enzo, *La purità della razza quale fattore di sviluppo demografico* (Città di Castello, 1940).
Rummo, G., and Ferrannini, L., "La campagna antimalarica in prov. di Napoli: Relazione a S.E. Il Ministro dell'Interno," *Giornale della malaria,* II (1908), 37–47.
Russell, Paul F., "Italy in the History of Malaria," *Rivista di parassitologia,* XIII (1952), 93–104.
——, *Malaria: Basic Principles Briefly Stated* (Oxford, 1952).
——, *Man's Mastery of Malaria* (New York, 1955).
Russell, Paul F., West, Luther S., and Manwell, Reginald D., *Practical Malariology* (Philadelphia, 1946).
Salaman, Redcliffe N., *The History and Social Influence of the Potato* (Cambridge, England, 1949).
Salapietra, F., "La malaria," *Rivista sanitaria siciliana,* XIV, no. 21 (Nov. 1926), 1034–1041.
Sanarelli, Giuseppe, *Lo stato attuale del problema malarico: Rilievi e proposte* (Rome, 1925).
——, "L'Agro Pontino nelle sue condizioni sanitarie," *Annali d'igiene,* XLIV (1934), 536–542.
Sanfelice, Francesco, and Calvino, V. E. Malato, "Le miniere della Sardegna: Ricerche sperimentali sull'aria e statistiche sugli operai," *Annali d'igiene sperimentale, nuova serie,* XII (1902), 1–49.
Santori, Saverio, "La malaria nella provincia di Roma nel decennio 1888–1897," *Atti della Società per gli Studi della Malaria,* I (1899), 110–132.
Scalzi, Francesco, *La meteorologia in rapporto alle febbri malariche e alle flogosi polmoniche studiate negli ospedali di Santo Spirito e del Laterano nell'anno 1878* (Rome, 1879).
Schindler, John R., *Isonzo: The Forgotten Sacrifice of the Great War* (Westport, Conn., 2001).
Schlichtherle, I. M., Treutiger, C. J., Fernandez, V., Carlson, J., and Wahlgren, M., "Molecular Aspects of Severe Malaria," *Parasitology Today,* XII (1996), 329–332.
Schoenbaum, David, *Hitler's Social Revolution: Class and Status in Nazi Germany, 1933–1939* (Garden City, N.Y., 1966).
Schreiber, Gerhard, *La vendetta tedesca, 1943–1945: Le rappresaglie naziste in Italia,* trans. Marina Buttarelli (Milan, 2000).
Scott, James Brown, *The Hague Peace Conferences of 1899 and 1907,* 2 vols. (Baltimore, 1909).
Scuola Superiore di Malariologia, *Lezioni del Prof. A. Missiroli* (Rome, 1929).
Scuole per I contadini dell'Agro Romano e delle Paludi Pontine, *Relazione (1913–1928)* (Rome, 1929).
——, *Relazione (1929–1931)* (Rome, 1931).
Selmi, Antonio, *Il miasma palustre: Lezioni di chimica igienica* (Padua, 1870).
Sergi, Antonio, "Sulla profilassi chininica scolastica," *Malariologia,* Serie II, I (1915), 59–63.
Sergi, Giuseppe, *Da Alba Longa a Roma: Inizio dell'incivilimento in Italia* (Turin, 1934).

——, *Specie e varietà umane* (Turin, 1900).
Serpieri, Arrigo, *La guerra e le classi rurali italiane* (Bari, 1930).
——, *La legge sulla bonifica integrale nel quinto anno di applicazione* (Rome, 1935).
Snowden, Frank M., *The Fascist Revolution in Tuscany, 1919–1922* (Cambridge, England, 1989).
——, *Naples in the Time of Cholera, 1884–1911* (Cambridge, England, 1995).
——, *Violence and Great Estates in the South of Italy: Apulia, 1900–1922* (Cambridge, England, 1984).
Società per gli Studi della Malaria, *Istruzioni popolari per difendersi dalla malaria* (Rome, 1904).
Sombart, Werner, *La Campagna Romana*, trans. F. C. Jacobi (Turin, 1891).
Sontag, Susan, *Illness as Metaphor* (New York, 1978).
Soper, Fred L., and Wilson, D. Bruce, *Anopheles Gambiae in Brazil, 1930–1949* (New York, 1943).
Sori, Ercole, *L'emigrazione italiana dall'Unità alla seconda guerra mondiale* (Bologna, 1979).
Strozza, Francesco, *Giovanni Cena e le scuole per I contadini* (Rome, 1992).
Swellengrebel, Nicholas H., and Buck, A. De, *Malaria in the Netherlands* (Amsterdam, 1938).
Tassinari, Giuseppe, *La bonifica integrale nel decennale della legge Mussolini* (Rome, 1939).
Tognotti, E., *Americani, comunisti e zanzare: Il piano di eradicazione della malaria in Sardegna tra scienza e politica negli anni della guerra fredda, 1946–1950* (Sassari, 1995).
——, *La malaria in Sardegna: Per una storia del paludismo nel Mezzogiorno, 1880–1950* (Milan, 1996).
Tommasi-Crudeli, Corrado, *The Climate of Rome and the Roman Malaria*, trans. Charles Cramond Dick (London, 1892).
Torelli, Luigi, *Carta della malaria dell'Italia illustrata* (Florence, 1882).
——, *Il curato di campagna e la malaria dell'Italia: Quindici dialoghi* (Rome, 1884).
Trambusti, Arnaldo, *La lotta contro la malaria in Sicilia* (Palermo, 1910).
Treves, A., *L'emigrazione interna nell'Italia fascista* (Turin, 1976).
Tropeano, Antonio, "Contro l'esclusivismo della dottrina zanzaro-malarica," *Giornale della malaria*, II (1908), 483–509.
——, "Febbre ittero-ematurica da chinina e febbre ittero-ematurica spontanea nei malarici," *Giornale della malaria*, III (1909), 15–37.
——, "La profilassi della malaria con l'uso quotidiano del chinino: Relazione all'Assemblea dell'Ordine dei Sanitari di Catanzaro e Provincia (Dicembre 1906)," *Giornale della malaria*, II (1908), 261–279.
Tropeano, Antonio, and Tropeano, Giuseppe, "Ragioni e scopo di uno studio critico-sperimentale sulla profilassi chininica," *Giornale della malaria*, III (1909), 55–75.
Tropeano, Giuseppe, "Il programma della nostra campagna nel 1909," *Giornale della malaria*, III (1909), 5–7.
——, "La bancarotta della profilassi chininica," *Giornale della malaria*, II (1908), 510–518.

——, "La campagna antimalarica nel Mezzogiorno (verso la nazionalizzazione)," *Giornale della malaria,* I (1907), 268–279.
——, *La clinica della malaria nel Mezzogiorno d'Italia* (Naples, 1909).
——, "La malaria," *Giornale della malaria,* II (1908), 4–36.
——, *La malaria nel Mezzogiorno d'Italia* (Naples, 1908).
——, "La storia clinica della Capitanata," *Giornale della malaria,* I (1907), 129–139.
——, "L'educazione igienica popolare e le conferenze antimalariche nel Mezzigiorno," *Giornale della malaria,* III (1909), 193–226, 241–273, 433–473.
——, "Per la lotta contro la malaria (la scheda C)," *Giornale della malaria,* I (1907), 31–47.
——, "Profilassi sperimentale e profilassi sociale," *Giornale della malaria,* II (1908), 241–255.
United Nations Relief and Rehabilitation Administration: Italian Mission, *Survey of Italy's Economy* (Rome, 1947).
Vellauro, Carlo, ed., *Fascio e aratro* (Rome, 1985).
Verdone, Luca, *I film di Alessandro Blasetti* (Rome, 1989).
Verga, Giovanni, *Little Novels of Sicily,* trans. D. H. Lawrence (New York, 1953).
——, *Mastro-Don Gesualdo* (Milan, 1979).
Vitullo, Donato, "Andamento dell'endemia malarica nell'Agro Romano in relazione ai metodi di lotta usati," *Rivista di malariologia,* XXXI (1952), 27–39.
Voltaire, *Candide et autres contes* (Paris, 1992).
Wernsdorfer, Walter H., and McGregor, Ian, *Malaria: Principles and Practice of Malariology* (Edinburgh, 1988).
Woodbridge, George, *UNRRA: The History of the United Nations Relief and Rehabilitation Administration,* 3 vols. (New York, 1950).
World Health Organization, *The World Health Report 2000: Health Systems: Improving Performance* (Paris, 2001).
World Health Organization, Regional Office for Europe, *Prevention of the Reintroduction of Malaria in the Countries of the Western Mediterranean: Report on a WHO Meeting, Erice (Italy), 23–27 October 1979* (Geneva, 1979).
Zangheri, Renato, *Lotte agrarie in Italia: La Federazione dei Lavoratori della Terra, 1901–1926* (Milan, 1960).
Zappi, Elda Gentili, *If Eight Hours Seem Too Few: Mobilization of Women Workers in the Italian Rice Fields* (Albany, 1991).
Zola, Emile, *Rome* (Paris, 1907).
Zulueta, J. de, "The End of Malaria in Europe: An Eradication of the Disease by Control Measures," *Parassitologia,* XL (1998), 245–246.

Index